2005 YEAR BOOK OF ORTHOPEDICS®

The 2005 Year Book Series

Year Book of Allergy, Asthma, and Clinical Immunology™: Drs Rosenwasser, Boguniewicz, Milgrom, Routes, and Spahn

Year Book of Anesthesiology and Pain Management™: Drs Chestnut, Abram, Black, Gravlee, Mathru, Lee, and Roizen

Year Book of Cardiology®: Drs Gersh, Cheitlin, Graham, Kaplan, Sundt, and Waldo

Year Book of Critical Care Medicine®: Drs Dellinger, Parrillo, Balk, Bekes, Dries, and Dorman

Year Book of Dentistry®: Drs Zakariasen, Hatcher, Horswell, McIntyre, Scott, Victoroff, and Zakariasen

Year Book of Dermatology and Dermatologic Surgery™: Drs Thiers and Lang

Year Book of Diagnostic Radiology®: Drs Osborn, Birdwell, Dalinka, Gardiner, Levy, Maynard, and Oestreich

Year Book of Emergency Medicine®: Drs Burdick, Cydulka, Hamilton, Handly, Werner, and Quintana

Year Book of Endocrinology®: Drs Mazzaferri, Rubin, Molitch, Leahy, Kennedy, Kannan, Bessesen, Rogol, and Meikle

Year Book of Family Practice®: Drs Bowman, Apgar, Dexter, Miser, Neill, and Scherger

Year Book of Gastroenterology™: Drs Lichtenstein, Dempsey, Drebin, Faust, Ginsberg, Katzka, Kochman, Morris, Reddy, and Stein

Year Book of Hand and Upper Limb Surgery®: Drs Berger and Ladd

Year Book of Medicine®: Drs Barkin, Frishman, Klahr, Loehrer, Mazzaferri, Phillips, Pillinger, and Snydman

Year Book of Neonatal and Perinatal Medicine®: Drs Fanaroff, Maisels, and Stevenson

Year Book of Neurology and Neurosurgery®: Drs Gibbs and Verma

Year Book of Nuclear Medicine®: Drs Coleman, Blaufox, Royal, Strauss, and Zubal

Year Book of Obstetrics, Gynecology, and Women's Health®: Dr Shulman

Year Book of Oncology®: Drs Loehrer, Arceci, Glatstein, Gordon, Hanna, Morrow, and Thigpen

Year Book of Ophthalmology®: Drs Rapuano, Cohen, Eagle, Grossman, Hammersmith, Myers, Nelson, Penne, Sergott, Shields, Tipperman, and Vander

Year Book of Orthopedics®: Drs Morrey, Beauchamp, Peterson, Swiontkowski, Trigg, and Yaszemski

Year Book of Otolaryngology-Head and Neck Surgery®: Drs Paparella, Otto, and Keefe

Year Book of Pathology and Laboratory Medicine®: Drs Grzybicki, Raab, Bejarano, Bissell, and Stanley

Year Book of Pediatrics®: Dr Stockman

Year Book of Plastic and Aesthetic Surgery™: Drs Miller, Bartlett, Garner, McKinney, Ruberg, Salisbury, and Smith

Year Book of Psychiatry and Applied Mental Health®: Drs Talbott, Ballenger, Buckley, Frances, Jensen, and Markowitz

Year Book of Pulmonary Disease®: Drs Phillips, Barker, Dunlap, Lewis, Maurer, and Willsie

Year Book of Rheumatology, Arthritis, and Musculoskeletal Disease™: Drs Panush, Hadler, Hellmann, Hochberg, Lahita, and Seibold

Year Book of Sports Medicine®: Drs Shephard, Alexander, Cantu, Feldman, McCrory, Nieman, Rowland, Sanborn, and Shrier

Year Book of Surgery®: Drs Copeland, Bland, Cerfolio, Daly, Eberlein, Fahey, Mozingo, Pruett, and Seeger

Year Book of Urology®: Drs Andriole and Coplen

Year Book of Vascular Surgery®: Dr Moneta

2005

The Year Book of ORTHOPEDICS®

Editor-in-Chief
Bernard F. Morrey, MD
Professor of Orthopedic Surgery, Mayo Medical School; Emeritus Chairman, Department of Orthopedics, Mayo Clinic, Rochester, Minnesota

ELSEVIER
MOSBY

ELSEVIER
MOSBY

Vice President, Continuity Publishing: Timothy M. Griswold
Publishing Director, Continuity: J. Heather Cullen
Associate Developmental Editor: Timothy Maxwell
Senior Manager, Continuity Production: Idelle L. Winer
Senior Issue Manager: Pat Costigan
Illustrations and Permissions Coordinator: Kimberly E. Denando

2005 EDITION

Printed in the United States of America
Composition by Thomas Technology Solutions, Inc
Printing/binding by Sheridan Books, Inc.

Editorial Office:
Elsevier, Inc.
Suite 1800
1600 John F. Kennedy Blvd
Philadelphia, PA 19103-2899

International Standard Serial Number: 0276-1092
International Standard Book Number: 0-323-02114-X

Editorial Board

Table of Contents

Journals Represented

Journals represented in this YEAR BOOK are listed below.

Acta Orthopaedica Scandinavica
American Journal of Roentgenology
American Journal of Sports Medicine
American Surgeon
Anesthesia and Analgesia
Annals of Surgery
Archives of Physical Medicine and Rehabilitation
Archives of Surgery
Arthroscopy
British Journal of Cancer
Clinical Orthopaedics and Related Research
Clinical Radiology
Diabetes Care
European Journal of Surgical Oncology (London)
Foot & Ankle International
Journal of Arthroplasty
Journal of Athletic Training
Journal of Bone and Joint Surgery (American Volume)
Journal of Bone and Joint Surgery (British Volume)
Journal of Bone and Mineral Research
Journal of Hand Surgery (American)
Journal of Hand Surgery (British)
Journal of Neurosurgery: Spine
Journal of Orthopaedic Research
Journal of Orthopaedic Trauma
Journal of Pediatric Orthopaedics
Journal of Pediatric Surgery
Journal of Reconstructive Microsurgery
Journal of Spinal Disorders & Techniques
Journal of Trauma: Injury, Infection, and Critical Care
Journal of the American Geriatrics Society
Journal of the American Medical Association
Neurosurgery
Orthopedics
Plastic and Reconstructive Surgery
Radiology
Skeletal Radiology
South African Orthopaedic Journal
Spine
Spine Journal
Transfusion

STANDARD ABBREVIATIONS

The following terms are abbreviated in this edition: acquired immunodeficiency syndrome (AIDS), anterior cruciate ligament (ACL), anteroposterior (AP), avascular necrosis (AVN), cardiopulmonary resuscitation (CPR), central nervous system (CNS), cerebrospinal fluid (CSF), computed tomography (CT), deoxyribonucleic acid (DNA), electrocardiography (ECG), health maintenance organization (HMO), human immunodeficiency virus (HIV), intensive care unit (ICU), intramuscular (IM), intravenous (IV), magnetic resonance (MR) imaging (MRI), range of motion (ROM), ribonucleic acid (RNA), total hip arthroplasty (THA), total knee arthroplasty (TKA), ultrasound (US), and ultraviolet (UV).

NOTE

The YEAR BOOK OF ORTHOPEDICS® is a literature survey service providing abstracts of articles published in the professional literature. Every effort is made to assure the accuracy of the information presented in these pages. Neither the editors nor the publisher of the YEAR BOOK OF ORTHOPEDICS® can be responsible for errors in the original materials. The editors' comments are their own opinions. Mention of specific products within this publication does not constitute endorsement.

To facilitate the use of the YEAR BOOK OF ORTHOPEDICS® as a reference tool, all illustrations and tables included in this publication are now identified as they appear in the original article. This change is meant to help the reader recognize that any illustration or table appearing in the YEAR BOOK OF ORTHOPEDICS® may be only one of many in the original article. For this reason, figure and table numbers will often appear to be out of sequence within the YEAR BOOK OF ORTHOPEDICS®.

Introduction

The interesting and exciting feature of reviewing the orthopedic literature is that it allows us to observe first hand a dynamic and ever-changing specialty. Yet, even with the fast-moving reality of change, it is equally interesting to observe the stability and the common truths that continue to be expressed in each year's series of articles. In this year's edition, we have constantly considered the general practicing orthopedic surgeon as opposed to the individual with specialty training.

In this context, the question that is asked is, "What does the practicing orthopedic surgeon need to know about this subset of our discipline?" For the most part, articles are picked on this basis so that, at the end of the review of this year's selections, an individual will have a comfortable grasp of what is new, what works, and what doesn't.

The perspective of the basic scientific studies is to select those that have a direct or immediate impact on one's practice or decision making. The clinical material is more and more being selected on the basis of the scientific rigor of the assessment as well as our opinion of the "impact factor" of the findings. In some instances, we are comfortable to simply reaffirm what we realize the orthopedic community already perceives or knows to be true. In other instances, articles will challenge accepted thought and if felt to be conclusive, these are accepted as well.

At the end of the day, the hope and expectation is that the busy orthopedic surgeon who reads this little text will feel as though this has been a valuable and effective refresher of our specialty, demonstrating where we have been, where we are, and where we are going. With this as a goal, it is a pleasure to serve as editor of the YEAR BOOK OF ORTHOPEDICS.

Bernard F. Morrey, MD

1 Basic Science

Introduction

The Basic Science chapter this year covers a spectrum of investigations that have been chosen on the basis of clinical relevance. Several articles continue to address the issues of prosthetic joint articulation, the impact of wear particles, and further discussion of the relevance of ion release from metallic bearing surfaces. Insights into wound and bone healing, as well as clinically relevant markers to possibly predict the development of ectopic ossification, are exciting initiatives that have direct relevance to a broad spectrum of orthopedic practice. Finally, this chapter touches on computer-based navigation tools for knee, hip, and spine surgery. This topic is also addressed in the anatomic-specific chapters. Overall, it is hoped that this chapter will have a direct relation to the current practice or at least provide insight into potential practice applications in the future.

Bernard F. Morrey, MD

Biochemical Markers of Bone Turnover and Development of Heterotopic Ossification After Total Hip Arthroplasty

Wilkinson JM, Stockley I, Hamer AJ, et al (Univ of Sheffield, England; Northern Gen Hosp, Sheffield, England)

J Orthop Res 21:529-534, 2003 1–1

Background.—Heterotropic ossification (HO) of severity sufficient to impair joint function occurs in approximately 5% of patients after THA. Risk factors for this significant complication include previous heterotropic ossification, male sex, hypertrophic osteoarthritis, ankylosing spondylitis, and diffuse idiopathic skeletal hyperostosis. However, most patients with HO have no identifiable risk factors. The pathogenesis of HO is unclear but may involve inappropriate differentiation of pleuripotent mesenchymal cells under the influence of skeletal growth factors.

Several serum and urine assays have been developed that provide sensitive and specific quantification of bone formation and resorption activity. These assays are used increasingly as a noninvasive adjunct in the diagnosis of metabolic bone disease and in the evaluation of response to therapy. Changes in bone marker activity has also been correlated with changes in bone mass, although this has not been a universal finding. The changes in bone turnover markers over the first 26 weeks after THA were studied to determine whether preoperative levels and postoperative patterns of activity differ in persons in whom HO develops compared with those in whom it does not.

Methods.—Biochemical markers of bone turnover were studied in 20 men and women over 26 weeks after THA to characterize the changes in bone metabolism associated with development of HO.

Results.—There were transient increases in biochemical markers of both osteoclast and osteoblast activity after surgery. The 9 study subjects in whom HO developed had greater increases in the osteoclast marker C-telopeptide of type I collagen and the osteoblast markers N-terminal propeptide of type I procollagen and osteocalcin than those who did not have HO. A rise of more than 42% in C-telopeptide of type I collagen at 1 week after surgery had a sensitivity of 89% and a specificity of 82% for predicting HO development at week 26. Rises of greater than 57% in N-terminal propeptide of type I procollagen and more than 13% in osteocalcin at week 6 had sensitivities of 89% and 56%, and specificities of 82% and 91%, respectively, for the development of HO.

Conclusion.—Transient increases in osteoblast and osteoclast activity occur after THA, and these changes are greater in patients in whom HO develops than in those in whom it does not. The markers have the potential for use as a noninvasive, radiation-free tool for the investigation of the pathogenesis of HO and as an early outcome marker for the development of HO in clinical trials of novel prophylaxis regimes for its prevention.

► This is a very important topic. An increase in C-telopeptide type I collagen and terminal peptide type I protocollagen, as well as osteocalcin, is not surprising since these products are associated with bone metabolism. The finding that C-telopeptide of type I collagen had statistically significant sensitivity for predicting the development of HO is a noteworthy finding. The percentage in osteoblast markers N-terminal propeptide of type I procollagen and osteocalcin also showed a similar sensitivity and specificity, thus providing insight to the potential prediction for this complication.

It should be noted that the differences were negated 1 week after the surgery. The authors do point to a possible strategy for treatment based on these data. One might also wonder whether or not this provides any opportunity for the all-important question of preoperative screening to determine who is at risk for developing the complication to begin with.

B. F. Morrey, MD

The Effect of Growth Factors on Biomechanical Properties of the Bone-Patellar Tendon-Bone Graft After Anterior Cruciate Ligament Reconstruction: A Canine Model Study

Yasuda K, Tomita F, Yamazaki S, et al (Hokkaido Univ, Sapporo, Japan)

Am J Sports Med 32:870-880, 2004 1–2

Background.—The structural properties of the femur-tendon autograft-tibia complex are reduced after reconstruction of the ACL, and these reduced properties are not restored even at 12 months after surgery. It is likely that the deterioration of the autograft is induced by extrinsic fibroblast proliferation and ingrowth along with revascularization, which occur after intrinsic fibroblast necrosis. Investigated was the hypothesis that application of exogenous transforming growth factor–β and epidermal growth factor may affect the structural properties and histology of the bone-patellar tendon-bone autograft after ACL reconstruction.

Methods.—Reconstruction of the ACL was performed in 20 dogs by means of the autogenous bone-patellar tendon-bone graft in bilateral knees. In 10 animals, 12 ng of transforming growth factor–β and 300 ng of epidermal growth factor mixed with fibrin sealant of 0.6 mL were applied to the left knee. Fibrin sealant alone was applied to the left knee in the remaining 10 dogs. No additional treatments were applied to the right knee.

Results.—Application of the growth factor increased the stiffness and maximum failure load of the femur-graft-tibia complex at 12 weeks, with no significant effect from the sham treatment. Histologically, most of the cells in the grafts treated with growth factors had spindle-shaped nuclei, while cells in the other grafts had round nuclei.

Conclusion.—The application of growth factors has shown the potential for prevention of graft deterioration in ACL reconstruction. In this canine model, application of transforming growth factor–β and epidermal growth factor improved the structural properties of the autograft and ACL reconstruction.

▶ This basic investigation is relevant in that it does provide objective data of the value of growth factors on the bone-patella bone-graft mechanical characteristics. It is a practical matter to know that increased strength is demonstrated with such a strategy. What is not answered is whether or not there is long-term value in this approach. In addition, the implication of a faster rehabilitation period and the opportunity to return to sport in a more abbreviated period are logical questions that are not answered by this study. Nonetheless, it does point out the future direction of basic investigations and their potential value for both long-term benefit and short-term rehabilitative efficiency with such treatment strategies. The cost effectiveness of such an approach will not be answered in the near future.

B. F. Morrey, MD

Serum Zinc as a Prognostic Tool for Wound Healing in Hip Hemiarthroplasty

Zorrilla P, Salido JA, López-Alonso A, et al (Complejo Hospitalario Ciudad Real, Spain; Univ of Alcalá, Madrid)

Clin Orthop 420:304-308, 2004 1–3

Background.—Malnutrition is a common state in patients with hip fracture, and the most immediate postsurgical consequence of this condition is delayed wound healing. Among the sequelae of delayed wound healing are increased health care costs because of extended hospital stays and a higher incidence of prosthetic infection. Zinc is an essential nutritional element that directly influences wound healing. Perioperative serum zinc levels and other nutritional parameters were investigated to establish criteria that would be predictive of delayed wound healing.

Methods.—This prospective study was conducted from January 1, 1998, to September 28, 1999, among 97 consecutive patients who had hemiarthroplasty for hip fracture. Preoperative serum zinc levels (micrograms per deciliter) were determined in all of the patients by means of atomic absorption spectrophotometry. The preoperative nutritional status of the patients was evaluated by determining the levels of serum albumin (grams per deciliter), serum transferrin (milligrams per deciliter), and total lymphocyte count (cells per millimeter^2).

Demographic variables, duration of surgery, and concomitant diseases also were analyzed. Cefamandol was given preoperatively and postoperatively for prophylaxis. Vancomycin was used in patients with an allergy to penicillin. Calcium nadroparin was administered for thromboembolic prophylaxis.

Results.—Univariate and multivariate analyses showed a significant correlation between impaired wound healing and serum zinc levels. The logistic regression equation for probability of delay was $P = 1/[1 + e^{-(10.88-0.12 \cdot \text{Zinc})}]$. Serum zinc levels less than 95 μg/dL were found to increase the risk of delayed healing 11.76 times.

Conclusion.—Serum zinc levels are predictive of delayed wound healing in patients who have hemiarthroplasty for hip fracture.

► Most surgeons have been faced with a difficult and perplexing issue of lack of wound healing, usually in an older patient, often felt to be related to malnutrition. This study was, therefore, accepted for this year's YEAR BOOK to demonstrate the value of simple serum zinc assessment as a predictor for wound healing. The fact that these were shown to have a predictive value may be of value to the orthopedic surgeon when facing this difficult clinical management problem.

B. F. Morrey, MD

Cell-Based Therapy for Meniscal Repair: A Large Animal Study

Peretti GM, Gill TJ, Xu J-W, et al (Harvard Med School, Boston; Universitá Vita-Salute, Milan, Italy; Fudan Univ, Shanghai, People's Republic of China)
Am J Sports Med 32:146-158, 2004 1–4

Background.—The knee meniscus is not fully vascularized, with a blood supply present only in the outer third of the meniscus. Thus, the healing capacity of cartilaginous meniscal tissue is limited. The reparative process can-

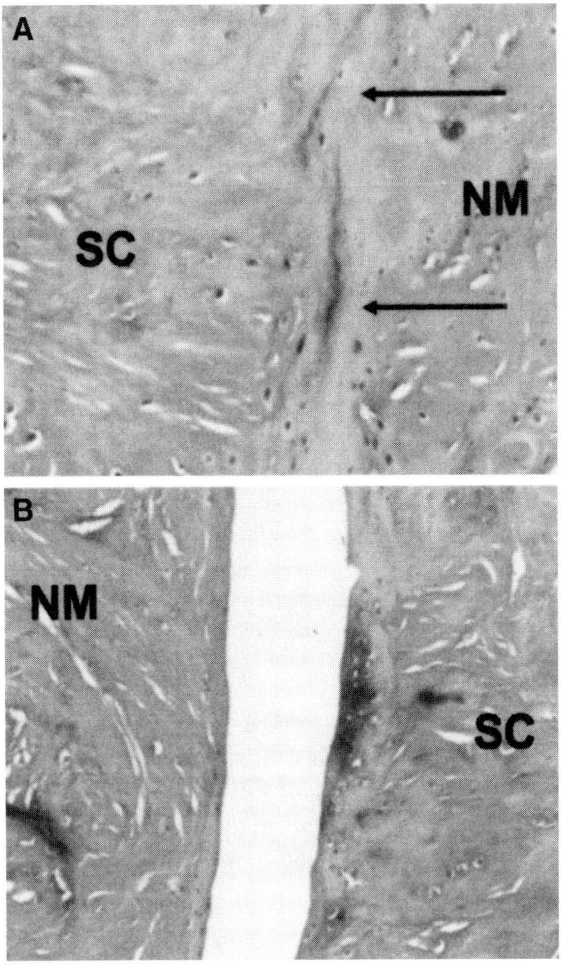

FIGURE 5.—Histologic example for histomorphometric analysis of a group 1 specimen treated with the seeded meniscal scaffold. The images showed a nonhomogeneous result at the interface between the native meniscus and the seeded scaffold. Some healing was noted in various specimens (**A**) with good integration (*arrows*) between the cell-loaded meniscal scaffold and the native meniscus. However, the repair was not achieved in other samples (**B**). Analysis judged as "repaired" the sample in **A** and as "not repaired" that of **B**. *SC* indicates meniscal scaffold; *NM*, native meniscus. (Courtesy of Peretti GM, Gill TJ, Xu J-W, et al: Cell-based therapy for meniscal repair: A large animal study. *Am J Sports Med* 32:146-158, 2004.)

not occur when a lesion involves the avascular portion of the meniscus, because this process is initiated by bleeding and subsequent inflammation. Previous studies have demonstrated the ability of isolated chondrocytes to adhere to a devitalized cartilage matrix in vitro and produce an immature cartilaginous tissue that can bond cartilage matrices together after in vivo transplantation.

More recently, this adhesive ability has been translated into a meniscus repair model by documenting the ability of chondrocytes to adhere to a meniscal matrix and to repair a lesion in the inner third of a devitalized meniscus heterotopically in a murine model. The hypothesis that cell-based therapy can repair a lesion in the swine meniscus was investigated.

Methods.—Sixteen Yorkshire pigs were divided into 4 groups in this controlled laboratory study. A longitudinal tear was created in the avascular portion of the left medial meniscus of 4 pigs. Autologous chondrocytes were seeded onto devitalized allogenic meniscal slices and then secured inside the lesion with 2 sutures.

Identical incisions were created in 12 other pigs, which were used as 3 separate control groups. One control group included 4 animals treated with an unseeded scaffold; a second group had 4 animals that were simply sutured; and the third control group consisted of 4 animals that were left untreated. Meniscal samples were collected after 9 weeks, and the samples were subjected to gross, histologic, and histomorphometric analysis (Fig 5).

Results.—The gross analysis showed bonding of the lesion margins in the specimens of the experimental group, while no repair was observed in any of the control group specimens. Histologic and histomorphometric analysis showed multiple areas of healing in the specimens in the experimental group.

Conclusion.—Seeded chondrocytes have the capacity to heal a meniscal tear in a swine model of meniscal tear.

► The increasing awareness of the critical importance of meniscal function to prevent knee arthrosis, particularly in those with ACL deficiency, clearly increases the importance of these observations. If applicable to human conditions, the ability of healing meniscal tears in avascular segments would be an important consideration in the patient with an ACL with such a meniscus tear. The mechanical integrity and strength of the repair—particularly in an in vivo circumstance—is yet to be determined, but this concept is interesting and these findings are encouraging. The process requiring culture of the articular cartilage does raise practical issues referable to clinical applications.

B. F. Morrey, MD

Computed Tomography-Based Navigation for Hip, Knee, and Spine Surgery

Amiot L-P, Poulin F (Université de Montréal; ORTHOsoft Inc, Montreal)

Clin Orthop 421:77-86, 2004 1–5

Background.—Intraoperative surgical navigation was originally developed for neurosurgery and ear, nose, and throat surgery, but this technology has been adapted to orthopedic procedures with the development of systems for installation of pedicle screws. Many different orthopedic applications have been proposed to address various surgical procedures such as THA, TKA, periacetabular osteotomy, ACL reconstruction, sacroiliac screw insertion, long bone fracture reduction, and distal radius osteotomy.

At present, there is no consensus on the methodology for laboratory testing of these applications, and the array of different test methods has made comparisons of the published results difficult. The state of CT-based clinical orthopedic navigation was reviewed, with specific emphasis on arthroplasty for the hip and the knee. In addition, basic issues regarding the laboratory and clinical validation of the applications were addressed.

Methods.—The ability to compute the position and orientation of an acetabular implant using a postoperative CT scan was evaluated. Angle deviations relative to known positions were computed with an error of less than 1°, and the system accuracy for 3-dimensional reconstruction and registration of 2 cadaveric pelvis specimens was measured with more than 350 registrations.

Results.—A maximal inclination error of 5° was observed in 99% of cases, and a maximal anteversion error of 5° was observed in 97% of cases. The accuracy of the 3-dimensional reconstruction and registration for knee arthroplasty was measured and computed with an angular accuracy of 0.5° in the AP plane and accuracy of 3° in the lateral plane.

Conclusion.—CT-based navigation for orthopedic surgery was found to provide greater accuracy and reproducibility than conventional surgery. However, software improvements are needed to bring this technology into daily clinical practice.

▶ This article reviews the question of the value of navigation in the 3 potential areas that are beneficial to the orthopedic community: hip, knee, and spine surgery. There is no question, based on this study and others, that navigation systems do allow more accurate execution of desired technique. Since this has been proven to be true for the hip, the knee, and the spine, what remains to be answered is whether or not this incremental improvement in positioning will offer a translatable benefit or advantage to the patient, usually in a long-term survival mode. In addition, the considerable expense in time and cost for such strategies remains to be demonstrated. An additional observation of this particular presentation is the fact that investigation of the value of this navigation system is not unique to the United States. It is being carried out around the globe.

B. F. Morrey, MD

The Effect of Mixing on Gentamicin Release From Polymethylmethacrylate Bone Cements

Neut D, van de Belt H, van Horn JR, et al (Univ Hosp Groningen, The Netherlands; Univ of Groningen, The Netherlands)
Acta Orthop Scand 74:670-676, 2003 1–6

Introduction.—The sustained release of antibiotics from bone cements is greatly affected by the penetration of fluids into the polymer matrix, which requires a certain porosity of the cement. Vacuum mixing diminishes the porosity of bone cement with a concurrent increase in mechanical properties. It is not known to what degree this action affects the release of antibiotics from the cement. It is also not known if the preoperative manual addition of antibiotics to the polymer powder will produce a bone cement with antibiotic release properties comparable to those of industrially manufactured, commercially available antibiotic-loaded bone cement. The release of antibiotics from 6 commercially available gentamicin-loading bone cements was compared after vacuum mixing and hand mixing.

Findings.—The 6 gentamicin-loaded bone cements that were evaluated were Palacos R and Palamed (both with 2.1 w/w% gentamicin sulfate); and CMWI, CMW3, CMWendurance, and CMW2000 (all 4 with 4.2 w/w% gentamicin sulfate). Porosity of cements was reduced in each vacuum-mixed cement, compared to that of hand-mixed cements, concurrently with a statistically significant decrease (3/6) or increase (1/6) in the total amounts of gentamicin released. The total gentamicin release was evaluated in 3 of the brands after the manual addition and mixing of the antibiotics. The release of antibiotics was less, compared to samples made from industrial mixing.

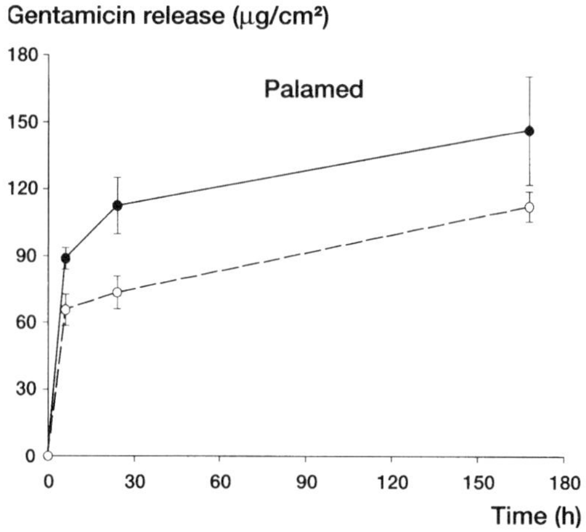

FIGURE 1.—Cumulative gentamicin release (μg/cm²) of Palamed antibiotic-loaded bone cement as a function of time during exposure to phosphate-buffered saline. The findings are given as averages of 3 experimental runs, with *bars* indicating the SD. The *dotted lines* represent vacuum-mixed cements, while the *continuous lines* represent hand-mixed ones. (Courtesy of Neut d, van de Belt H, van Horn JR, et al: The effect of mixing on gentamicin release from polymethylmethacrylate bone cements. *Acta Orthop Scand* 74:670-676, 2003.)

After a high initial release, all cements demonstrated a rapid reduction in their release rates after 24 hours and decreased below the detection level after 168 hours. The initial rates varied slightly in each brand and were highest for Palamed (Fig 1).

Conclusion.—The manual addition and mixing of gentamicin in polymethylmethacrylate bone cements produces a lower release of antibiotics, compared to corresponding commercially available antibiotic-loaded cements; vacuum-mixing only produces a minor decrease in antibiotic release, compared to hand-mixing.

▶ This study is elegant in its simplicity. Similar questions have been asked in the past, but the article is included here to emphasize the irrationality of the Food and Drug Administration (FDA). The FDA continues to disapprove commercially mixed antibiotic cement, although there is little question of the efficacy of this treatment. Hence, the surgeon is forced to mix this by hand, resulting in a poorer efficacy than that resulting from a commercial process. It would be helpful to also define the mechanical properties that may be altered by hand mixing. It has been demonstrated that the use of current concentrations of gentamicin and other antibiotics currently available do not adversely effect the mechanical properties of the cement. This would be a worthwhile line of investigation.

B. F. Morrey, MD

Comparison of the Wear Rates of Twenty-eight and Thirty-two-Millimeter Femoral Heads on Cross-linked Polyethylene Acetabular Cups in a Wear Simulator

Hermida JC, Bergula A, Chen P, et al (Scripps Clinic Ctr, La Jolla, Calif)

J Bone Joint Surg Am 85-A:2325-2331, 2003

1–7

Introduction.—The use of larger femoral head sizes in THA decreases the rate of dislocation and increases the ROM. The larger femoral head components have been linked with unacceptably high polyethylene wear rates. Dramatic differences in wear rates have been observed between nominally cross-linked polyethylene (ie, polyethylene that is cross-linked during radiation sterilization) and increased cross-linked polyethylene (ie, polyethylene that is cross-linked to a higher extent than that obtained by radiation sterilization alone). The effects of increased cross-linking and increased head size on polyethylene wear rates were evaluated.

Methods.—Four groups of acetabular liners were obtained from a single manufacturer (Howmedica Osteonics; Rutherford, NJ) and included in the study as follows: 28-mm-diameter nominally cross-linked, 32-mm-diameter nominally cross-linked, 28-mm-diameter elevated cross-linked, and 32-mm-diameter elevated cross-linked. Three implants from each group were evaluated in a 12-station hip wear simulator that used 90% bovine serum as a lubricant. The liners were articulated with an appropriately-sized Co-Cr femoral head. Additional liners from every design underwent the same load without motion to act as load-soak controls to account for any weight gain caused by fluid absorption. Gravimetric analysis was conducted every 500,000 cycles for 5 million cycles.

Results.—Nominally cross-linked liners for the 28-mm and 32-mm head sizes had mean wear rates of 14.97 and 16.92 mg per million cycles, respectively. Both of the elevated cross-linked liners had significantly lower wear rates, compared to the nominally cross-linked liners, with a mean of 1.51 and 2.57 mg per million cycles for the 28-mm and 32-mm head sizes, respectively ($P < .001$).

Conclusion.—The dramatic decrease in wear rates with polyethylene cross-linking, even with the larger head size, may increase the potential for use of 32-mm head components in total hip arthroplasty.

▶ This study complements the other (Abstract 1–8) in which the cross-linked polyethylene has been shown to decrease wear compared to that of traditional polyethylene. The fact that there is no difference in the 28- and 32-mm head size is of some value. Yet, there are few data that indicate there is any particular value to a 32-mm head to begin with. The critical thickness for the new cross-linked polyethylene has not been accurately defined but has been suggested as being as little as 5 mm or less. The author continues to use the intermediate to 28-mm head size in hip replacement to ensure the greatest possible thickness of the polyethylene, whether it be standard or cross-linked.

B. F. Morrey, MD

Short-term In Vivo Wear of Cross-linked Polyethylene

Heisel C, Silva M, Dela Rosa MA, et al (Orthopedic Hosp, Los Angeles)

J Bone Joint Surg Am 86-A:748-751, 2004 1–8

Introduction.—Cross-linked polyethylene was created to decrease volumetric wear in prosthetic joints. Hip simulator trials have demonstrated promising results concerning wear reduction. The short-term in vivo wear of a moderately cross-linked polyethylene (Marathon) was compared with that of a conventional polyethylene (Enduron).

Methods.—Linear head penetration, as an indicator of in vivo polyethylene wear, was measured in 2 groups of patients who underwent total hip replacement. Twenty-four hips received a conventional polyethylene insert, and 34 received a polyethylene liner. Both inserts were manufactured by DePuy (Warsaw, Ind). Linear and volumetric wear rates were measured on radiographs via a computer-assisted technique and were adjusted for patient-associated factors. Patient activity was evaluated via a computerized 2-dimensional accelerometer worn on the ankle.

Results.—Patients with a conventional polyethylene insert demonstrated a mean linear wear rate of 0.13 mm/y and a mean volumetric wear of 87.6 mm^3/y. The cross-linked polyethylene liner group had a mean linear wear rate of 0.02 mm/y and a mean volumetric wear rate of 17.0 mm^3/y. Wear in the cross-linked polyethylene group was 81% less than in the conventional polyethylene group ($P < .00001$). Accounting for variations in patient activity, the adjusted wear rates per million cycles for a patient weight of 70 kg were 50 mm^3 per million cycles in the conventional polyethylene group and 15 mm^3 per million cycles in the cross-linked polyethylene group; this represented a 72% decrease in the wear rate ($P = .0002$). No factor, other than the types of polyethylene, influenced the between-group differences in wear rates.

Conclusion.—Compared with conventional polyethylene, cross-linked polyethylene had an 81% decrease in the clinical wear rate and a 72% decrease in wear per million cycles. The in vivo wear reduction in the cross-linked polyethylene was consistent with predictions from hip simulator studies.

▶ This is a level of evidence type 2 prospective cohort study, and thus, it has considerable clinical validity. It is impressive to note the simple outcome that cross-linked polyethylene is associated with a statistically and apparently clinically significant decreased wear compared to that of conventional polyethylene. As other alternate bearing surfaces become available, data such as these that support the basic investigation continue to be of critical importance. Long-term follow-up, of course, is required to attribute complete certainty that the cross-linked polyethylene will behave in vivo as is demonstrated in the laboratory.

B. F. Morrey, MD

Metal Degradation Products: A Cause for Concern in Metal-Metal Bearings?

Jacobs JJ, Hallab NJ, Skipor AK, et al (Rush Univ, Chicago)
Clin Orthop 417:139-147, 2003 1–9

Introduction.—Implants fabricated from nonbiological engineering material are important tools in the orthopedic surgeon's armamentarium. These implants have proved successful with few serious short-term and long-term clinical sequelae. However, concern is increasing that permanent orthopedic implants may experience adverse local and remote tissue responses in some individuals and may impact long-term outcome. The characterization of the bioavailability and bioreactivity of the metal species that have been released from the prosthetic materials is important to understand. A literature review was performed to determine whether the metal degradation products originating from the current generation of metal-on-metal bearings are associated with adverse, clinically significant toxicologic sequelae.

Metal Degradation Products.—Particulate debris makes up a substantial portion of metal degradation products produced by joint replacement prostheses. It has been shown that tissues from patients with metal-on-metal bearings have more extensive and severe ulceration of the synovial surface with a predominant lymphocytic infiltrate accompanied by abundant plasma cells, along with a striking pattern of perivascular inflammation. Metallic implants, or wear debris produced from implants may release chemically active metal ions into surrounding tissues. These ions may stay bound to local tissues or bind to protein moieties that are transported in the bloodstream and/or lymphatics to remote organs. Multiple trials have demonstrated chronic increases in serum and urine Co and Cr after total joint replacement. The incidence of metal sensitivity in patients with well- and poorly-functioning implants is about twice as high as that of the general population. The association between metal release from orthopedic implants and carcinogenesis is conjectural; causality has not been definitely established in humans.

Conclusion.—Longer-term, multicenter, epidemiologic investigations are needed to fully address the issues concerning metal implants associated with carcinogenesis, hypersensitivity, and remote toxicity.

▶ This question has been asked for many years among orthopedic investigators, but the increasing interest in using metal-on-metal resurfacing procedures has increased interest once again in this topic. We rarely include review articles in the YEAR BOOK, but this was a well- written summary that lent itself to effective condensation. The many variables that come into play when considering metal degradation products are of greater concern in those with resurfacing devices. Issues, such as the absolute volume, the manner in which the assay is carried out, and whether the metallic product is in an active, an inactive, or a protein-bound form are all important considerations. An additional feature is whether a steady state or a plateauing of the concentration occurs with time. The underlying issue, of course, is cell toxicity and oncogenesis. There is no evidence in the orthopedic literature of any definite cell toxicity or oncogenesis associated with artificial implants. However, ongoing and constant surveillance is necessary to ensure that this perception is, in fact, a reality.

B. F. Morrey, MD

2 General Orthopedics

Introduction

This section was expanded slightly this year since so many relevant topics have appeared in this year's literature. By intent, the titles cover a diversity of subjects. The common theme is the hope that each selection will be of some relevance to a large number of orthopedic practitioners. Some contributions in this section include developments in information technology to enhance diagnostic techniques. We have made a particular effort to consider prospective and, when possible, randomized studies or those that involve large populations, all of which enhance the reliability of the conclusions. Functional rating scores as well as consensus survey material are included as methodologies in this potpourri of topics.

Bernard F. Morrey, MD

Adoption of Information Technology by Resident Physicians
Parekh SG, Nazarian DG, Lim CK (Univ of Pennsylvania, Philadelphia; Pennsylvania Hosp, Philadelphia; Permanente Med Group, Redwood City, Calif)
Clin Orthop 421:107-111, 2004 2–1

Introduction.—The Internet is positioned to revolutionize health care in the United States. In the health care industry, physicians have been depicted as slow adopters of information technology. The younger physicians have been brought up in a computer-prevalent society and may be more likely to use technology. The use and acceptance rates of the Internet and information technology tools and services were examined, along with concerns regarding the security, privacy, and credibility of information on the Internet by resident physicians at a large academic medical center.

Findings.—Of 150 surveys (41 questions) distributed to pediatric, medical, and surgical residents at an urban academic medical center, 135 were completed (90% response rate). Most resident physicians had adopted the tools of information technology. The Internet and e-mail were used by 98% and 96%, respectively, of resident physicians. Two thirds of residents used the Internet for health care–associated purposes. A similar proportion reported they thought the Internet had affected their practice of medicine positively.

Most respondents indicated they thought Internet health care services—including electronic medical records, peer-support websites, and remote patient monitoring—would be beneficial for the health care industry. They indicated concern regarding the credibility, privacy, and security of health and medical information online.

Conclusion.—Most responding resident physicians use the Internet and information technology in their practice of medicine. Most indicate that the Internet will continue to have a beneficial role in the health care industry.

▶ The descriptions and assessment of this topic continue to be important and continue to emerge. The significant increase in various Internet technology comes, of course, as no surprise. This article simply quantifies this effect. The relative use of the various Internet options also comes as no surprise, with computer, Internet, and e-mail being used by almost 100% of residents. Similarly, the use for health care–related issues mostly consists at this time of accessing the literature.

An additional trend not mentioned in this work is the adaptation of technology as a function of age. It goes without saying that Internet technology is the standard whereby resident physicians learn. The challenge for the editor and for the "mature" generation is to similarly adopt these powerful tools as much as we are able.

B. F. Morrey, MD

Unremitting Health-Care-Utilization Outcomes of Tertiary Rehabilitation of Patients With Chronic Musculoskeletal Disorders

Proctor TJ, Mayer TG, Gatchel RJ, et al (Productive Rehabilitation Inst of Dallas for Ergonomics (PRIDE), Dallas)

J Bone Joint Surg Am 86-A:62-69, 2004 2–2

Introduction.—Unremitting behaviors seeking health care are rarely addressed in the literature as an outcome of treatment for chronic disabling work-associated musculoskeletal disorders. A focus has never been placed on the patient as the "driver" of health-care use. Thus, little attention has been paid to the differences between treated patients who do and do not seek additional health care from a new provider. The demographic and socioeconomic outcome variables that characterize patients with a chronic disabling work-associated disorder who pursue additional health-care services from a new provider after completion of a tertiary rehabilitation program were evaluated. The characteristics and outcomes of these patients, all of whom were treated using an identical interdisciplinary protocol, were investigated prospectively.

Methods.—A cohort of 1316 consecutively treated patients from a rehabilitation program for functional restoration was grouped according to whether they had sought treatment from a new health-care provider in the years after completion of treatment. The 966 patients in group 0 did not visit a new health-care provider for treatment of their original occupational injury; the 350 patients in group 1 visited a new provider on at least 1 occasion. A structured clinical interview was performed to evaluate socioeconomic outcomes at 1 year postdischarge from the treatment program. The interview addressed pain, health-care use, work status, recurrent injury, and whether the Workers' Compensation case had been closed.

Results.—The percentage of group 0 patients who underwent prerehabilitation surgery was significantly less than that of group 1 patients who underwent surgery before rehabilitation (12% vs 21%; odds ratio [OR], 1.9; 95% confidence interval [CI], 1.3-2.7; $P < .001$). At 1 year posttreatment, 90% and 78% of group 0 and group 1 patients, respectively, had returned to work (OR, 2.6; 95% CI, 1.9-3.6; $p < .001$). Similarly, 88% and 62% of patients in group 0 and group 1, respectively, were still working at 1 year (OR, 4.5; 95% CI, 3.3-6.0; $p < .001$). The percentage of patients in group 0 and group 1 who had resolved all related legal and/or financial disputes by 1 year were 96% and 77%, respectively (OR, 6.9; 95% CI, 4.5-10.5; $p < .001$). Only a negligible percentage of group 0 patients had undergone a new surgery at the site of the original injury, compared to group 1 patients (0.4% vs 12%; OR, 31.0 (95% CI, 11.0-87.3; $p < .001$). When the previously mentioned outcome variables were assessed by dividing group 1 according to the number of visits to a new service provider, a trend was noted for poorer socioeconomic outcomes to be linked with an increasing number of health-care visits.

Conclusion.—About 25% of patients with a chronic, disabling work-associated musculoskeletal disorder pursue new health-care services after completing a course of treatment; this subgroup accounts for a significant proportion of lost worker productivity, unremitting disability payments, and excess health-care consumption.

▶ This is an extremely interesting level 1 evidence prospective study. The authors have documented what most clinicians intuitively know to be true; that is, a certain group of patients unnecessarily and irrationally consume health-care resources due to real or perceived musculoskeletal dysfunction. The authors introduce the topic emphasizing the burden of disease associated with musculoskeletal disorders. It is particularly important to note that surgery was the most discriminating factor selecting the group that had a significant increase in health-care usage.

B. F. Morrey, MD

Long-term Deterioration of Joint Evaluation Scores

Ritter MA, Thong AE, Davis KE, et al (St Francis Hosp, Mooresville, Ind)

J Bone Joint Surg Br 86-B:438-442, 2004 2–3

Introduction.—Despite the widespread acceptance of the Harris Hip and Knee Society Scores (HHS and KSS) in the assessment of the long-term outcome of total joint arthroplasty, they have recognized limitations. During long periods of follow-up. patients without any identifiable medical complications or radiologic reason for a reduction in their joint evaluation score will experience diminished function because of the effects of aging. Long-term changes in HHS and KSS were assessed to ascertain whether they result from overall functional decline rather than actual changes in the condition of the prosthesis.

Methods.—The HHS for 106 THAs with a minimum follow-up of 12 years and no medical complications after surgery or signs of radiographic loosening and the KSS for 264 TKAs with a minimum follow-up of 12 years and no medical complications postoperatively or signs of radiographic loosening were assessed.

Results.—Statistically significant reductions in functional scoring components of the joint evaluation systems were observed, despite no loosening of the prosthesis or other significant medical complications. The HHS decreased an average of 0.67 points per year from between 3 and 10 years postoperatively ($P < .0001$) (Fig 1). Contributing to this were worsening in gait and limp ($P < .0004$), use of support aids ($P < .0001$), the distance walked ($P < .0001$), and the ability to climb stairs ($P < .0455$). The functional component of KSS decreased significantly at an average of 0.88 points/y between years 3 and 12 postoperatively ($P < .0001$). Significant reductions were noted in every component of the functional scores, including distance walked ($P < .0001$), the ability to climb stairs ($P < .0001$), and the use of support aids ($P < .0001$). The knee score component of the KSS did not decrease significantly ($P < .9750$).

Conclusion.—The combination of functional and pain scores within the HHS and HKS system leads to an inaccurate reduction in the entire score. The reduction in HHS and HKS functional score in total joint arthroplasties, in the absence of implant-associated problems, indicates that deterioration

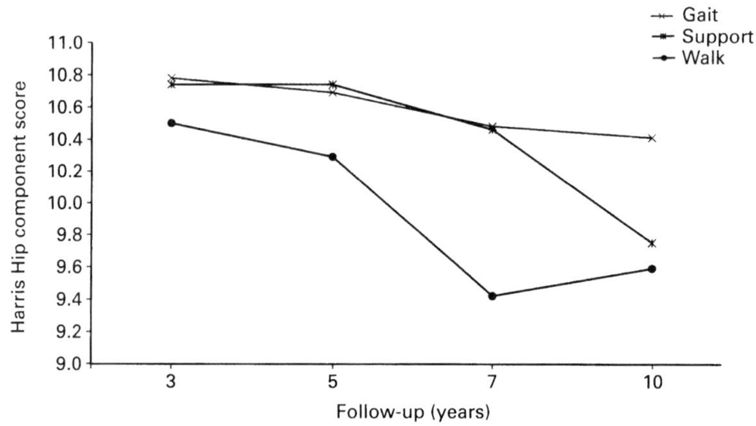

FIGURE 1.—Progression of the average gait (11 points maximum), support (11 points maximum) and walking (11 points maximum) components of the HHS score at follow-up visits. *Abbreviation: HHS*, Harris Hip Society score. (Courtesy of Ritter MA, Thong AE, Davis KE, et al: Long-term deterioration of joint evaluation scores. *J Bone Joint Surg Br* 86-B:438-442, 2004.)

in the functional capacity of aging patients is an important consideration in longitudinal investigations using these scoring systems.

▶ This is not the first study that has demonstrated that the deterioration of joint function after replacement is, to a great extent, simply related to the aging process. These survival curves might serve as a baseline. Any additional deterioration might logically be related to implant-related problems. Information such as this is helpful for the clinician to put into perspective the long-term outcome of otherwise successful joint replacement.

B. F. Morrey, MD

How Accurate Is Partial Weightbearing?

Dabke HV, Gupta SK, Holt CA, et al (Univ Hosp of Wales, Cardiff; Cardiff Univ, Wales)

Clin Orthop 421:282-286, 2004 2–4

Introduction.—Partial weight-bearing is often recommended as a means of avoiding excessive or premature loading that may inhibit healing after fracture or surgery. A limited degree of early loading stimulates fracture healing, whereas full weight-bearing can result in tissue damage. The accuracy of partial weight-bearing was assessed in 6 volunteers and 23 patients.

Methods.—The volunteers (4 men, 2 women; mean age, 30 years) were free of any visual, sensory, or motor impairment. All had a below-knee plaster walking cast applied to the right leg. Patients (12 men, 11 women; mean age, 41 years) were in good health except for the orthopedic condition for which they were being treated.

Ten underwent uncemented hip replacement, 7 had nailing for a comminuted fracture of the tibia, 3 had fixation of a comminuted ankle fracture, 2 had a comminuted hip fracture fixed with a dynamic hip screw, and 1 had revision of an ACL reconstruction. All participants were trained by a physiotherapist to weight bear partially, using the bathroom scale technique. Weight-bearing was subsequently tested in 6 separate walks using force platforms. The extent of weight-bearing was expressed as a percentage of body weight.

Results.—Four volunteers were weight-bearing a mean of 27% of body weight more than required, and 2 exerted a mean of 8.5% of body weight less than required. In the patient group, 21 exerted a mean of 35.3% of body weight more than prescribed, and 2 exerted a mean of 11.97% of body weight less than prescribed. Neither volunteers nor patients could reproduce the extent of partial weight-bearing that they had been trained for.

Conclusion.—The bathroom scale technique of instructing patients in partial weight-bearing proved inaccurate, both when healthy volunteers and when patients with fracture of a lower limb or surgery were studied. Volunteers did better than patients, perhaps because pain compromises a patient's ability to bear weight partially.

▶ This article investigates one of the most common practical issues in orthopedics, the recommendation for protected or partial weight-bearing. This simple but interesting study demonstrates what the orthopedist knows intuitively: specifically, the ability to quantify partial weight-bearing is difficult if not impossible. The observation that the majority of patients exerted more than one third more body weight than was expected and an occasional patient more than 10% less objectifies this observation.

From a practical standpoint, the message might be to recommend a less amount of weight than is desired. The article does not address the true issue, which is the lack of scientific basis for protected weight-bearing to begin with. Nonetheless, this does offer interesting insight for further discussion and the basis for more detailed discussion with our patients regarding this issue.

B. F. Morrey, MD

Abstinence From Smoking Reduces Incisional Wound Infection: A Randomized Controlled Trial

Sorensen LT, Karlsmark T, Gottrup F (Bispebjerg Univ, Copenhagen)

Ann Surg 238:1-5, 2003 2–5

Introduction.—The rate of postoperative wound complications is higher in smokers than in nonsmokers. Wound hypoxia predicts wound infection. Perioperative supplemental oxygen increases tissue oxygen tension and reduces incisional wound infection. The effect of abstinence from smoking on incisional wound infection was examined in 78 healthy research subjects, 48 of whom were smokers and 30 of whom were never-smokers.

Methods.—The participant age range was 18 to 40 years. All smokers had a history of smoking 20 cigarettes/d for at least 2 years. Never-smokers acted as control subjects. During the first week of the 15-week evaluation period, smokers smoked 20 cigarettes/d. Subsequently, they were randomly assigned to continuous smoking, abstinence with a transdermal nicotine patch (25 mg/d), or abstinence with a placebo patch.

At completion of the first week and 4, 8, and 12 weeks after randomization, incisional wounds were made lateral to the sacrum to excise punch biopsy wounds. Identical wounds were made in the 6 participants who were never-smokers. A wound was made once in 24 never-smokers. All wounds were evaluated for 2 weeks for development of wound complications.

Results.—Two hundred twenty-eight wounds were assessed. The wound infection rates were 12% (11/93 wounds) and 2% (1/48 wounds), respectively, for smokers and never-smokers ($P < .05$). Wound infections were significantly fewer in abstaining smokers than in continuous smokers at 4, 8, and 12 weeks after randomization.

Conclusion.—Smokers have a higher wound infection rate than never-smokers. Four weeks of abstinence from smoking decreases the incidence of wound infections.

► Almost every year, we attempt to feature 1 or 2 articles that highlight the adverse affect of smoking in virtually every orthopedic circumstance. This interesting randomized controlled study clearly documents the increased wound infection rate among those who smoke compared with those who do not. The fact that the incisions were standardized and placed in an area with good vascularity is an important strength of the methodology of this contribution. Although this may not be of particular surprise, an important correlating observation is that 4 weeks of abstinence tends to reduce the risk factor. The increasing use of nicotine patches and similar approaches to help decrease pulmonary complications of surgery have no protective effect regarding bone or soft tissue healing; thus, they do not provide viable alternatives to abstinence.

B. F. Morrey, MD

Changes in Bacterial Skin Colonisation During Hospital Admission for Elective Surgery

Lindeque BGP, Botha JL, Wessels W, et al (Univ of Pretoria, South Africa)

SA Orthopaedic Journal Feb:24-29, 2004 2–6

Introduction.—Development of a surgical site infection (SSI) is estimated to increase a patient's hospital stay by approximately 10 days, with a concomitant increase in costs. Although numerous studies have examined potential etiologic factors, risk factors, and preventive measures, many questions regarding SSIs remain unanswered. In a prospective cohort study of patients admitted to 2 hospitals for elective orthopedic surgery, changes in bacterial colonization of the skin were examined.

Methods.—The 48 patients (24 men, 24 women; mean age, 48 years) included in the study had swabs taken from the intended operative site within 2 hours of admission and from the same area within 24 hours postoperatively for routine culture. All patients received IV prophylaxis (cefazolin or clindamycin) and were cleaned and draped according to the usual protocol.

Results.—Fifty-six sites were cultured. There were 27 from the lower limb, 20 from the upper limb, 4 from the head and neck, and 5 from other anatomical regions. Coagulase-negative staphylococcus (CNS) was the most prevalent organism cultured and the most common causative organism found in SSI. Skin colonization did not change in a statistically significant manner during hospitalization.

The overall incidence of preoperative skin colonization with CNS was 68%; the overall incidence of postoperative cultures for CNS was 61%. Preoperative methicillin resistance of CNS was 6%, whereas postoperative resistance was 49% (a statistically significant difference). Resistance of CNS to cefazolin increased from 11% to 37%. Both augmentin and gentamicin also showed a statistically significant change in sensitivity. At both hospitals, vancomycin had 100% sensitivity preoperatively and postoperatively.

Conclusion.—Multiple drug-resistant organisms colonize the skin of healthy individuals during hospital admission. Practices recommended to limit the risk of SSI caused by skin colonization include same-day patient admission, nasal swabs for *Staphylococcus aureus*, chlorhexidine showers and scrubs, cefazolin prophylaxis (or an alternative when patients are admitted more than 24 hours before surgery), and coverage of wound sites with occlusive dressing until suture removal.

▶ As patients are being dismissed from the hospital with shorter lengths of stay, one justification is lessening the potential for nosocomial infection. This very simple study clearly documents justification for this concern and practice. The documentation of the colonization of drug-resistant organisms on the skin during hospitalization is an important observation. The authors discuss this finding in the context of current length of stay and 1-day admission practices.

B. F. Morrey, MD

A Survey of Orthopedic Surgeons' Attitudes and Knowledge Regarding Regional Anesthesia

Oldman M, McCartney CJL, Leung A, et al (Univ of Toronto; Toronto Western Hosp)

Anesth Analg 98:1486-1490, 2004 2–7

Background.—Surgeon preference is an important factor influencing patient anesthetic choice. There is much research in the literature regarding patient preferences, but there is little information available that examines surgeons' attitudes toward general anesthesia versus regional anesthesia. The attitudes and preferences of orthopedic surgeons toward regional anesthesia were reported.

Methods.—A survey was conducted among 76 Canadian orthopedic surgeons identified from publicly available membership databases available on the Royal College of Physicians and Surgeons of Canada and the American Association of Orthopedic Surgeons. Exposure to and attitudes toward regional anesthesia were recorded. Anesthetic preferences (general anesthesia alone, general anesthesia and regional anesthesia, regional anesthesia alone, or no preference) were determined for hypothetical surgical procedures, both for a healthy patient and for the surgeon.

Results.—Surveys were returned by 61% of the surgeons. Forty-eight percent of these respondents indicated that they directed their patients' choice of anesthetic. Over one third of surgeons (40%) directed their patients to selection of regional anesthesia. The main reasons for favoring regional anesthesia were less postoperative pain (32%), decreased nausea and vomiting (12%), and safety (14%). Reasons for not favoring regional anesthesia were delays in the induction of anesthesia (43%), and an unpredictable success rate (12%).

Conclusion.—These findings suggest that orthopedic surgeons are supportive of regional anesthesia. The barriers to increasing use of regional anesthesia are perceived delays and unreliability.

► Simple observations noted in this report were attractive since it seems to provide an objective basis for one's intuition. Most surgeons favor regional anesthesia due to the assistance in postoperative pain and complications associated with general anesthesia, specifically nausea and vomiting. It is recognized that one of the major reasons to avoid regional anesthesia is the delay in surgery. This problem can be addressed by more effective planning and the anesthesiologist's willingness to begin the case somewhat earlier.

The unreliability of regional anesthesia is decreasing as techniques are improving. Similarly, the incidence of nausea and vomiting is likewise decreasing after general anesthesia, with improved general anesthetic agents. In the final analysis, selection of either of these anesthetics remains that of patient or surgeon preference.

B. F. Morrey, MD

Microbiological Culture Results for the Femoral Head: Are They Important to the Donor?

James LA, Ibrahim T, Esler CN (Univ Hosps of Leicester, England)

J Bone Joint Surg Br 86-B:797-800, 2004 2–8

Background.—Osteolysis is a major impediment to the long-term survival of arthroplasties. The success of arthroplasty in improving the quality of life for younger patients has led to an increase in the number arthroplasty patients who require revision for osteolysis. Bone stock may be restored by the impaction of cancellous allografts. After initial reports of the use of this technique in cases of protrusion in primary THA, the use of this technique has not been expanded through the use of allografts for femoral revision arthroplasty in the presence of poor bone stock.

Femoral heads donated at the time of primary THA have provided a supply of bone that is suitable for grafting. However, contamination of donated femoral heads can result in infection after THA. The rate of contamination of donated femoral heads at primary hip arthroplasty within a single region from July 1992 to July 2001 was investigated. Also investigated was whether or not microbial contamination was predictive of early infection in the donor arthroplasty.

Methods.—A null hypothesis was established that culture results had no role in the prediction of early failure of the joint because of infection. The study was based on prospectively obtained data from all primary THA patients at a single institution who consented to donation of their femoral heads. The detached femoral head was cleaned and subjected to microbiological screening before storage. Patients were also asked to participate in an ongoing audit of primary and revision hip and knee surgery.

Results.—A total of 4045 femoral heads were donated during the study period. Of these, 367 (9%) were contaminated. The organism isolated in a majority of the positive cases (77%) was coagulase-negative staphylococcus. At a minimum follow-up of 1 year, there was no statistically significant difference in the rate of complications or of revision in age-matched patients whose femoral heads had a positive culture compared with those whose femoral heads were sterile.

Conclusion.—The culture of the femoral head was found to have no role in the prediction of future failure of joint replacement in the recipient of THA.

▶ This simple study confirms that which has been previously documented but becomes increasingly relevant in the era of cost containment. The fact of almost a 10% contamination rate of femoral head cultures certainly serves to confuse the value of this practice. The conclusion that culture of the femoral head plays no role in determining the expected outcome of the donor has been recognized at our clinic for many years; hence, the practice of culturing the femoral head has long since been abandoned. When we were culturing femoral heads, there was wide disagreement among the staff with regard to the value and whether or not patients with positive cultures should be treated with antibiotics. This article should put that issue to rest.

B. F. Morrey, MD

Lower Limb Arthroplasty Complicated by Deep Venous Thrombosis: Prevalence and Subjective Outcome

Cordell-Smith JA, Williams SC, Harper WM, et al (Glan Clwyd Hosp, Rhyl, Wales; Glenfield Gen Hosp, Leicester, England; Middlesborough Gen Hosp, England)

J Bone Joint Surg Br 86-B:99-101, 2004 2–9

Background.—Deep venous thrombosis (DVT) is a common complication after total hip or knee replacement. DVT is not always symptomatic, and the late effects of asymptomatic DVT have not been fully discerned. Chronic venous insufficiency may be precipitated by perioperative DVT, but this is a difficult condition to evaluate clinically because both the postphlebitic limb and leg ulceration are common afflictions among elderly persons and are most likely multifactorial. The prevalence of DVT after lower limb arthroplasty was investigated, and whether it adversely affected satisfaction, relief from pain, or the level of mobility as perceived by patients was determined.

Methods.—Routine postoperative venography was performed in 610 consecutive recipients of primary total hip replacement (THR) or total knee replacement (TKR). The functional outcome in these patients had already been assessed at 1 year by using the Regional Arthroplasty Database questionnaire, with results of this questionnaire correlated to venographic records.

Results.—The combined prevalence of DVT after THR and TKR in the patients who did not receive chemical thromboprophylaxis was 46.4%. Thrombus was identified in 57.6% of patients with a TKR and in 33.5% of patients with a THR. Proximal thrombus was identified in 11% of patients with a TKR and in 14.8% of patients with a THR. At 1 year after surgery, patients who had a DVT established by venography did not report higher levels of immobility, discomfort, or dissatisfaction when compared with patients with patent venous systems.

Conclusion.—The prevalence of DVT after TKR or THR without chemical thromboprophylaxis may be high, and the findings of this study were consistent with the literature. However, the patients did not perceive thrombosis to compromise their overall outcome. These findings challenge the view that DVT is associated with morbidity and are indicative of a need for additional comprehensive research in this area. The low morbidity of the lower limb associated with DVT in these patients does not support the use of chemical thromboprophylaxis.

▶ This study is included in the YEAR BOOK to provide a perspective of opinions related to this perennial subject of intense investigation. The philosophy of thromboembolic prophylaxis management is not universal. The conclusion of these investigators that chemical thromboprophylaxis is not necessary is an uncommon opinion of surgeons in the United Kingdom. While the orthopedic community in the United States accepts chemical prophylaxis, the specific clinical protocol varies dramatically. In our judgment currently, the most important issue is the protection for several weeks after the patient is dismissed from the hospital. As length of stay continues to be abbreviated, this will be an area of continued investigation for some time to come.

B. F. Morrey, MD

MRI Diagnosis of Tears of the Hip Abductor Tendons (Gluteus Medius and Gluteus Minimus)

Cvitanic O, Henzie G, Skezas N, et al (Southwest Oklahoma MRI, Oklahoma City)

AJR 182:137-143, 2004 2–10

Introduction.—Abductor tendon tears are increasingly recognized as a cause of greater trochanteric pain syndrome. In a recent MRI study of 15 surgically confirmed abductor tendon tears, just 2 tears were correctly recognized, even though MRI was performed to exclude this diagnosis. Some secondary signs of abductor tendon tears may be relatively less affected by field-of-view limitations. The accuracy of MRI for diagnosis of hip abductor tendon tears was analyzed, focusing on signs of tendon disruption.

Methods.—In a series of MRI scans of 74 hips in 45 patients, 15 had surgically confirmed tears of the hip abductor tendons. The patients (mean age, 70 years) generally had clinical signs and symptoms similar to those of trochanteric bursitis. The MRI findings were compared with those of 6 hips with surgically confirmed intact tendons and 48 hips of asymptomatic ambulatory volunteers. The main MRI findings considered were tendon discontinuity, elongation of the gluteus medius tendon, atrophy of the gluteus medius and minimus muscles, and high-signal intensity areas superior and lateral to the greater trochanter on T2-weighted images.

Results.—The MRI finding most frequently associated with hip abductor tears was an area of high-signal intensity superior to the greater trochanter on T2-weighted images. This finding appeared as a focal area larger or smaller than 1 cm in diameter or as a thin sheet enveloping the lateral and superior aspects of the greater trochanter. For areas of high-signal intensity superior to the greater trochanter, the most sensitive MRI sequences were short tau inversion recovery (STIR) and fat-suppressed T2-weighted coronal images. The finding of muscle atrophy was associated with large tears, but not with small tears. On consensus interpretations, other MRI findings positively associated with abductor tendon tears were tendon elongation in the gluteus medius, tendon discontinuity, and areas of T2 hyperintensity later to the greater trochanter. For diagnosis of abductor tendon tears, MRI offered sensitivity of 93% and accuracy of 91%. Interobserver agreement was good for abductor tendon tears, as well as for areas of T2 hyperintensity superior and lateral to the greater trochanter.

Discussion.—MRI is an accurate test for the diagnosis of tears of the hip abductor tendons. The MRI finding of T2 hypersensitivity superior to the greater trochanter appears to be the sign with the highest predictive value. Particular with the use of STIR or fat-suppressed T2-weighted coronal sequences, a negative MRI scan may help to avoid surgery in patients with greater trochanteric pain but no abductor tear.

▶ This article was included to call attention to the diagnosis of this still not generally recognized condition. The main point is the distinction between this entity and chronic trochanteric bursitis is essential. In my judgment, this can be made by careful clinical assessment, but lacking that, the MRI is an effective and accurate means of making this diagnosis. Probably the most important point, however, is to emphasize the awareness of this condition so that the possibility of this diagnosis is considered, thus prompting the imaging procedure.

B. F. Morrey, MD

Twenty-Five Years Followup of Patients Who Had Valgus Osteotomy for Arthritis Hips

Kawate K, Tanaka Y, Ohmura T, et al (Nara Med Univ, Kashihara, Nara, Japan)

Clin Orthop 426:151-158, 2004 2–11

Introduction.—THA is now often done for young patients, but long-term outcomes of the procedure in this age group is unknown. A number of studies, however, report a high rate of revision surgeries in active young patients. Factors that influence the long-term effectiveness (more than 20 years after surgery) of intertrochanteric valgus ostomy were examined in a review of 106 patients with 127 arthritic hips.

Methods.—The average age of the patients at surgery was 42 years and the average duration of follow-up was 25 years. All operations were performed by the same surgeon between March 29, 1962, and September 5, 1980. Preoperative degenerative change was classified radiologically into 1 of 4 grades according to the criteria of Tönnis. Immediately after surgery, radiographs were taken to measure acetabular coverage. The Japanese Orthopedic Association hip score was used for clinical evaluation before surgery, during follow-up, and at the latest follow-up.

Results.—Thirty-eight patients (41 hips) had THA, with a 25-year survival rate of 69% for the procedure. Improvements over time were observed and good clinical outcomes obtained in patients with mild preoperative degenerative changes (Tönnis grade 1) and in those whose hips had better acetabular coverage (center-edge angle greater than 0°, sharp angle less than 50°, or acetabular head index greater than 60%). Radiologic measurements, however, did not influence clinical scores. The latest clinical scores differed significantly between patients younger than 50 years and patients older than 50 at surgery, with average scores of 61.8 and 53.1, respectively. Hips with unilateral involvement had significantly better latest clinical scores than hips with bilateral involvement (average, 64.2 and 58.2, respectively).

Conclusion.—The intertrochanteric valgus osteotomy is appropriate for younger patients, especially those with unilateral involvement. Ideal patients for this technique are younger than 50 years, with opening of the lateral edge of the joint space greater than 3 mm compared with radiographs taken with the hip in neutral position, or improvement of congruency seen on preoperative radiographs taken with the hip adducted. Ideal patients for a THA are older than 50 years with severe pain and arthritic change but without the above radiographic findings.

▶ This article is of some interest to those dealing in adult reconstructive issues but probably is of more value for the younger age group. This is one of the largest recent series of a long-term follow-up of a large cohort of patients. This study does provide a strong rationale for nonjoint replacement reconstruction in the younger age group with symptomatic dysplastic hips.

The authors carefully point out the outcome as a function of radiographic criteria. These selection factors along with specific surgical technique would seem to be important considerations for satisfactory outcome. The preoperative radiographic rate of joint space regeneration is also of importance. One issue that is not well addressed is the ease of converting a failed osteotomy to a total hip, which is the only major reservation one might offer regarding this approach to the young patient with early degenerative arthrosis.

B. F. Morrey, MD

Autologous Chondrocyte Implantation Compared WIth Microfracture in the Knee: A Randomized Trial

Knutsen G, Engebretsen L, Ludvigsen TC, et al (Univ Hosp Tromsø, Norway; Oslo Orthopaedic Univ Clinic, Norway; Univ Hosp Trondheim, Norway; et al)
J Bone Joint Surg Am 86-A:455-464, 2004 2–12

Background.—The outcomes of new methods for treating full-thickness cartilage defects have been promising. Autologous chondrocyte implantation was compared with microfracture in a randomized study.

Methods.—Eighty patients without general osteoarthritis but with a single symptomatic cartilage defect on the femoral condyle in a stable knee were enrolled in the study. Forty patients underwent autologous chondrocyte implantation, and 40 had microfracture. Follow-up assessments were done at 12 and 24 months. At 2 years after surgery, arthroscopy with biopsy was performed for histologic examination.

Findings.—The differences between groups were minimal (Fig 4). Both had significant clinical improvement at 2 years. On the SF-36 physical component score at 2 years, the microfracture group had significantly more im-

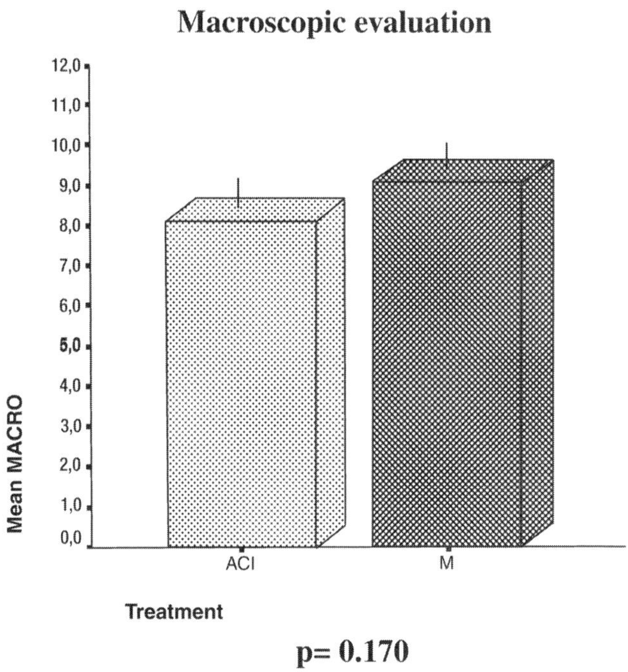

FIGURE 4.—Histogram showing the mean scores on the ICRS macroscopic evaluation (MACRO) at the second-look arthroscopy performed at 2 years postoperatively. The maximum score for the evaluation is 12 points. No significant difference between the autologous chondrocyte implantation (ACI) and microfracture (M) groups was detected. (Republished with permission of the Journal of Bone and Joint Surgery, Inc, from Knutsen G, Engebretsen L, Ludvigsen TC, et al: Autologous chondrocyte implantation compared with microfracture in the knee: A randomized trial. *J Bone Joint Surg Am* 86A:455-464, 2004. Reproduced by permission of the publisher via Copyright Clearance Center, Inc.)

provement than did the autologous chondrocyte implantation group. In both groups, younger and more active patients had better outcomes. Histologic evaluation of repair tissue in biopsy specimens, obtained in 84% of patients, demonstrated no significant between-group differences.

Conclusions.—The short-term results of both autologous chondrocyte implantation and microfracture in the knee are acceptable. Macroscopic and histologic findings did not differ between the treatment groups. Histologic findings did not appear to correlate with clinical outcome at 2 years.

▶ This is an excellent study and one of the best that we have recently seen. It is a level 1 evidence study, which is a randomized controlled trial. The article is important because the methodology is sound and the question is of great clinical relevance. Documentation that microfractures are not only as effective as autologous chondrocyte implantation but even more so at 2 years by most standards is I think an extremely important finding. The value of the technique is enhanced when it is considered that it is less expensive than the chondrocyte implant option. The authors did not mention in their methodology the postoperative course, but microfracture typically would be anticipated to be associated with less morbidity as well. Thus, in the editor's mind, this manuscript goes a long way to defining with considerable certainty the treatment of choice for the specific lesion defined in the inclusion criteria.

B. F. Morrey, MD

Reoperation After Autologous Chondrocyte Implantation: Indications and Findings

Henderson I, Tuy B, Oakes B (St Vincent's and Mercy Private Hosp, Melbourne, Australia; Monash Univ, Melbourne, Australia)

J Bone Joint Surg Br 86-B:205-211, 2004 2–13

Background.—Autologous chondrocyte implantation (ACI) has emerged in the last decade as a viable and effective treatment for injury to articular cartilage. Short-term results with ACI have been encouraging in regard to patient satisfaction and standard knee scores. Patients who have required additional surgery after ACI were evaluated, and the surgical findings, procedures required, the clinical outcome, and the results of biopsy were described.

Methods.—A review was conducted of 22 of 135 patients who were treated with ACI and who had undergone additional surgery for pain in the knee and mechanical symptoms after a mean of 10.5 months. There were 31 grafted lesions. At surgery, the findings included lifting (24 of 31) and detachment (4 of 31) of periosteal patches for which arthroscopic shaving was performed. Chondroplasty was undertaken on 2 new lesions, 1 lesion required and ACI, and another patient required trimming of a meniscus.

Results.—Resolution of the mechanical symptoms occurred within 2 weeks. At the last follow-up, which occurred at 2 to 14 months from reoperation, 68% had improved and 6% had normal or nearly normal International Knee Documentation Committee scores. Of the 31 lesions, 30 (97%) had normal or nearly normal visual repair scores.

Biopsy findings indicated good integration with subchondral bone and the marginal interface in all specimens, most of which showed hyaline or hyaline-like cartilage (70%). Persistent adverse mechanical symptoms required surgery in 13% of patients treated with ACI; these symptoms were attributed to periosteal extrusion. Simple arthroscopic debridement was curative in these cases.

Conclusion.—ACI is a relatively new treatment for defects of articular cartilage. In this series, only 14% of patients treated with ACI had further surgery for problems related to the graft; they were mainly mechanical symptoms.

► This study was of interest to demonstrate the intermediate-term outcome of a significant number of patients undergoing ACI. The overall favorable outcome is worth noting. Of additional and significant value is the insight gained by realizing those patients that had problems after the initial procedure could be managed with a subsequent operation in a high percentage of incidences. This and other studies are important to more clearly understand the value of cartilage transplantation and its role in the overall spectrum of managing the young patient with a localized cartilage problem.

B. F. Morrey, MD

Fatal Pulmonary Embolism After Knee Arthroscopy

Navarro-Sanz A, Fernández-Ortega JF (Málaga City Hall, Spain; Carlos Haya Hosp, Málaga, Spain)

Am J Sports Med 32:525-528, 2004 2–14

Background.—Venous thromboembolic disease (VTED) is relatively common in the general population. There are several predisposing factors, both congenital and acquired, involved in the pathophysiology of VTED. The most severe form of this disease is pulmonary thromboembolism (PTE), which can be life threatening. However, the occurrence of PTE in healthy young persons with no known risk factors is quite unusual. A case of PTE that developed as a complication of arthroscopy of the knee was described in a young man who suffered a lesion of the medial meniscus during a soccer game.

> *Case Report.*—Man, 46, was seen with pain on the inside of the left knee, occasional locking, and limitation of full extension of the knee. The man regularly participated in soccer games and was an avid hiker. He had no noteworthy medical history. Physical examination showed medial jointline tenderness, evidence of effusion, and a positive McMurray sign. A bucket-handle tear of the medial meniscus was confirmed by MRI. Arthroscopy was performed after limb

exsanguination under tourniquet ischemia. A partial meniscectomy was performed with no immediate complications.

The patient was walking in the street 1 week after the operation when he suffered a sudden episode of dyspnea, syncope, paleness, and low perfusion—all signs of low cardiac output. He suffered cardiopulmonary arrest in the form of electromechanical dissociation, which required advanced resuscitation. The presence of deep venous thrombosis with subsequent PTE was suspected on the basis of radiographic examination and a transthoracic electrocardiogram. After hemodynamic stabilization, the patient remained in a deep coma and died 3 days after admission.

Conclusion.—A review of the literature concerning VTED after knee arthroscopy found only 1 reference to another case of fatal PTE after arthroscopy. Included in this case report are recommendations for its prevention, a discussion of the clinical course of the disease and its potential severity, and recommendations for mechanical or pharmacologic measures to further reduce its incidence.

► The topic remains a major issue for the orthopedic surgeon in general. Typically, PTE is not felt to be a concern or significant risk after arthroscopy. We have certainly experienced thrombophlebitis following this relatively noninvasive procedure. The documentation of a fatal PTE was added to this year's YEAR BOOK to underscore the unlikely but possible event. The postoperative management program might be considered based on this report.

B. F. Morrey, MD

Surgical Reconstruction of Severe Patellofemoral Maltracking

Palmer SH, Servant CT, Maguire J, et al (Australian Inst of Musculo-Skeletal Research, Sydney, Australia)

Clin Orthop 419:144-148, 2004 2–15

Background.—Different realignment procedures in patients with dysfunction of the patellofemoral mechanism yield greatly variable outcomes. A surgical technique was developed in an attempt to correct all the abnormalities of patellofemoral maltracking.

Methods and Outcomes.—The procedure was performed in 117 knees in 84 patients. Fifty-five percent had frank dislocation, and the rest had anterior knee pain and abnormal patella tracking. The procedure involved a lateral release, vastus medialis (obliquus) tendon advancement, and tibial tubercle transfer. The tubercle was not only moved medially but distally to correct patella alta. The tubercle was also elevated anteriorly to decrease patellofemoral joint reaction forces. Patients were observed up for an average of 5.6 years. Functional outcomes were good to excellent in 79% of patients. Eighty-four percent said they would have the surgery again. Patellar dislocation recurred in 2 patients with marked generalized ligamentous laxity.

Conclusions.—Comprehensive patellofemoral reconstruction tailored to individual patients can yield a good to excellent outcome in 78%. Clinicians should inform patients of the possible postoperative restriction of flexion and need to remove metalwork.

► This retrospective study is important since it addresses the common problem of a subluxing or dislocating the patella. The outcome is one of the most impressive yet reported in the literature. The patient selection criteria are rather simple and basic. The important features are the 3 components of this technique: lateral release, medial advancement, and tibial tubercle translocation. The specific technique of the translocation may be important but the manuscript does not clarify this. It should also be noted that some follow-up is less than 1 year and an overall 5-year average may be considered limited. However, usually the outcome is measured by elimination of the subluxation, which can usually be documented within 6 months of surgery.

B. F. Morrey, MD

Surgical Management of Knee Dislocations

Harner CD, Waltrip RL, Bennett CH, et al (Univ of Pittsburgh, Pa)

J Bone Joint Surg Am 86-A:262-273, 2004 2–16

Background.—Several soft tissue stabilizing structures are damaged in traumatic dislocation of the knee. There have been reports of isolated injuries of the ACL or posterior cruciate ligament in these injuries, but in most cases both cruciate ligaments are completely disrupted. Strategies for the management of knee dislocation have been varied and controversial. Immobilization has generally resulted in poor outcomes, and most experienced surgeons have preferred surgical treatment. However, surgical management is controversial, particularly in regard to the timing of surgery, which structures to repair or reconstruct, and graft selection. One method of surgical treatment of knee dislocations with the use of a standardized protocol was described and the clinical results reported.

Methods.—The study group was composed of 47 consecutive patients with an occult (reduced) or grossly dislocated knee. Fourteen were excluded from this study because of confounding variables. The remaining 33 patients received surgical treatment for their knee dislocation with a standard approach. Anatomical repair and/or replacement was performed with fresh-frozen allograft tissue. Of these patients, 31 returned for subjective and objective evaluation with the use of 4 different knee rating scales at a minimum of 24 months after the operation.

Results.—Acute treatment was provided to 19 of 31 patients, and 12 were treated chronically. The mean Lysholm score was 91 points for the acutely reconstructed knees and 80 points for the chronically reconstructed knees. The Knee Outcome Survey Activities of Daily Living scores averaged 91 points for the acutely reconstructed knees and 84 points for the chronically reconstructed knees. The scores on the Sports Activity section of the survey averaged 89 points for the acutely reconstructed knees and 69 points for the chronically reconstructed knees.

The Meyers ratings showed that 23 patients had an excellent or good score and 8 had a fair or poor score. The Meyers score was good or excellent in 16 of 19 acutely reconstructed knees and 7 of 12 chronically reconstructed knees. The average loss of extension was 1° and the average loss of flexion was 12°. There was no difference in the ROM between the acutely and chronically treated patients. All patients demonstrated consistently improved stability on laxity tests, with more predictable results in the acutely treated patients.

Conclusion.—Surgical treatment of knee dislocations provided satisfactory subjective and objective outcomes at 2 to 6 years postoperatively. Almost all of the patients who were treated acutely had higher subjective scores and better objective restoration of knee stability than did the patients treated 3 weeks or more after the injury, and nearly all of the patients were able to perform activities of daily living with few problems. However, their ability to return to high-demand sports and strenuous manual labor was not so predictable.

▶ This retrospective study of level III evidence, reviews a large series of patients with a condition that has not been recently discussed in the literature. The article serves to outline a reasonable treatment protocol and demonstrates improved subjective and objective clinical outcomes compared with prior reports. The more aggressive repair and reconstruction of damaged tissues, particularly in the acute setting, is clearly the treatment of choice for this devastating injury.

B. F. Morrey, MD

3 Pediatrics

Introduction

This year, the Pediatrics chapter of the YEAR BOOK OF ORTHOPEDICS features trauma (with the usual emphasis on femoral shaft and elbow fractures) and elective surgery-related subjects. These are complemented with 2 articles on each of the following subjects: anatomy, epidemiology, deformities (developmental dysplasia of the hip and scoliosis), and Perthes disease.

Hamlet A. Peterson, MD, MS

Anatomy

Age-Related Vascular Changes in the Epiphysis, Physis, and Metaphysis: Normal Findings on Gadolinium-Enhanced MRI of Piglets
Jaramillo D, Villegas-Medina OL, Doty DK, et al (Harvard Med School, Boston)
AJR 182:353-360, 2004 3–1

Background.—Cartilaginous development in the immature skeleton is closely associated with changes in the epiphyseal and metaphyseal vessels. The cartilaginous epiphysis of human beings and other mammals contains numerous vessels at birth, most of which are lost with the progressive development of the secondary ossification center. The vessels disappear almost entirely by the end of the first year of life in human infants but persist to a greater extent in piglets. Gadolinium-enhanced MRI provides a depiction of the vascular canals of the cartilaginous epiphysis and the enhancement of the physeal and epiphyseal cartilage and vascularity of the marrow. However, the temporal sequence of and changes in gadolinium enhancement that occur with age are poorly understood. The normal enhancement patterns seen on MRIs of the epiphysis, physis, and metaphysis and the age-related vascular change in piglets with gadoteridol were investigated.

Methods.—Quantitative and qualitative analyses of the normal changes were performed on sequential T1-weighted images of the proximal and distal femurs of 26 piglets 1 to 6 weeks old after intravenous administration of gadoteridol. The enhanced images were correlated with findings on intermediate-weighted, T2-weighted, and gradient recalled echo images and at histologic examination.

Results.—Early enhancement of the epiphyseal vascular canals, the main physis, the physis of the secondary ossification center, and a metaphyseal band adjacent to the physis was observed (Fig 1). Enhancement was slower in the epiphyseal and metaphyseal marrow and in the epiphyseal cartilage. In the epiphyseal cartilage 3 phases of enhancement were observed: vascular, canalicular, and cartilaginous. There was a decline in the enhancement of the epiphyseal cartilage as the piglets matured, and the epiphyseal vascular canals became less conspicuous. Physeal enhancement was greatest during the first week of life, declined at 3 weeks, and increased again as the physis came to lie adjacent to a larger segment of the epiphyseal ossification center.

Conclusions.—Gadoteridol-enhanced MRI of the growing piglet skeleton demonstrated multiple cartilaginous and vascular structures. Epiphy-

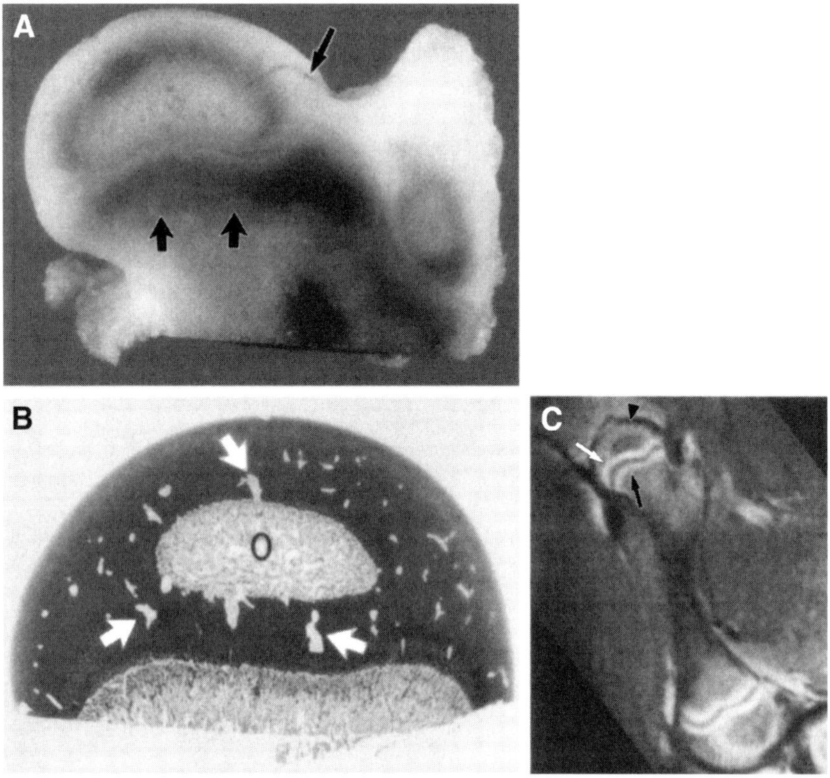

FIGURE 1.—Epiphysis of 3-week-old piglet. **A**, Photomicrograph of coronal macroscopic section of proximal femur shows major vascular canal (lateral epiphyseal vessel, *thin arrow*) within white epiphyseal cartilage. Dark area in metaphysis (*thick arrows*) corresponds to metaphyseal spongiosa. **B**, Photomicrograph of coronal histologic section of proximal femur reveals numerous vascular canals (*arrows*) within epiphyseal cartilage surrounding secondary center of ossification (O). (Toluidine blue, ×2.) **C**, Coronal T1-weighted spin-echo image (TR/TE, 300/25) of entire femur obtained 3 minutes after IV administration of gadoteridol. In both proximal and distal femoral epiphyses, marked enhancement is observed in physis (*white arrow*) and in band (*black arrow*) in juxtaphyseal metaphysis corresponding anatomically to metaphyseal spongiosa. Enhancement of vascular canals (*arrowhead*) within epiphyseal cartilage is less marked. (Courtesy of Jaramillo D, Villegas-Medina OL, Doty DK, et al: Age-related vascular changes in the epiphysis, physis, and metaphysis: Normal findings on gadolinium-enhanced MRI of piglets. *AJR* 182:353-360, 2004. Reprinted with permission from the American Journal of Roentgenology.)

seal cartilage enhancement decreased and physeal cartilage enhancement increased with skeletal maturity and progressive epiphyseal ossification.

► It is difficult to stay abreast of all the different facets of MRI that affect conditions important to pediatric orthopedists. Although this study was of a basic science nature, it vividly shows in vivo anatomic detail of unossified cartilage in the immature skeleton approaching that previously seen only with histologic sections. The implications for improved analysis of cartilage (for example, of physeal damage) are huge.

H. A. Peterson, MD, MS

The Natural History of Cervical Disc Calcification in Children

Dai L-Y, Ye H, Qian Q-R (Xinhua Hosp, Shanghai, China; Changzheng Hosp, Shanghai, China)

J Bone Joint Surg Am 86-A:1467-1472, 2004 3–2

Background.—When calcified intervertebral disks occurs in children, the lower cervical region is most frequently involved. Only about 200 cases of children having calcified intervertebral disks exist in the literature. Conservative treatment proves effective for most cases. Surgery may be required for patients with progressive neurologic deficits. Seventeen cases of children with symptomatic or asymptomatic cervical disk calcification were documented to determine the disorder's natural history and identify related factors.

Methods.—The symptoms of 10 boys and 7 girls (mean age, 7.7 years; range, 5-13 years) included a fever in 3 and a history of trauma in 2. One patient was asymptomatic and had been discovered by chance. The 16 others complained of neck pain. Calcification involved the central part of the cervical intervertebral disks, as determined radiographically. Symptoms had been treated, and periodic follow-up occurred until the symptoms and the calcific deposits were gone.

Results.—All patients had complete disappearance of the symptoms within 17 to 173 days (mean, 34.3 days), and none had a recurrence. The calcific deposits resolved completely in 3 to 60 months (mean, 15 months); these did not return either (Fig 4). No significant correlation was found for any of the factors (ie, age, sex, level of disk calcification, severity of symptoms, or degree of spinal canal compromise). In addition, no relationship was found between the time of resolution of symptoms and the calcification.

Conclusions.—In children, cervical disk calcification seems to be a self-limiting condition. The prognosis is excellent, and clinical symptoms and radiographic abnormalities completely resolve. Conservative treatment was effective, even when the symptoms were caused by nerve-root or spinal cord compression. Surgical intervention is rarely needed.

► It is generally accepted that cervical disk calcification in children is self-limiting and has an excellent prognosis. The etiology remains obscure, and this

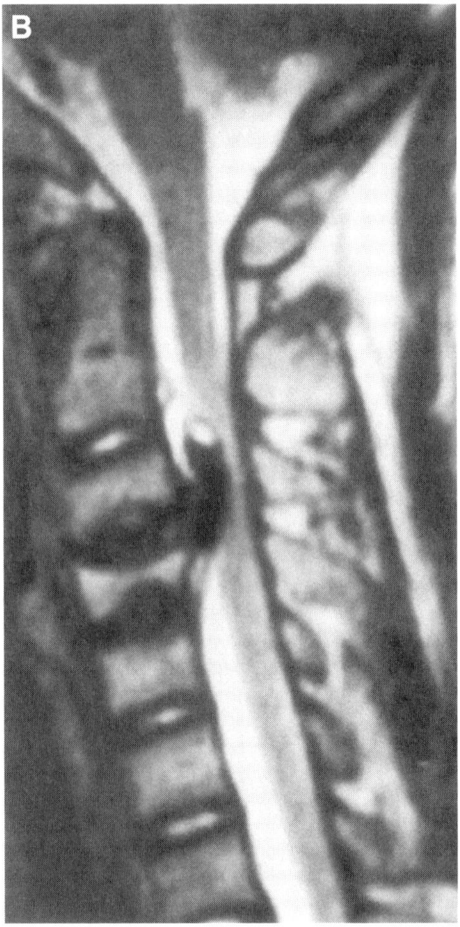

FIGURE 4B.—T2-weighted MRI showing a low-signal intensity in the spinal cord. The extent of spinal canal compromise was 64%. (Republished with permission of the Journal of Bone and Joint Surgery, Inc, from Dai L-Y, Ye H, Qian Q-R: The natural history of cervical disc calcification in children. *J Bone Joint Surg Am* 86-A:1467-1472, 2004. Reproduced by permission of the publisher via Copyright Clearance Center, Inc.)

article discusses various theories; however, it endorses none. This study is deficient in describing the treatment, stating only that the "treatment included analgesia, traction, and/or a cervical collar until the patients became asymptomatic." The article is, however, very significant in describing 16 patients, 11 who had CT scans, and 7 who had MRI. Some of these patients had marked compromise of the spinal canal and spinal cord, which resolved spontaneously without surgery. The authors concluded that surgical intervention for the treatment of nerve-root or spinal cord compression by a calcified cervical disk is rarely indicated.

H. A. Peterson, MD, MS

Epidemiology

Epidemiology of Childhood Fractures in Britain: A Study Using the General Practice Research Database

Cooper C, Dennison EM, Leufkens HGM, et al (Univ of Southampton, England; Univ of Utrecht, The Netherlands; Univ of Sheffield, England; et al)

J Bone Miner Res 19:1976-1981, 2004 3–3

Introduction.—Most data concerning the epidemiology of fractures in childhood come from Scandinavian trials, which have reported that the risk of sustaining a fracture from birth to 16 years of age is 42% among males and 27% among females. Fractures of the distal radius are the most common, followed by fractures of the phalanges of the hand. United States data, which are based on referral to secondary care, show annual rates of femoral shaft fractures to be 19 per 100,000, with a bimodal peak of incidence at 2 and 17 years of age. The age- and gender-specific incidence rates for fractures at various skeletal sites were obtained from the General Practice Research Database (a population-based British cohort that contains computerized medical records of about 7 million residents) between 1988 and 1998.

Results.—A total of 52,624 males and 31,505 females sustained 1 or more fractures during follow-up, for a rate of 133.1 per 10,000 person-years. Fractures occurred more frequently in males than in females (161.6/10,000 person-years vs 102.9/10,000 person-years). The most frequently occurring fracture in both sexes was the radius/ulna (30%). The incidence of fractures was greater in males versus females at all ages, with the peak incidence at 14 years in males and 11 years in females. Substantial geographic variation was seen in standardized fracture incidence. A significantly greater rate was seen in Northern Ireland, Wales, and Scotland, compared with southeast England.

Conclusion.—Fractures are common in childhood; about one third of males and females have at least 1 fracture before 17 years of age. The rates are higher among males than females; incidence rates peak later in males than females. The radius/ulna is the most frequently affected site in both sexes.

▶ This population-based British cohort study is a role model for determining the epidemiology of fractures in children. Almost all data on fracture epidemiology are the result of series reports of cases from centers which are subject to the vagaries of referral and without the benefit of denominator statistics. Thus, there are few places in the world that true population-based studies are undertaken, most notably Scandinavia, Britain, and Olmsted County, Minnesota. Population-based studies are essential for determining fracture rates for gender and age, which allows allocation of resources to study, prevent, and treat the fractures. In the study reported here, the authors acknowledge a coding system limitation, which may be the explanation for the absence of hand and foot metacarpal, metatarsal, and phalangeal fractures.

H. A. Peterson, MD, MS

Demographics of Traumatic Amputations in Children: Implications for Prevention Strategies

Loder RT (Shriners Hosp for Children, Minneapolis, Minn)
J Bone Joint Surg Am 86-A:923-928, 2004 3–4

Introduction.—Trauma is the leading cause of mortality and the second leading cause of morbidity in children in the United States. Among children who survive a severe injury, amputations account for a large component of trauma-associated morbidity. A retrospective review of patients seen at a referral center examined the demographics of traumatic amputations in children.

Methods.—Many children with traumatic amputations resulting from injuries are brought to the Shriners Hospital for Children/Twin Cities in Minnesota. The review included all children 18 years or younger with traumatic amputations who were cared for at the hospital between 1980 and 2000. Data collected from medical records consisted of the cause of the amputation, amputation level, age distribution of patients, and seasonal variations in the amputations.

Results.—A total of 256 amputations were performed in 235 children (177 boys and 58 girls). The amputation involved a single extremity in 217 children, 2 extremities in 16 children, and 3 and 4 extremities in 1 child each. A lower extremity was amputated in 147 children, an upper extremity was amputated in 84, and both the upper and lower extremity were amputated in 4. The most common causes of amputation were lawnmower injuries

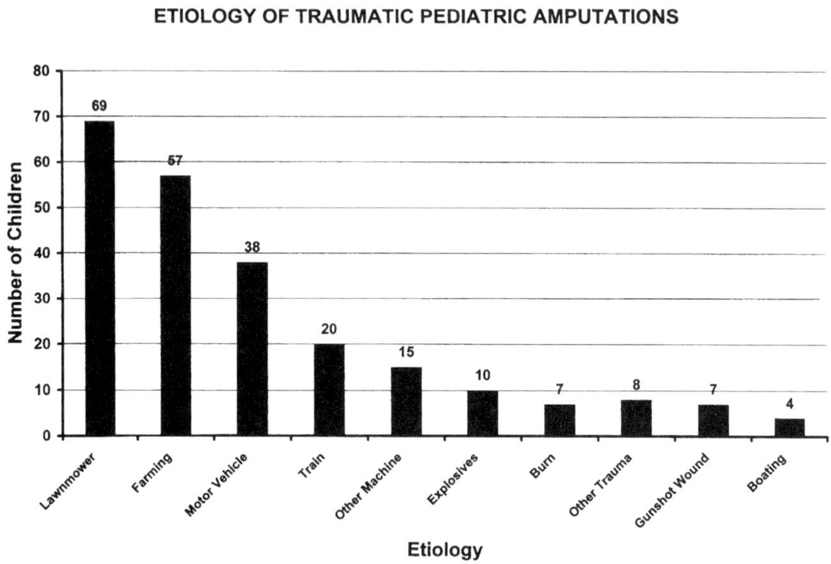

FIGURE 1.—The etiology of traumatic amputations in 235 children. (Republished with permission of the Journal of Bone and Joint Surgery, Inc, from Loder RT: Demographics of traumatic amputations in children: Implications for prevention strategies. *J Bone Joint Surg Am* 86-A:923-928, 2004. Reproduced by permission of the publisher via Copyright Clearance Center, Inc.)

(29%), farming injuries (24%), and motor vehicle collisions (16%). The mean age at the time of injury was 7.9 years, but most children (78%) with a lawnmower amputation were 5 years or younger. Significant seasonal variation was seen in amputations. The mean date was July 3, and amputations caused by lawnmower and motor vehicle accidents were most common in June and July, respectively. The mean date for farming-related amputations was September 2.

Conclusion.—In this review of traumatic amputations in children in the upper midwestern United States, common patterns emerged based on the mechanism of the injury (Fig 1), the season of the year, and the age of the child. Efforts to prevent lawnmower injuries, most of which involve young children, should be promoted in the spring and directed toward parents. Campaigns to prevent farming-related injuries should target both children and parents and should be conducted in spring and early fall.

► In addition to being a thorough collection and analysis of traumatic amputations in children, this superb epidemiologic study has also evaluated and recommended potential procedures to reduce these injuries in the future. Success in reducing these devastating injuries is dependent on the advocacy and support of these recommendations by pediatric orthopedists.

H. A. Peterson, MD, MS

Trauma

The Most Frequent Traumatic Orthopaedic Injuries From a National Pediatric Inpatient Population

Galano GJ, Vitale MA, Kessler MW, et al (Columbia Univ, New York)
J Pediatr Orthop 25:39-44, 2005 3–5

Introduction.—Pediatric trauma continues to be the leading cause of death and disability in children. It accounts for 11 million hospitalizations, 100,000 permanent disabilities, and 15,000 deaths yearly in the United States. The 1997 Kids' Inpatient Database (KID) was used to assess orthopaedic trauma as it occurred in a national pediatric inpatient population. A current descriptive picture of traumatic pediatric orthopedic injuries was presented.

Methods.—The Healthcare Cost and Utilization Project KID was used to retrospectively evaluate patients with a traumatic orthopedic condition as their primary diagnosis. The database has information for 1.9 million unweighted discharge records for patients whose age at admission was 18 years or younger from 2521 community hospitals in the United States in 1997.

Results.—More than 84,000 patients were admitted for orthopedic trauma; they accrued an estimated $932.8 million in hospital charges. The most common injury was femur fracture (21.5% of orthopaedic trauma), then tibia or fibula fracture or both (21.5%), humerus fracture (17.0%), radius or ulna fracture or both (14.8%), and vertebral fracture (5.2%). Most pediatric orthopedic trauma was treated at nonchildren's hospitals (70.4%). Patients with femur, humerus, vertebral, pelvic, or hand/finger fractures, or a back sprain/strain were directed to children's hospitals more often, compared with the total number of pediatric orthopedic trauma patients. Practice patterns varied for patients with femoral shaft fractures, depending on the type of hospital. Patients with a femoral shaft fracture in the 6- to 10-year age group were significantly more likely to receive internal fixation versus casting or traction if they were treated at a children's hospital. Pelvic fracture was associated with an average of 5.2 other diagnoses, followed by 5.0 for vertebral fracture; 3.8 for back sprains/strains; 3.7 for femoral fracture, hand/finger fracture, and foot/toe fracture; 3.3 for fractured tibia/fibula; 3.1 for knee/leg sprain/strain; and 3.0 for humeral fracture and radial/ulna fracture.

Conclusion.—Understanding the patterns in which pediatric trauma occurs is crucial to establishing effective injury prevention strategies and adapting treatment to optimize outcomes.

▶ This study indicates that pediatric orthopedic trauma represents a substantial amount of all pediatric hospitalizations. Understanding the patterns of the most common pediatric orthopedic trauma is critical for injury prevention. Orthopedists can be instrumental in preventing pediatric injuries by participating in patient education, research, and programs that promote safety.

H. A. Peterson, MD, MS

Spinal Cord Injury Without Radiographic Abnormality in Children, 2 Decades Later

Pang D (Univ of California, Davis)

Neurosurgery 55:1325-1343, 2004 3–6

Introduction.—Injuries to the spinal cord vertebral column are somewhat uncommon from birth to 17 years of age, thanks to the juvenile vertebral column being inherently malleable. This physiologic hypermobility of the vertebral segments is always at the expense of their protective function to the underlying spinal cord, which handles deformation poorly. Much data have emerged since 1982, when the original description of spinal cord injury without radiographic abnormalities (SCIWORA) as a self-contained syndrome was reported. New and old data on SCIWORA since its original description were reviewed, with an emphasis on the unique biomechanical properties of the juvenile spine, the mechanisms of injuries, the profound influence of age on injury pattern and outcome, MRI characteristics, and management of SCIWORA.

Findings.—The increasing use of MRI in SCIWORA has provided ample evidence concerning damage in nearly all nonbony supporting tissues of the juvenile vertebral column, including rupture of the anterior and posterior longitudinal ligaments, intervertebral disk disruption, muscular and interspinal ligament tears, tectorial membrane rupture, and shearing of the subepiphyseal growth zone of the vertebral endplates. This information provides the structural basis for the postulated "occult instability" in the spine of a patient after SCIWORA. Five classes of post-SCIWORA cord findings have been identified by MRI: complete transection, major hemorrhage, minor hemorrhage, edema only, and normal. These "neural" findings are highly predictive of patient outcome. Transection and major hemorrhage are linked with profoundly poor outcomes, but 40% of patients with minor hemorrhage improved to mild grades, whereas 75% with edema only became mild grades and 25% became normal. Complete recovery was observed in all patients with normal cord signals. Thoracic SCIWORA consists of 3 subtypes: high-speed direct impact, distraction from lap belts, and crush injuries by slow-moving vehicles. In the ICU, children with cervical spinal cord injuries are immobilized in a cervicothoracic brace for 3 months, midthoracic to low thoracic lesions are treated with a thoracolumbar orthosis, and those with upper thoracic lesions are fitted with a thoracolumbar orthosis with added chin and occiput supports.

Conclusion.—Injury prevention, prompt injury recognition, usc of MRI and electrophysiologic verification, and timely bracing of SCIWORA patients continue to be the primary measures used to improve outcome.

▶ This article is a re-review of SCIWORA by the author who first described the entity in 1982. It is followed by 3 critiques. The one by Michael Fehlings and Ross Gurgo is reproduced here.

"This article represents a comprehensive and thoughtful review of SCIWORA, a term that the author himself coined 2 decades ago and now has widespread use in adult and pediatric clinical setting. MRI, which was not available when the concept of SCIWORA was initially described, does allow a far better visualization of injury to neural and soft tissue structures. However, the correlation of MRI findings with appropriate treatment is more controversial; that is, one must consider possible 'instability' of the spine owing to soft tissue disruption and consequently the need and time required for bracing. The author describes well his treatment algorithm based on MRI and SSEP findings and, of course, the clinical examination. The emphasis placed on evaluating pediatric spinal injury—always with SCIWORA in mind—is valuable and is now, thanks to the author's work over the past 2 decades, commonplace in clinical practice."

H. A. Peterson, MD, MS

Analysis of 51 Tibial Triplane Fractures Using CT With Multiplanar Reconstruction

Brown SD, Kasser JR, Zurakowski D, et al (Children's Hosp, Boston)

AJR 183:1489-1495, 2004 3–7

Background.—The triplane fracture accounts for 6% to 10% of distal tibial epiphyseal fractures in adolescents. All triplane fractures involve the epiphysis, physis, and metaphysis; however, these fractures seem to conform to different Salter-Harris configurations, depending on the location within the distal tibia and the plane that is being studied, which makes the evaluation of the anatomy of these complex multiplanar fractures even more confusing. The most common patterns of triplane fractures were determined, and the risk of epiphyseal separation was assessed for each pattern.

Methods.—CT was performed in 51 children with tibial triplane fractures, and the resultant scans underwent multiplanar reconstruction. Epiphyseal and physeal involvement was categorized, as was the number of fragments, the appearance of the Salter-Harris fracture in each plane, and the degree of separation of the epiphyseal fragments.

Results.—The most frequent type of fracture in this group was the classic 2-fragment type of fracture with medial epiphyseal extension (33 of 51 patients). All 3-fragment types (8 of 51 fractures) resulted in a separate anterolateral fragment. Extension to the medial malleolus was a common finding (12 of 51 patients). None of the 5 reported fracture types involving anteromedial physeal separation were found in this study group. Children with epiphyseal separation requiring surgery were older and had plafond involvement.

Conclusion.—CT and multiplanar reconstruction of triplane fractures can provide an improved understanding of the patterns of injury in triplane fractures and their relative prevalence.

► CT scans have been known for some time to give superior visualization of comminuted and difficult-to-visualize fractures of epiphyses, particularly the triplane fracture. This article demonstrates the added benefits of improving CT multiplanar reconstruction technology when analyzing triplane fractures of the distal tibia, as well as attempting to clarify terminology and classification of these complex fractures.

H. A. Peterson, MD, MS

Compartment Syndrome Following Intramedullary Fixation of Pediatric Forearm Fractures

Yuan PS, Pring ME, Gaynor TP, et al (Children's Hosp, San Diego, Calif; Univ of California, San Diego)

J Pediatr Orthop 24:370-375, 2004 3–8

Introduction.—Compartment syndrome (CS) is one of the most challenging complications associated with fractures and fracture management. This complication is rare in isolated fractures of the forearm. CS of the forearm after intramedullary fixation of the radius has been reported; its true risk in children has not been thoroughly investigated. The incidence and associated risk factors of CS after forearm fracture treatment with either closed reduction or intramedullary fixation were examined in a large series of consecutive patients from a single institution.

Methods.—A retrospective review was performed of 285 consecutive children treated for diaphyseal both-bone forearm fractures between May 1997 and December 1999. Medical records, including emergency department evaluation and treatment, radiographs, operative reports, anesthesia records, and intraoperative fluoroscopy times were examined.

Results.—Of 235 closed fractures, 205 were treated with closed reduction and casting; none developed CS. Of 30 patients treated with closed reduction and intramedullary fixation, 3 (10%) had CS develop. Fifty patients underwent debridement and open reduction with intramedullary pinning; 3 (6%) of these patients had CS develop. The 80 patients treated with intramedullary fixation had an increased rate of CS compared with the 205 patients treated with closed reduction and castings ($P < .001$). Among patients who underwent surgery, those with longer operative times and more use of intraoperative fluoroscopy were at increased risk of having CS develop.

Conclusion.—Excellent results have been reported with intramedullary fixation of both-bone forearm fractures, but the surgeon, patient, and patient's family need to understand the risk involved: 7.5% of patients treated with intramedullary fixation subsequently had signs and/or symptoms of CS and needed formal fasciotomy, whereas none of the 205 patients treated with closed reduction and casting subsequently had CS.

▶ The incidence of CS after fractures of forearm bones in children treated by closed reduction and casting, closed reduction and intramedullary (IM) fixation of both bones, and open reduction and IM fixation is nicely compared in this article. Knowledge of the 10% incidence of CS in patients treated by closed reduction and IM fixation of both bones could cause a reduction in the future use of this method. An alternative for unstable fractures might be closed reduction and IM fixation of either the radius or the ulna rather than both. Hopefully, the authors will consider analyzing this alternative and determine which situations would benefit the most from fixation of the radius and which would benefit from fixation of the ulna.

H. A. Peterson, MD, MS

Healing of a Chondral Fragment of the Knee in an Adolescent After Internal Fixation: A Case Report

Nakamura N, Horibe S, Iwahashi T, et al (Osaka Rosai Hosp, Japan)
J Bone Joint Surg Am 86-A:2741-2746, 2004 3–9

Introduction.—Articular cartilage lacks a blood supply and is considered to have poor healing potential. A case was reported in which successful fixation of a partial-thickness chondral fracture of the subchondral bone was achieved in the knee of an adolescent. This is the first known report in which the healing of a chondral fragment to the lesion base has been established histologically.

Case Report.—Boy, 11 years, was seen for persistent swelling 19 days after twisting the left knee while kicking a soccer ball. The left knee had full extension and a slight loss of flexion to 120°. Joint effusion was observed. There was no ligamentous laxity. MRI (Fig

2) and subsequent arthoplasty identified an intra-articular free cartilage fragment. The free fragment on macroscopic examination looked like normal cartilage; with higher magnification, the substance of the fragment was composed of normal cartilage with apparently viable cells. There was degeneration of the cartilage matrix in the deep zone, along with some proliferation of chondrocytes. Spindle-shaped (fibroblast-like) cells were clustered in a layer covering the detached surface, and the matching defect on the lateral femoral condyle was covered with white tissue. The surface tissue was curetted away; histologic examination showed it consisted of hyaline cartilage matrix with underlying subchondral bone. The cartilage matrix contained clusters of chondrocytes. The lesion was repaired. The knee was immobilized postoperatively for 3 weeks in an above-the-knee cast at 45° flexion. The patient gained full range of motion at 4 months follow-up, with no ligamentous laxity. He was asymptomatic performing activities of daily living. Six months after surgery, MRI revealed the reattached cartilage fragment was

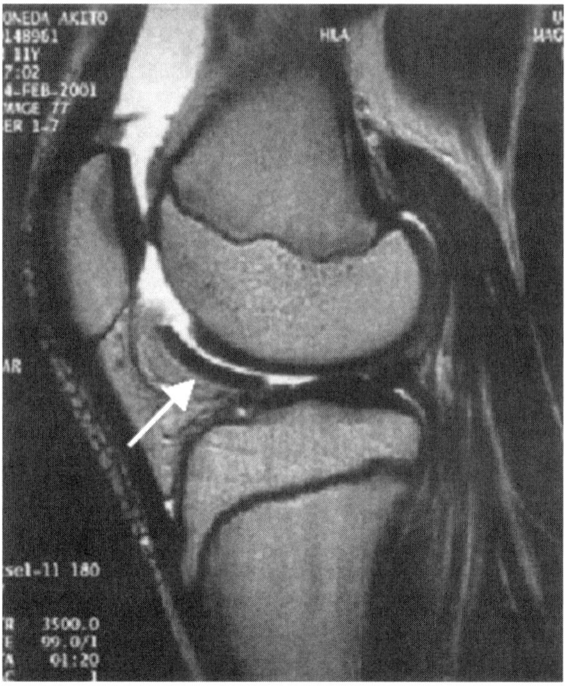

FIGURE 2.—Preoperative magnetic resonance image of the injured knee, showing the free cartilage fragment within the joint (*arrow*). Magnetic resonance imaging was accomplished with use of a Seimens 1.0 T Impact Expert unit (Seimens, Erlangen, Germany). Scans were obtained with a 16-cm field of view, a 256 × 224 matrix, and a 4.0-mm slice thickness with a 0.8-mm interslice gap. Fast-spin-echo images were obtained with a repetition time of 3500 ms and an echo time of 99 ms. (Republished with permission of the Journal of Bone and Joint Surgery, Inc, from Nakamura N, Horibe S, Iwahashi T, et al: Healing of a chondral fragment of the knee in an adolescent after internal fixation: A case report. *J Bone Joint Surg Am* 86-A:2741-2746, 2004. Reproduced by permission of the publisher via Copyright Clearance Center, Inc.)

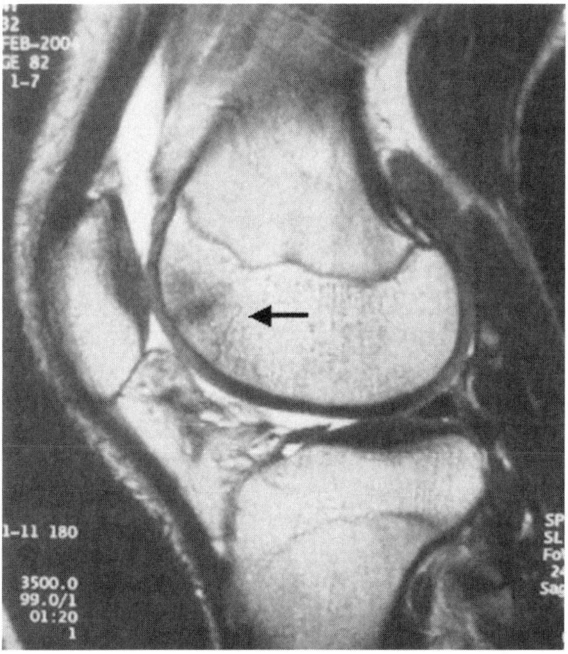

FIGURE 9.—Magnetic resonance imaging scan of the knee, made 2 years and 9 months postoperatively with the use of the same technique as described in Figs 2 and 6. Note that the cartilage fragment appears to be completely healed to the femoral condyle and that the boundary with the adjacent cartilage is smooth and indistinguishable. The *arrow* indicates where the degraded fixation pin had been. (Republished with permission of the Journal of Bone and Joint Surgery, Inc, from Nakamura N, Horibe S, Iwahashi T, et al: Healing of a chondral fragment of the knee in an adolescent after internal fixation: A case report. *J Bone Joint Surg Am* 86-A:2741-2746, 2004. Reproduced by permission of the publisher via Copyright Clearance Center, Inc.)

indistinguishable from the adjacent cartilage tissue. Core biopsy obtained from the center of the fragment included subchondral bone. The reattached cartilage was indistinguishable from normal hyaline cartilage tissue. At follow-up at 2 years 9 months, MRI showed the cartilage fragment was completely healed to the femoral condyle. The boundary with the adjacent cartilage was smooth and indistinguishable (Fig 9).

Conclusion.—A unique case of chondral fracture healing in the knee of an adolescent was described. Of significance, the injury occurred in the deep zone of the cartilage.

► This case report is beautifully illustrated and demonstrates adequate fixation of a large chondral fragment and absorbability of bioabsorbable pins. MRI now allows excellent assessment of acute and chronic chondral fractures as well as healing of the cartilage after treatment. For all pediatric orthopedists who have been slow to embrace the use of bioabsorbable pins, this case demonstrates their superiority to metal pins or bone pegs and suggests that bioabsorbable pins be included in everyone's armamentarium, if for no other reason than the treatment of chondral fractures.

H. A. Peterson, MD, MS

The Bryan-Morrey Triceps-Sparing Approach to Open Reduction of T-Condylar Humeral Fractures in Adolescents: Cybex Evaluation of Triceps Function and Elbow Motion

Remia LF, Richards K, Waters PM (Cleveland Clinic Florida, Weston; Children's Hosp, Boston)

J Pediatr Orthop 24:615-619, 2004 3–10

Introduction.—T-condylar fractures of the distal humerus are rare in adolescents. In this age group, the periosteum may be thin; considerable displacement of fracture fragments may occur. Several series have reported good results with open reduction. A series of 9 adolescent patients in whom T-condylar fractures of the distal humerus were treated with the use of the Bryan-Morrey approach were followed for determination of postoperative triceps functioning and elbow motion.

Methods.—The clinical and operative notes, along with current follow-up examination records, were reviewed. The average age of 5 males and 4 females at the time of injury was 14 years 5 months (range, 13 years 3 months-16 years 3 months). The average time to the follow-up evaluation was 3 years 5 months. Functional outcomes were assessed with the use of the Objective Functional Elbow Index, and points were assigned on a weighted scale that reflected motion, strength, pain, and stability. The outcome was regarded as satisfactory if the result was rated as good or excellent and unsatisfactory if it was rated fair or poor.

Results.—The average ROM at follow-up was –8° to 136°. Cybex testing revealed that the average triceps deficit, compared with the uninvolved arm, was 6% at 60°/s and 10% at 180°/s. Seven patients were pain free (0/10 intensity level on the visual analog scale) and 2 scored 1/10 for pain intensity at the latest follow-up (average pain intensity level, 0.2/10). There were no reports of functionally limiting pain, and none required analgesic. All patients reported satisfaction with their results. None reported activity restriction, including competitive sports. All patients had full supination and pronation. One patient who had an ulnar nerve neuropraxia postoperatively had complete resolution of symptoms at 2 months and normal 2-point discrimination. Functional outcomes were satisfactory in all 9 patients. The average functional rating index was 96 points. Six patients (67%) had an excellent functional rating, and 3 had a good rating (33%).

Conclusion.—The Bryan-Morrey triceps-sparing approach may be used with good results in children and adults who need open reduction for T-condylar distal humeral fractures.

▶ The advantages and disadvantages of various surgical exposures of the elbow for a variety of problems are frequently debated; usually a single technique is analyzed. In this article, the Bryan-Morrey triceps-sparing approach was compared with the triceps splitting approach with the use of 2 studies, both performed on adolescent patients with T-condylar humeral fractures in the same institution. The 2 studies used similar postoperative regimens, similar testing techniques, and had 1 common author but were from 2 different time periods. This study represents as close a representation of the scientific method as possible when small patient populations are analyzed. The authors concluded that the 2 surgical approaches yielded similar results and are both satisfactory for treatment of T-condylar humeral fractures in adolescents.

H. A. Peterson, MD, MS

Lateral-Entry Pin Fixation in the Management of Supracondylar Fractures in Children

Skaggs DL, Cluck MW, Mostofi A, et al (Children's Hosp Los Angeles)

J Bone Joint Surg Am 86-A:702-707, 2004 3–11

Background.—In managing supracondylar humeral fractures in children, controversy surrounds optimal pin configuration. The configuration that is more stable mechanically is a crossed-pin configuration. However, it is associated with an increased risk for iatrogenic injury of the ulnar nerve. Inserting pins through the lateral condyle alone avoids ulnar nerve injury and is claimed to be as clinically effective as the crossed-pin configuration. Lateral-entry pins, which, when properly placed, are maximally separated at the fracture site, engage the medial and lateral columns just proximal to the fracture site and engage sufficient bone in both the proximal and distal frag-

FIGURE 1

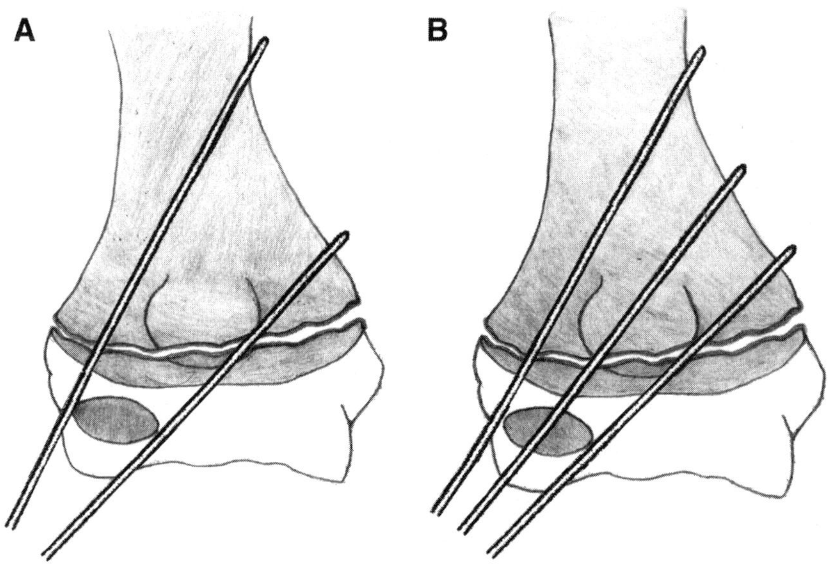

(*Continued*)

FIGURE 1 (cont.)

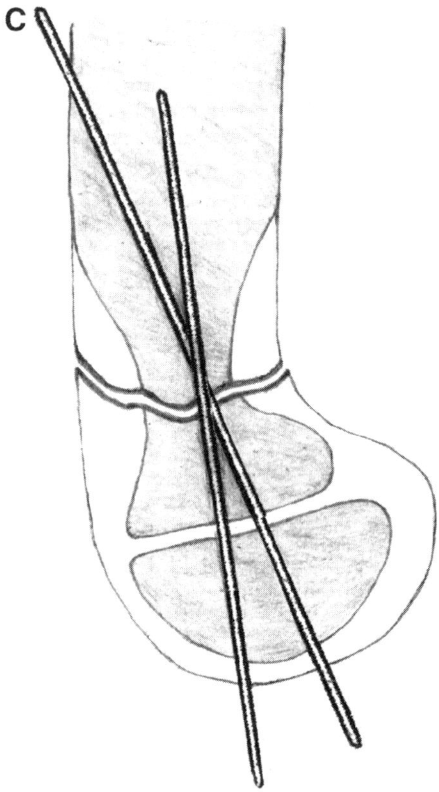

FIGURE 1.—A, B, C, Correct positioning of lateral-entry pins. A, In the anteroposterior plane, the pins should be maximally separated at the fracture site, should engage the medial and lateral columns just proximal to the fracture, site, and should engage an adequate amount of bone in both the proximal and the distal fragment. B, Positioning when three pins are used. C, In the lateral plane, the pins should incline slightly in an anterior-to-posterior direction in accordance with normal anatomy. (Republished with permission of the Journal of Bone and Joint Surgery, Inc, from Skaggs DL, Cluck MW, Mostofi A, et al: Lateral-entry pin fixation in the management of supracondylar fractures in children. *J Bone Joint Surg Am* 86-A:702-707, 2004. Reproduced by permission of the publisher via Copyright Clearance Center, Inc.)

ments. The efficacy of lateral-entry pins for displaced supracondylar humeral fractures in children was assessed. In addition, guidelines were formed for the placement of lateral-entry pins by documenting problems with the technique in cases where the fixation failed.

Methods.—The study included 124 consecutive patients (ages 8 months to 14 years; mean age, 4 years) with displaced supracondylar humeral fractures that were fixed with lateral-entry pins regardless of fracture stability. Patients' medical records and radiographs were assessed to reveal complications that occurred. The causes of 8 failed cases were analyzed to reveal shortcomings in the method, so that guidelines for correct placement could be formulated.

Results.—Of the 124 fractures, 121 were treated with closed reduction and percutaneous pinning (Fig 1). Twelve suffered preoperative nerve palsies, 6 of which resolved immediately after surgery and the other 6 within 10 weeks of injury. No iatrogenic nerve injuries occurred. Preoperatively, 117 patients had a palpable radial pulse. Doppler US found the pulse in 5 additional patients; 2 patients had no pulse detected. All vascular injuries occurring before surgery were associated with a type 3 fracture. None of the patients suffered an iatrogenic vascular injury. An infection developed in 1 patient 7 days after surgery that responded to antibiotics and an additional week of cast immobilization. In most patients, pins were removed 3 weeks postoperatively, and a follow-up evaluation was conducted 6 weeks after their removal. A minimum follow-up of 9 weeks was observed. No patients required additional surgery linked to the supracondylar fracture. The maximum change in the Baumann angle was 7°. The findings on radiographs of failed fixation noted that pins were too close together, engaged only the lateral column, permitted the distal fragment to rotate around the 2 pins, crossed at the fracture site, and failed to engage the distal fragment. The use of 3 lateral-entry pins achieved fracture fixation in all cases.

Conclusions.—Lateral-entry pins alone were sufficient to successfully treat all of the fractures. The Baumann angle changed a maximum of only 7°, which is comparable to the case following cross-pinning. Technical errors in pin placement can produce failure. The use of 3 lateral-entry pins was always associated with success, so this method should be chosen more often. Care must be taken to space the pins well and to ensure that all fragments are appropriately engaged.

▶ The strategy of pin placement to stabilize distal humeral supracondylar fractures has been an important issue for decades. This study basically supports the insertion of 2 pins laterally, with "a low threshold" to add a third pin, also from laterally. Even so, the authors had a loss of reduction in 11.6% of patients, suggesting that the technical points of pin placement are highly important and that a significant learning curve exists.

H. A. Peterson, MD, MS

Treatment of Supracondylar Humeral Fractures in Children Using External Fixation

Gris M, van Nieuwenhove O, Gehanne C, et al (Universitaires de Bruxelles, Belgium)

Orthopedics 27:1146-1150, 2004 3–12

Background.—Displaced supracondylar humeral fractures are the most common pediatric fractures requiring surgery. Among the conservative measures used to treat these fractures are closed reduction and collar and cuff or cast immobilization and traction with or without prior closed reduction. Surgical treatment has ranged from closed reduction and percutaneous Kirschner-wire (K-wire) fixation (crossed, lateral, or transarticular) to open reduction with external fixation. The use of humeroulnar external fixation for the treatment of displaced supracondylar fractures in children has not been reported. The outcomes of humeroulnar external fixation in the treatment of complex (A2-3, C2-3 of the AO classification, or type III after Gartland) supracondylar humeral fractures in children (Figure) were reported.

Methods.—A 12-year-old patient was seen in 1992 with a severe posteriorly displaced open supracondylar fracture of the left humerus, which was anatomically reduced under direct control through the wound. Two S40

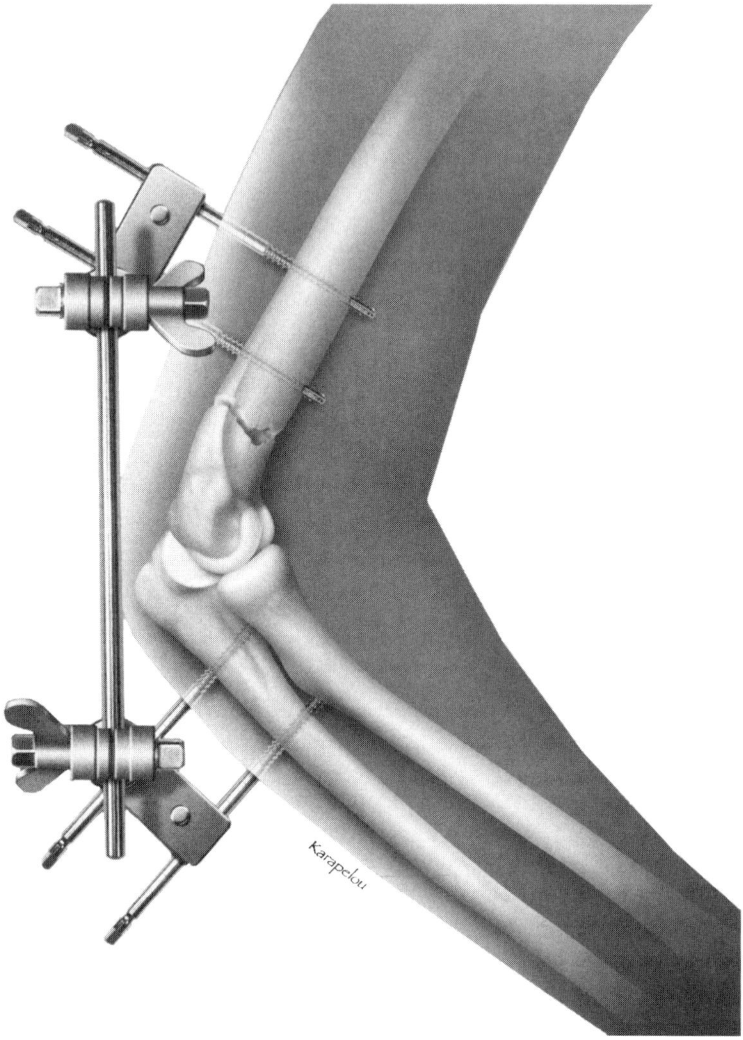

FIGURE.—(Courtesy of Gris M, Van Nieuwenhove O, Gehanne C, et al: Treatment of supracondylar humeral fractures in children using external fixation. *Orthopedics* 27:1146-1150, 2004. Copyright John Karapelou.)

Apex pins were inserted posteriorly in the distal humerus, and 2 were inserted in the proximal ulna; all pins were fixed by a Hoffmann II half frame in distraction, in the axis of the ulna with the elbows gently flexed (35°-50°). After this patient recovered with good ROM in the affected elbow, a prospective study was conducted.

Results.—A total of 13 patients (7 boys and 6 girls) with supracondylar humeral fractures were treated between 1992 and 2002. The patients ranged in age from 3 to 12 years (average age, 7.8 years). All patients were treated with a half frame external fixation bridging the elbow and the use of Apex S30 or S40 pins. The mechanism of injury was a fall from a height in 6 patients, and a sports-related injury in 7 patients. The fixator was removed after 30 days on the basis of radiologic healing. The mean follow-up was 58 months (range, 4-125 months). No serious complications and no infections occurred. At the last follow-up, the patients had normal functioning, full functional ROM, and no significant radiologic alteration of the carrying angle. The reduction was anatomical in all patients.

Conclusions.—Supracondylar humeral fractures are a frequent occurrence in children and account for 60% of all elbow fractures. External fixation of this pediatric fracture is a simple and versatile method that provides the advantages of both traction and surgical fixation.

► External fixation in the treatment of fractures traditionally stabilizes the 2 ends of a diaphyseal fracture. Stabilizing a fracture involving a joint by external fixation is uncommon. The technique described in this article adds another choice to the existing numerous choices of treatment of supracondylar fractures, most of which are also discussed in the article. This method obviates the controversies over the placement and the number of pins needed to stabilize a supracondylar fracture. The authors' claim that "this method combines the advantages of traction and surgical fixation" is rhetorical and not scientifically proven.

H. A. Peterson, MD, MS

Management of Closed Femoral Shaft Fractures in Children, Ages 6 to 10: National Practice Patterns and Emerging Trends

Heyworth BE, Galano GJ, Vitale MA, et al (Columbia Univ, New York)

J Pediatr Orthop 24:455-459, 2004 3–13

Background.—Femur fractures are among the most common traumatic pediatric orthopedic injuries that require inpatient care in the United States and result in significant morbidity and direct and indirect expenditures annually. Closed fractures of the femoral diaphysis are caused mainly by high-impact trauma from falls, vehicle–pedestrian accidents, and motor vehicle accidents. The treatment of femoral shaft fractures varies significantly by age group and by complexity of the fracture. Although it is generally agreed that children less than 6 years of age are best treated with spica casting and that adolescents generally benefit from internal or external fixation, controversy exists regarding the appropriate management of closed femoral shaft fractures in children 6 to 10 years of age (intermediate ages). Practice patterns and emerging trends in the management of these fractures were elucidated by review of a national pediatric inpatient database.

Methods.—A review was conducted of the Kids Inpatient Database, a national database that contains volumes for all inpatient pediatric admissions in about half of the states in the United States. The review was focused on the years 1997 to 2000 and included a total of 18,256 children younger than 19 years.

Results.—For the study period, femur fractures accounted for 21.7% of all traumatic orthopedic conditions requiring hospitalization. Surgical treatment, most commonly internal fixation, increased significantly during the study period, while the frequency of spica casting decreased. This change in practice was significantly greater at pediatric hospitals than at general hospitals. The overall cost of treatment and hospital length of stay were significantly lower at pediatric hospitals than at general hospitals, regardless of the treatment modality.

Conclusions.—Closed femoral shaft fractures are the most common type of femur fractures managed by inpatient care in the United States. Children of intermediate age (5-10 years) are increasingly being treated by internal fixation rather than by traditional spica casting, traction with delayed casting, or external fixation techniques. Operative treatment is also performed more frequently at specialized pediatric care centers than at general hospitals. These findings may have relevance for the issue of pediatric orthopedic trauma care.

▶ Study of the ongoing controversy of the optimal treatment of femoral shaft fractures in children ages 6 to 10 years requires analysis of multiple variables, always including the length of hospitalization, the time to union, complications, and the cost. In addition to being a large study from multiple sites, this study is unique in that it introduces the variable of children treated at a children's hospital versus a general hospital. It also documents a significant increase in the use of operative treatment, most commonly consisting of internal fixation, and a decrease in the frequency of spica casting during the study period 1997 to 2000.

H. A. Peterson, MD, MS

Comparison of Titanium Elastic Nails With Traction and a Spica Cast to Treat Femoral Fractures in Children

Flynn JM, Luedtke LM, Ganley TJ, et al (Children's Hosp of Pennsylvania, Philadelphia; Univ of Pennsylvania, Philadelphia)

J Bone Joint Surg Am 86-A:770-777, 2004 3–14

Introduction.—Titanium elastic nails are often used to stabilize femoral fractures in school-aged children. Few trials have examined the risks and

TABLE 2—Recovery Outcomes and Charge Data for Each Treatment Group

	Titanium Elastic Nails	Traction and Spica Cast	*P* Value
Outcomes			
No. of days until:			
Discharge	5	24	<0.0001
Walking with aids	14	70	<0.0001
Walking independently	67	106	<0.0001
Return to school	48	103	<0.0001
Average charges			
Surgical	$18,990.00	$13,338.49	<0.0001
Room	$ 5,005.15	$12,942.61	<0.001
Total	$23,995.15	$26,281.10	Not significant

(Reprinted with permission of the Journal of Bone and Joint Surgery, Inc, from Flynn JM, Luedtke LM, Ganley TJ, et al: Comparison of titanium elastic nails with traction and a spica cast to treat femoral fractures in children. *J Bone Joint Surg Am* 86-A:770-777, 2004. Reproduced by permission of the publisher via Copyright Clearance Center, Inc.)

benefits of this procedure, compared with traditional traction and application of a spica cast. Titanium elastic nails were compared with traction and a spica cast in a prospective cohort investigation, with a focus on the initial year after injury in which the treatment method should have the greatest impact.

Methods.—The age range of 83 consecutive children evaluated was 6 to 16 years. Clinical and radiographic data, complications, hospital charges, and outcome data were examined. Outcome and recovery were evaluated both with the American Academy of Orthopaedic Surgeons Pediatric Outcomes Data Collections Instrument, version 2.0, and according to a series of important recovery milestones including the time to walking with aids, the time to independent walking, the time absent from school, and the time until full activity was permitted.

Results.—Thirty-five children (35 fractures) with a mean age of 8.7 years were treated with traction and application of a spica cast; 48 children (49 fractures) with a mean age of 10.2 years underwent treatment with titanium elastic nails. All fractures healed. There were no complications expected to cause permanent disability. At 1 year postfracture, 80 children had acceptable alignment and no inequality between the lengths of the lower extremities. Three children had an unsatisfactory result; all 3 had been treated with traction and a spica cast. Twelve patients (34%) treated with traction and a cast had a complication, compared with 10 (21%) treated with titanium elastic nails. Compared with children treated with traction and a cast, those treated with titanium elastic nails had a shorter hospitalization, walked with support sooner, walked independently sooner, and returned to school earlier ($P < .0001$). There were no significant between-group differences in hospital charges (Table 2).

Conclusion.—These findings concur with those of earlier reports that children with femoral fractures treated with titanium elastic nails achieve recovery milestones significantly faster, compared with children treated with traction and a spica cast. Hospital charges and complication rates for the 2 treatment approaches were similar.

▶ The optimal treatment of femoral shaft fractures in children continues to elicit debate. This prospective study comparing skeletal traction with intramedullary flexible rods is as well done as any comparative study can be. The conclusions drawn by the authors appear neither overstated nor understated. The limitations of the study are well stated.

H. A. Peterson, MD, MS

Bilateral High Upper Limb Replantation in a Child

Koul AR, Cyriac A, Khaleel VM, et al (Medical Trust Hosp, Cochin, India)
Plast Reconstr Surg 113:1734-1738, 2004 3–15

Background.—Rarely are there bilateral high amputations of the upper limbs in a child. The reported case was challenging because of the anticipated systemic effects of reperfusion but also carried a hopeful long-term prognosis.

Case Report.—Girl, 6 years, had her dress become entangled in a rapidly rotating machine shaft that tore both of her arms from her body. She was immediately resuscitated, then taken to a microvascular center 2.5 hours after the accident. Evaluation revealed amputation of both upper limbs 3 cm below the shoulder on the right side and at midarm on the left side. Soft tissue avulsion was considerable, especially on the left side, but the rest of her body and the 2 amputated limbs had no other significant injuries. The right limb appeared to be in better shape, so it was quickly debrided, and the main vessels and nerves were identified. The distal bony stump was shortened by about 4 cm, and the 2 bone ends were fixed with Kirschner wires. The left side was debrided and shortened by about 5 cm and fixed. Vascularity was restored to both sides; the brachial artery and the basilic vein were reconstructed on each side. The total ischemic time was 4 hours 45 minutes for the right arm and 5 hours 20 minutes for the left arm. Direct repair on the right side was undertaken for the median, ulnar, radial, and musculocutaneous nerves and the long head of the biceps and deltoid muscles. Only the median nerve and triceps muscle were able to be directly repaired on the left side. The avulsed radial and ulnar nerves were tagged and buried. Over a surgical time of 7 hours 40 minutes, wounds were repaired and closed, and bilateral forearm fasciotomies and lower arm fasciotomy of the right arm were completed. The estimated total blood loss was 1250 mL.

Continuous monitoring of the child's vital signs and bilateral limb vascularity was carried out. She was given IV mannitol to prevent kidney failure, and blood transfusions were given to maintain a 30% hematocrit level. Thrombocytopenia and hypoproteinemia were corrected with administrations of fresh frozen plasma and platelets. Fluid balance was maintained. Antibiotic coverage (ie, piperacillin, amikacin, and metronidazole) was given for 2 weeks. Thrombocytopenia for the first 4 days postoperatively and a transient fever were the only clinical or laboratory variables not within the normal range. Arterial insufficiency signs developed on the left side on the sixth day postoperatively, leading to replacement of an occluded vein graft. No other circulatory problems developed. She began gentle passive exercises of the upper limb joints 2 weeks after surgery, with active and passive mobilization of the shoulders beginning 2 months postoperatively. Over the next few months, the left humerus was restored with cancellous bone grafting, and active elbow flexion and good muscle coverage were obtained for the left humeral fracture site. Evaluations at 4.5, 9, and 15 months showed good progress. Both humeral fractures showed sound unification, and the Kirschner wires were removed. Claw-hand correction was performed at 23 months for the left hand. At that point, all muscle groups showed good recovery.

Conclusion.—A closely coordinated team of anesthesiologists, intensivists, and orthopedists as well as a microvascular surgery team was able to successfully manage bilateral high avulsion-amputation of the upper limbs in a child.

► This case report of a bilateral high upper limb replantation is included as a reminder of what can be accomplished in complex and challenging cases, provided that the appropriate team of physicians is available and prepared. The age of the child, the level of amputation, and the amount and nature of tissue damage are factors that cannot be controlled but that do influence the outcome. A discussion by Fu-Chan Wei, MD, accompanying the article thoroughly covers the subject.

H. A. Peterson, MD, MS

Elective Surgery

C-Reactive Protein Response Following Pediatric Orthopaedic Surgery

Limpisvasti O, Yandow SM, Raney EM (Univ of Hawaii, Honolulu)
J Pediatr Orthop 24:574-575, 2004 3–16

Background.—The C-reactive protein (CRP) level is used primarily in orthopedic patients for detection, confirmation, or exclusion of infection or inflammatory disease. The CRP level is often used in the postoperative period to detect infectious complications. Studies have shown that late or continued elevation of the CRP level may be indicative of infectious complications. This is clinically useful information for following up patients after surgery, but the available studies have focused on adults; there is no information in the literature to suggest that the postoperative CRP response in adults is the same in children. The pediatric CRP response after orthopedic surgery was described in terms of whether CRP values in children return to normal within 3 weeks as they do in adults.

Methods.—CRP levels were obtained before surgery and then on postoperative days 3, 7, and 21 in 22 children (12 boys, 10 girls; average age, 11 years 9 months) undergoing elective orthopedic procedures. These intervals were selected to evaluate the rise, fall, and return to normal of CRP levels.

Results.—Preoperative prophylactic cefazolin was administered in 16 of 22 patients. The average operative time was 4.8 hours, and the average estimated blood loss was 792 mL. The CRP levels on day 3 varied from normal to 22.2 mg/dL (mean, 7.3 mg/dL); on day 7, they averaged 2.2 mg/dL; and at 3 weeks after surgery, all values had returned to normal. No postoperative infections occurred in any of the patients.

Conclusions.—The rise in CRP values in children may be more varied than in adults. CRP levels in children will return to normal within 3 weeks after surgery. These findings are of potential value in the identification of postoperative infections in children undergoing orthopedic surgery.

▶ This study conclusively documents that CRP levels returned to normal within 21 days of orthopedic surgery in 22 children 5 to 18 years of age. Despite the small numbers and other variables, the results suggest that a lack of return to normal CRP levels can be helpful in identifying postoperative infections in children. The article made no recommendation concerning the propriety of a routine preoperative CRP baseline determination.

H. A. Peterson, MD, MS

Treatment of Adolescent Hallux Valgus With the First Metatarsal Double Osteotomy: The Denver Experience

Johnson AE, Georgopoulos G, Erickson MA, et al (Army Med Ctr (MCHE-SDR), Fort Sam Houston, Tex; Children's Hosp, Denver)

J Pediatr Orthop 24:358-362, 2004 3–17

Introduction.—The lack of consensus regarding the causative factors for adolescent hallux valgus (AHV) accounts for much of the controversy concerning optimal treatment. The experience with first metatarsal double osteotomy in the treatment of moderate to severe AHV was described.

Methods.—The medical records of all patients (9 patients; 14 feet) treated with first metatarsal double osteotomy for moderate to severe AHV between 1999 and 2001 were reviewed. The preoperative and postoperative hallux valgus (HVA), first, second intermetatarsal (IMA), and distal metatarsal articular angles (DMAA) were reviewed, and the average angular correction was calculated. Functional outcome was determined with the use of the American Orthopedic Foot and Ankle Society Hallux Metatarsophalangeal-Interphalangeal (HMI) scale, along with the duPont Bunion Rating Score (BRS).

Results.—The average patient was 15 years old at the time of surgery; the average follow-up was 27 months. The mean angular correction at follow-up was 21.54°, 9.25°, and 6.21° for HVA, IMA, and DMAA, respectively. Good to excellent results were reported in 90% of participants. Two (14%) complications occurred.

Conclusion.—The first metatarsal double osteotomy is effective and reliable in the treatment of severe AHV. Stiffness of the first metatarsophalangeal joint is the most important determinant of patient satisfaction.

▶ This article correctly notes that the incidence of AHV and the criteria for selection of patients for surgical correction varies widely among reports in the literature. These factors coupled with the large number of operative procedures available and the various techniques of reporting results makes the deformity a challenge for the treating physician. Nevertheless, this article effectively combines the literature review, parameters of severity, and rating score scales with their results and concludes that the first metatarsal double osteotomy is an effective treatment for severe AHV. The major objection of the double osteotomy is stiffness of the first metatarsophalangeal joint, which is attributed to the intramedullary wire used to maintain alignment, but which has never been compared with other corrective bunion operations. Because of this review, the authors state they "have abandoned the longitudinal pin fixation," leaving the reader to assume that in the future, no internal fixation will be used. Hopefully, they will report a subsequent cohort of patients using the double osteotomy without internal fixation.

H. A. Peterson, MD, MS

Correction of Madelung's Deformity by the Ilizarov Technique

Houshian S, Schrøder HA, Weeth R (Odense Univ, Denmark)

J Bone Joint Surg Br 86-B:536-540, 2004 3–18

Background.—The cause of Madelung's deformity is arrest of growth on the ulnar side of the distal epiphysis of the radius. The result of this arrested growth is palmar and ulnar tilt of the articular surface, volar transition of the hand and wrist, shortening of the radius, and dorsal subluxation of the ulnar head with incongruity of the distal radio-ulnar joint. The result of these anatomical changes is an alteration in the kinematics of the wrist, causing decreased range of movement, particularly supination and extension, decreased grip strength, and pain. A nonoperative approach to management has been recommended in most cases, but in the past decade surgery has been proposed in selected cases. The experience of one group with correction of Madelung's' deformity by the Ilizarov technique was presented.

Methods.—Seven patients with 8 deformities were treated by osteotomy of the radius with subsequent lengthening and angular correction. Outcomes for these patients were reviewed at a mean of 30 months (range, 1.5-5.5 years). The mean age of the patients at surgery was 19 years (range, 9-44 years).

Results.—At follow-up, all of the patients were free from pain, and supination had improved by a mean of 34 inches and pronation by 9 inches. Flexion was increased in most patients, with a median increase of 15 inches, but only 1 patient gained further extension. Radial and ulnar deviation were increased by a mean of 6 inches and 9 inches, respectively. Radiographic measurements demonstrated that the mean volar angulation had been reduced from 25 inches to 11 inches, ulnar inclination from 45° to 30°, and carpal malalignment (volar translation) from 7 to 2 mm. The mean lengthening of the radius was 12 mm (range, 6-25 mm). All patients expressed satisfaction with the functional and cosmetic results.

Conclusion.—The use of the Ilizarov technique should be considered for the surgical treatment of Madelung's deformity for patients suffering persistent pain when correction of a large angle and/or length is indicated.

▶ This article addresses the treatment of symptomatic Madelung's deformity in older children after the entire distal radial physis is closed. The gradual correction of angular deformity and deficient length of the distal radial articular surface can be well controlled using the Ilizarov apparatus as described by the authors.

This is a significant improvement over previous procedures of distal radial osteotomy, with or without accompanying resection of the distal ulna, the Darrach procedure, the Kapandji procedure, etc. In a child whose distal radial physis has sufficient potential of growth—say, for example, age 12 years and less—the Vickers procedure (resection of the tether band combined with inserting a fat graft adjacent to the exposed surface of the distal ulnar physis) has the potential to restore growth and ultimately more normal anatomy. If this is unsuccessful, the gradual distraction technique described here could still be used.

H. A. Peterson, MD, MS

Treatment of Congenital Muscular Torticollis in Patients Older Than 8 Years

Shim JS, Noh KC, Park SJ (Sungkyunkwan Univ, Seoul, Korea)

J Pediatr Orthop 24:683-688, 2004 3–19

Introduction.—The postoperative prognosis in patients with congenital muscular torticollis is affected by the timing of surgery; an early diagnosis and treatment are important. The clinical outcomes of treatment of congenital muscular torticollis in patients older than 8 years who had not received prior medical treatment or in whom torticollis had recurred since initial treatment were examined.

Methods.—Between October 1994 and December 2000, 86 patients with congenital muscular torticollis were given diagnoses and treated at a single institution. Of these, 34 were older than 8 years at the time of surgery. The average age of these 13 males and 19 females was 14 years (range, 8-24 years). Three patients underwent prior surgical treatment. A uniform surgical method of distal unipolar or bipolar (lower and upper) open release was used. Stretching exercises were initiated 5 days after surgery. A neck brace was applied 1 week postoperatively and was used for an average of 8 weeks (range, 4-16 weeks). Patients were followed up for an average of 39 months (range, 24-74 months). At the final follow-up visit, neck motion, craniofacial asymmetry, the head tilt angle, cosmetic and functional satisfaction, scarring, and lateral band formation were assessed. A new way of quantitatively assessing the head tilt angle was used: the cervicomandibular angle was measured between the line of the lower border of the C7 upper vertebral body and the line connecting the lower borders of both mandibles. Patients were divided into 2 groups: those who were still in the growing period (group 1; 19 patients) and those who had finished growth (group 2, 19 patients) at the time of surgery.

Results.—The overall clinical results according to the score table of Cheng et al (which includes motion deficits, craniofacial asymmetry, scarring, band formation, head tilt angles, and subjective assessment) were excellent in 13 patients and good in 6 group 1 patients; 2 excellent, 8 good, and 3 fair results were observed in group 2 patients ($P < .05$). Most patients experienced a substantial improvement in neck motion and head tilt angle and had satisfactory functional and cosmetic results.

Conclusion.—In patients older than school age, even for those who have finished growth, adequate unipolar or bipolar release of the sternocleidomastoid muscle and intensive postoperative care can be expected to provide satisfactory treatment results.

▶ This article is noteworthy for introducing a verifiable record of the head tilt angle relative to the torso measured roentgenographically both before and after surgery. Surgical release of congenital muscular torticollis has been known to give gratifying results for decades. With this method of documentation, a comparison of different operative and postoperative regimens can be analyzed more scientifically.

H. A. Peterson, MD, MS

Inferior Subluxation of the Fibular Head Following Tibial Lengthening With a Unilateral External Fixator

Hatzokos I, Drakou A, Christodoulou A, et al (Aristotelian Univ of Thessaloniki, Greece)

J Bone Joint Surg Am 86-A:1491-1496, 2004 3–20

Background.—After tibial lengthening by distraction osteogenesis with the use of a unilateral external fixator, subluxation of the proximal tibiofibular joint can occur. This inferior subluxation of the fibular head is a common radiographic finding that arouses little interest clinically. A clinical and radiographic assessment of inferior subluxation of the proximal fibula after tibial lengthening with a unilateral external fixator was carried out, with a special focus on symptoms or functional disorders.

Methods.—Seventeen patients (10 female and 7 male patients) with various conditions had tibial lengthening of 30 tibias with the use of distraction osteogenesis and a unilateral external fixator. The patients ranged in age from 8 to 25 years (mean age, 17 years). Clinical and radiographic evaluations were continued for 2 to 4 years (mean, 2 years 10 months). Tibias were lengthened 3.5 to 13 cm (mean, 8.1 cm).

Results.—The amount of subluxation of the fibular head detected radiographically ranged from 0.4 to 3.3 cm (mean, 1.6 cm). Symmetrical fibular subluxation was found in all but 1 case. A radiographic study found early reossification of the left fibular osteotomy site (4 months postoperatively) in that 1 case. No radiographic evidence of union was found in 40% of the 30 fibulas. A linear correlation was found between the degree of inferior subluxation of the fibula and the amount of tibial lengthening. No change in the amount of tibiofibular subluxation occurred once it was established. Clinical assessment found no symptoms in any of the knees preoperatively and no swelling, localized tenderness of the proximal tibiofibular joint, or pain or discomfort of the proximal tibiofibular syndesmosis. Rotation of the tibia or eversion or inversion of the foot was also accomplished without pain on the lateral side of the knee. Abnormal movement of the fibular head occurred in only 1 patient, who had achondroplasia with asymptomatic bilateral proximal tibiofibular instability. Neither peroneal nerve involvement nor muscle weakness was found in these patients. The limited knee extension that occurs during lengthening procedures resolved promptly with physiotherapy by the end of the follow-up period. During distraction, flexion and valgus deformities of the tibial axis were found, but the external fixator corrected these problems. None of the deformities remained after the fixator was removed, nor were there symptoms or tenderness at the osteotomy site with nonunion.

Conclusions.—No clinical signs or symptoms accompanied the finding of subluxation of the fibula detected radiographically over the approximately 3-year follow-up period. Fibular subluxation up to 3.3 cm produced no clinical problems. Thus, no surgical or other special treatment is needed for this situation, and it is not a contraindication for the use of a unilateral fixator.

▶ The relative lengths of the tibia and fibula, the amount and percentage of growth provided by the proximal and distal tibial and fibular physes, and the phenomenon of sliding of the proximal or distal epiphyses of the fibula relative to the tibia have all been studied extensively in normal growth and in clinical conditions. This study is significant for documenting a relative inferior position of the proximal fibula head after tibial lengthening and, more importantly, for determining that this occurrence resulted in no morbidity in the short term.

H. A. Peterson, MD, MS

Hydroxyapatite-Coated External-Fixation Pins: The Effect on Pin Loosening and Pin-Track Infection in Leg Lengthening for Short Stature

Pizà G, Caja VL, González-Viejo MA, et al (Universitari Germans Trias i Pujol, Badalona, Spain; Hosp Universitari Vall D'Hebron, Barcelona)

J Bone Joint Surg Br 86-B:892-897, 2004 3–21

Background.—Leg lengthening in patients of short stature is associated with long periods of pin implantation and high mechanical loads, and pin loosening and infection are inherent complications of external fixation. The complications are, in some cases, related to a lack of stability of the construct or a loosening of the pins. There have been many attempts to improve the mechanical characteristics of the pins, but the only biological approach to improving the bone–pin interface has been the use of a bioceramic coating such as hydroxyapatite (HA). Whether the use of HA-coated pins could produce clinical, mechanical, and radiologic improvements compared with standard uncovered pins was determined in patients being treated for short stature by bilateral leg lengthening.

Methods.—HA-coated pins were used on 1 side, and uncoated pins were used on the other side in 28 bilateral lengthening procedures in 23 patients. The location of the pins was randomly determined.

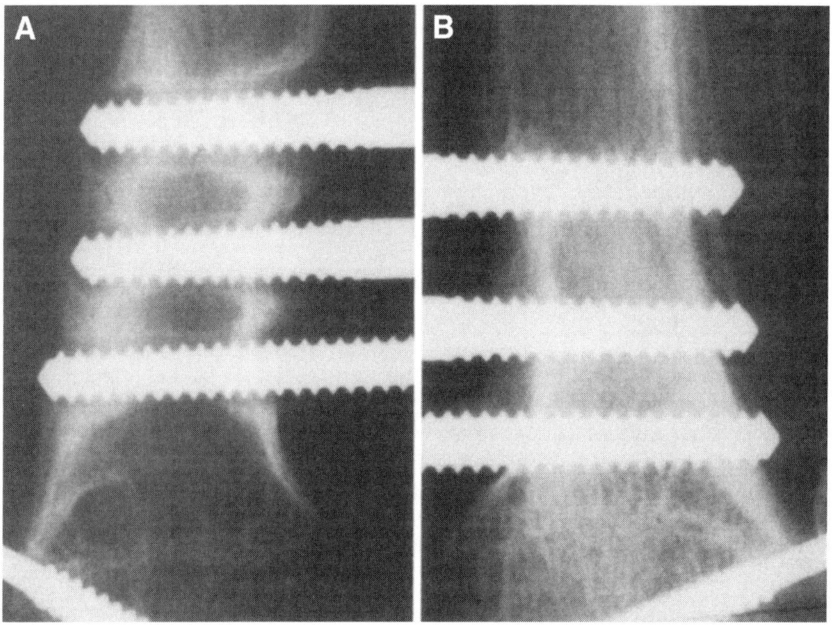

FIGURE 2.—Plain radiographs of a boy with achondroplasia (case 5) showing the distal group of tibial pins. (**A**) The right side; uncoated pins showing bicortical osteolysis. (**B**) The left side; HA-coated pins showing no osteolysis but endosteal and periosteal bone apposition. (Courtesy of Pizà G, Caja VL, González-Viejo MA, et al: Hydroxyapatite-coated external-fixation pins: The effect on loosening and pin-track infection in leg lengthening for short stature. *J Bone Joint Surg Br* 86-B:892-897, 2004.)

Results.—A total of 322 pins were used. The mean implementation time was 530 days, and the mean lengthening achieved was 78% of the initial bone length. The mean extraction torque was 7611.6 Newton millimeters per degree for HA-coated pins and 85.4 Newton millimeters per degree for uncoated pins (Fig 2). The rate of pin loosening was 4% for HA-coated pins and 80% for uncoated pins. No statistically significant difference in the incidence of pin-track infections was observed between the 2 groups.

Conclusion.—The use of HA coating seems to be an effective method for reducing the incidence of pin loosening in patients undergoing external fixation with a long implantation time and for mechanically highly stressed procedures such as leg lengthening in patients of short stature.

▶ Pins used in conjunction with bone lengthening procedures must remain in place for protracted periods of time. Pin loosening frequently occurs and results in a need for readjustment or reinsertion of the pins or premature discontinuation of the lengthening. This study conclusively demonstrates a marked reduction in loosening when pins coated with HA are used. Associated factors including skin necrosis, insertion torque, extraction torque, Pettine index, osteolysis at the entry cortex, bicortical osteolysis, and endosteal and periosteal bone apposition were all significantly superior with the use of HA-coated pins compared with the use of similar uncoated pins. Interestingly, these superior features did not significantly reduce the occurrence of pin-track infections. This supports the unconventional theory that pin loosening and pin-track infections are 2 different complications. However, even in the presence of infections, HA-coated pins were associated with less loosening.

H. A. Peterson, MD, MS

Deformities

Radiographic Measurements in Developmental Dysplasia of the Hip: Reliability and Validity of a Digitizing Program

Pedersen DR, Lamb CA, Dolan LA, et al (Univ of Iowa, Iowa City)
J Pediatr Orthop 24:156-160, 2004 3–22

Background.—Identifying radiographic factors that quantitatively indicate long-term outcome has been an important part of research surrounding developmental dysplasia of the hip (DDH). A poor anatomical result can often be detected considerably before clinical symptoms appear. A digitizing program was developed to automatically obtain measurements of 12 standard radiographic parameters, which would lessen the time required in taking the measurements and allow the creation of a measurement database. Evidence was collected concerning the reliability and validity of the digitizing program in comparison with those of traditional hand measurement.

Methods.—A random selection of 20 DDH cases was made of 119 cases of participants in a 30-year follow-up. For each patient an AP pelvic radiograph was chosen for evaluation. The specific aspects assessed were the acetabular angle of Sharp; the center-edge (CE) angle of Wiberg; articulotrochanteric distance (ATD); acetabular depth, width, and quotient; femoral head sphericity (FHS) and its width and height; percentage covering of the femoral head; femoral head-to-head ratio; and maximum width of the teardrop. Radiographs were scanned for use in the digitizing program, and the on-screen coordinates of the various landmarks were used to calculate the radiographic measures. The 2 raters measured the 20 radiographs in 1 sitting.

Results.—Except for a few values for acetabular width, FHS width, femoral head coverage, head-to-head ratio, and teardrop width and all or almost all FHS values, all coefficients were more than 0.85. In 2 cases, the interrater reliability and intermethod validity coefficients for FHS were essentially 0.000. Interrater reliability coefficients for the digitizer method were exceeded or equivalent to corresponding interrater coefficients for the traditional hand method. One exception was the value for acetabular width. The hand and digitizer methods were highly correlated except for FHS and its 2 components.

Conclusions.—The digitizing method proved to have high intrarater and interrater reliability coefficients, suggesting that it is an acceptable alternative to the taking of hand measurements. Femoral center and its components were the only parameters that were unreliable or invalid with the digitizing method. The hand method has similar problems with these measurements, with errors related to a lack of specific landmarks in defining FHS. Thus, these particular measurements may be unreliable with either method. The digitizing method produced rapid and reliable measurements of the radiographic parameters of DDH.

▶ There are many obvious benefits of a digitizing program for radiographic measurements of the hip. With any system of measurement, physician experience and the precise position of the landmarks is essential, particularly since comparison of serial data of the individual subject may be separated by years or decades entailing different raters. Neither the financial cost of implementing or maintaining this system, nor comparison of cost of this system with traditional methods of measurement, data accumulation, data storage, and data retrieval were mentioned.

H. A. Peterson, MD, MS

A Tale of Two Brothers: Ultra-Long-term Follow-up of Juvenile Idiopathic Scoliosis

Winter RB (Univ of Minnesota, Minneapolis; Gillette Children's Specialty Healthcare, St Paul, Minn)

J Spinal Disord Tech 17:446-450, 2004 3–23

Introduction.—Outcomes analysis has become of increasing interest to the medical profession. Reported is a "capsule" controlled series of 2 brothers: 1 who did and 1 who did not undergo appropriate spinal fusion at age 11 years. Presented is a true outcomes analysis with lifetime follow-up.

Case 1.—Boy, 11 years, was seen at a local crippled children's hospital in 1929. He had progressive spine deformity over the previous 3 years. There was no family history of scoliosis. The neurologic examination was normal. He had right thoracic scoliosis at T6 to L2 (apex, T10; 48°), for which spinal fusion was recommended and was performed in March 1929. Posterior exposure at T8 to L3 was used with posterior laminar decortication and insertion of autogenous tibial bone grafts. The postoperative course was complicated by multiple episodes of vomiting and a probable electrolyte imbalance. After stabilization, he was placed in a corrective cast, and bedrest was initiated for 6 months. The fusion appeared solid (curve, 42°). At age 16 years, the curvature measured 100°. The increased curvature was caused by a short fusion proximally plus crankshafting. There was no pseudoarthrosis. He was seen again at age 60 years (1978) requesting early retirement due to low back problems (no radicular or stenotic symptoms). He had worked at various office-type jobs. A radiograph at age 67 years revealed a solid arthrodesis at T8 to L3, and some degenerative changes at L3 to S1, and no findings of listhesis. In a telephone interview at age 84 years (73 years postoperatively), he stated that elimination of work stresses alleviated his low back pain; it never recurred. He stated he was having no problems.

Case 2.—Boy, 7 years (brother to the patient in case 1), was seen in 1929 6 months after his older brother's surgery. He had a T5 to T12 right thoracic scoliosis of 18°; it progressed to 46° by age 10 years. Bracing was recommended and was unsuccessful. At age 15 years, the curve progressed to 103°. Fusion surgery was recommended. The family declined because of the difficult postoperative course of the older brother. They requested continued nonsurgical treatments. Intensive physical therapy, suspension therapy, and bracing were performed; the curve continued to worsen. He underwent surgery at age 17 years, but it was unsuccessful. When last seen in 1940 at age 18 years, his curve was 126°. At age 45 years, he died of cor pulmonale.

Conclusion.—Properly performed spinal fusion can save the life of children who have progressive juvenile idiopathic scoliosis.

► It is frequently said that the greatest deficiency in the practice of pediatric orthopedics is a lack of long-term (decades) outcomes. Although lacking scientific statistical data, this article addresses the issue of long-term follow-up and is unique because it compares different outcomes in brothers with similar spinal abnormalities.

H. A. Peterson, MD, MS

Perthes

Legg-Calvé-Perthes Disease and Thrombophilia

Balasa VV, Gruppo RA, Glueck CJ, et al (Cincinnati Children's Hosp Med Ctr, Ohio)

J Bone Joint Surg Am 86-A:2642-2647, 2004 3–24

Introduction.—Thrombophilia may be a potential etiologic factor in Legg-Calvé-Perthes disease. The link between Legg-Calvé-Perthes disease and coagulation abnormalities was evaluated by comparing 72 affected children with 197 healthy controls.

Methods.—The mean age of a nonselected consecutive series of patients with Legg-Calvé-Perthes disease was 6.6 years; the mean age of controls was 7.6 years. Assays were performed for factor-V Leiden, prothombin G20210A, methylenetetrahydrofolate reductase C677T, and plasminogen activator inhibitor-1 4G/5G gene mutations. Levels of anticardiolipin antibodies immunoglobulin G and M (IgG and IgM), homocysteine, protein C, protein S, antithrombin III, and plasminogen activator inhibitor-1 were also determined.

Results.—The factor-V Leiden mutation was observed more often in patients (8/72) compared with controls (7/197) ($P = .017$). After controlling for the false-discovery rate, the case-control difference remained significant ($P = .017$). The odds ratio for development of Legg-Calvé-Perthes disease in the presence of the factor-V Leiden mutation was 3.39 (95% confidence interval [CI], 1.18-9.73). A high level of anticardiolipin antibodies (IgG, IgM, or both) was observed in 19 patients versus 22 controls ($P = .002$). After controlling for the false-discovery rate, the case-control difference continued to be significant ($P = .002$). The odds ratio of patients with Legg-Calvé-Perthes disease having one or more abnormalities in factor V, anticardiolipin antibody IgG, or anticardiolipin antibody IgM versus having normal values for all 3 variables was 3.29 (95% CI, 1.73-6.24; $P = .0003$).

Conclusion.—Factor-V Leiden mutation and anticardiolipin antibodies are associated with Legg-Calvé-Perthes disease. This association may reflect causality.

▶ This study is well constructed and well controlled and is noteworthy for attempting to advance the science of the relationship of thrombophilia to Legg-Calvé-Perthes disease. The identification of risk factors and the development of tests to identify and quantify these factors are essential to the eventual eradication of this disabling condition.

H. A. Peterson, MD, MS

Endocrine Profile and Physical Stature of Children With Perthes Disease
Kealey WDC, Lappin KJ, Leslie H, et al (Musgrave Park Hosp, Belfast, Northern Ireland; Royal Victoria Hosp, Belfast, Northern Ireland)
J Pediatr Orthop 24:161-166, 2004 3–25

Background.—Perthes disease is a form of avascular necrosis that affects the capital femoral epiphysis and occurs primarily in boys aged 4 to 8 years. The etiology of Perthes disease is obscure, but the disease appears to be multifactorial in origin, with environmental, genetic, metabolic, and hematologic factors all appearing to have a role. It is thought that children with Perthes disease are of smaller stature than their peers, but conclusions have differed in regard to the role of the endocrine system as a etiologic factor in this disease.

Northern Ireland has a high incidence of Perthes disease, with a cumulative risk of 1 in 607 and a relatively static population. The levels of thyroid-stimulating hormone (TSH), free thyroxine (T4), insulin-like growth factor 1 (IGF1), and the urinary cortisol/creatinine ratio were measured in a cohort of children in Northern Ireland with Perthes disease and the findings compared with those of a control group of healthy age- and sex-matched children.

Methods.—The study group was composed of 139 children with Perthes disease. Height and weight in these children were recorded and compared with standardized growth charts. A blood sample from each patient was analyzed for TSH, T4, and IGF1. Two urine samples were collected at 8 am and 8 pm within 24 hours, and a cortisol/creatinine ratio was calculated from these samples. Findings were compared with those from 40 healthy matched control subjects.

Results.—There were no significant differences between the study and control children for levels of TSH, T4, IGF1, or cortisol. A review of the height and weight results showed that the study children were of normal body habitus compared with a general pediatric population and did not experience a period of growth acceleration after active stages of Perthes disease.

Conclusion.—The results of this study are contradictory to findings of previous studies. The children with Perthes disease in this study were of normal stature. There was no evidence in this cohort of an increased growth velocity, as has been previously reported.

► This study, although not without imperfection, helps to dispel the contentions that Perthes disease is related to body habitus, hormonal abnormality, or social status and should provide a stimulus for subsequent researchers to look elsewhere for the etiology.

H. A. Peterson, MD, MS

4 Trauma and Amputation

Introduction

This year's group of selections is a bit different than the last 5 to 6 years. We do not see the continued rise in the number of well-done randomized control trials in the field of orthopedic trauma and amputation surgery. However, there is continued expansion in the use of optimal clinical research methods in analyses of existing databases, meta-analyses, and well-conducted prospective research. This year's group of selections has a particularly outstanding and influential group within the general consideration category as well as in amputation surgery. Multicenter efforts continue to be expanded. Because of the breadth of the field of musculoskeletal traumatology and the number of confounding variables, multicenter design is our future for improving the knowledge base on which we practice orthopedic trauma and amputation surgery.

Marc F. Swiontkowski, MD

Basic Science

Effect of COX-2-Specific Inhibition on Fracture-Healing in the Rat Femur
Brown KM, Saunders MM, Kirsch T, et al (Pennsylvania State Univ, Hershey)
J Bone Joint Surg Am 86-A:116-123, 2004 4–1

Introduction.—Nonsteroidal anti-inflammatory medications delay fracture-healing. Three COX-2-specific inhibitors have recently been approved for human use (celecoxib [Celebrex], rofecoxib [Vioxx], and valdecoxib [Bextra]). The impact of COX-2-specific inhibition on bone-healing was assessed mechanically, histologically, morphologically, and radiographically.

Methods.—A nondisplaced unilateral fracture was produced in the right femur of 57 adult male Wistar rats. Rats received either no drug, indomethacin (1 mg/kg/d), or celecoxib (3 mg/kg/d) beginning postoperative day 1. The femurs were examined at 4, 8, and 12 weeks after fracture. Radiographs were obtained to evaluate callus and bridging bone formation. Amounts of fibrous tissue, cartilage, woven bone, and mature bone formation were analyzed histologically. Morphological changes were evaluated to ascertain fibrous healing, callus formation, and bone-remodeling. Callus strength and stiffness were evaluated biomechanically, using 3-point bending tests.

Results.—At the 4-week follow-up, only the indomethacin group demonstrated biomechanical and radiographic evidence of delayed healing. Femurs from rats treated with celecoxib seemed to have more fibrous tissue, compared with that from untreated animals at 4 and 8 weeks, yet radiographic signs of callus formation, mechanical strength, and stiffness did not vary significantly between groups. By week 12, no significant between-group differences were noted among the 3 groups.

Conclusion.—The postoperative administration of celecoxib did not delay healing, as demonstrated at 12 weeks after fracture in adult rat femurs. At 4 and 8 weeks, fibrous healing was greatest in the celecoxib-treated group, compared with that of the untreated group, yet mechanical strength and radiographic signs of healing were not significantly inhibited.

▶ In addition to the recent controversy with the cardiovascular effects of the COX-2 inhibitors, the orthopedic community has been carrying on a dialog over the past 3 to 5 years regarding their impact on bone healing. In this well-done basic science study in rats, the postoperative administration of celecoxib did not delay healing. The orthopedic community will continue to await a well-done prospective randomized clinical trial in a consistent injury such as femoral shaft fractures managed with reamed interlocking nails.

M. F. Swiontkowski, MD

General Considerations

Older Women With Fractures: Patients Falling Through the Cracks of Guideline-Recommended Osteoporosis Screening and Treatment

Feldstein AC, Nichols GA, Elmer PJ, et al (Kaiser Permanente Ctr for Health Research, Portland, Ore)

J Bone Joint Surg Am 85-A:2294-2302, 2003 4–2

Introduction.—Evidence-based clinical guidelines for osteoporosis are not followed by many older patients with fractures. Guidelines recommend that patients receive treatment for clinically apparent osteoporosis or undergo bone mineral density (BMD) measurements followed by treatment when appropriate. The gap between guidelines and actual practice concerning BMD measurements and treatment of older females after fracture was characterized.

Methods.—The study included 3812 women members of a not-for-profit group-model health maintenance organization who were 50 years or older (average age, 71.3 years) and who had a diagnosis of a new fracture. Administrative databases and clinical electronic medical records were used to obtain data about demographics, diagnoses, drugs dispensed by the pharmacy, and measurement of BMD.

Results.—Less than 12% of the cohort had a diagnosis of osteoporosis before the index fracture; about 11% had an increased risk for secondary osteoporosis, and 39% were at increased risk for falls caused by a diagnosis of disease (Parkinson's disease, rheumatoid arthritis, etc) or medication. It was determined that 46.4% of the population was managed as specified by clinical guidelines. Patients managed according to clinical guidelines were younger and less likely to have the risk factor of a weight less than 127 lb (58 kg), a hip fracture or a wrist fracture; they were more likely to be taking steroids on a chronic basis, and to have had a vertebral fracture. The percentage of females who underwent measurement of BMD increased during the study from 1.3% in 1998 to 10.2% in 2001. Among patients who underwent treatment for osteoporosis, 73.6% adhered to the treatment regimen.

Conclusion.—Adherence to guidelines for assessment and treatment of osteoporosis after a patient experienced a fracture did not improve between 1998 and 2001, despite access to evidence-based guidelines. Methods to enhance education and facilitate care are needed. It may be useful to target high-risk subgroups for tailored interventions for prevention of refracture.

▶ The orthopedic community is being challenged to provide better screening for patients with osteoporosis with appropriate referral for screening and treatment. This well-done study from a large HMO serves as a baseline for our community to measure improvement against. Over a 3-year period of time from 1998 to 2001, the percentage of individuals who underwent measurement of bone mineral density increased from 1.3% to 10.2%. Our community has a long way to go in helping lead efforts to promote appropriate screening and treatment of women with fragility fractures.

M. F. Swiontkowski, MD

Acute Compartment Syndrome in the Absence of Fracture

Hope MJ, McQueen MM (Edinburgh Orthopaedic Trauma Unit, Scotland)

J Orthop Trauma 18:220-224, 2004 4–3

Introduction.—Delay of treatment of an acute compartment syndrome (ACS) can lead to muscle necrosis and nerve damage. Some cases of ACS occur without a fracture, spontaneously, as the result of a soft-tissue injury, or in the "well leg." Data were collected prospectively and retrospectively from patients with a diagnosis of ACS to determine how the absence of a fracture may influence presentation, referral patterns, and outcomes.

Methods.—A total of 164 patients with a diagnosis of ACS were admitted to an orthopedic trauma unit over an 8-year period. Thirteen patients with a diagnosis of crush syndrome were excluded, which left 151 cases of ACS for analysis: 113 with a fracture and 38 without a fracture. None of the cases involved ACS complicating vascular surgery. The fracture and no fracture groups were compared for patient demographics and operative findings.

Results.—Patients with ACS without fractures were significantly older and had significantly more medical comorbidities than did those with ACS and fractures. A greater proportion of men were in the fracture group, but this difference was not statistically significant. Most patients in both groups were referred by the accident and emergency department, had ACS in the lower leg, and had a sporting injury as the underlying cause. Patients without a fracture had a significantly greater mean delay from hospital admission to fasciotomy (34.0 hours vs 21.6 hours for the fracture group). Muscle necrosis requiring debridement at fasciotomy occurred in 20% of patients without fractures but in only 8% with fractures.

Conclusion.—Patients with ACS who do not have fractures are more likely than patients with ACS and fractures to have muscle necrosis at fasciotomy. Fasciotomy is often delayed in those without fractures, and these patients tend to be older and less fit. Patients with a swollen limb but no fracture should have compartment monitoring or prompt referral to an orthopedic unit for diagnosis.

▶ Over the past decade, the entity of ACS and the absence of fracture in hypotensive individuals has been increasingly recognized. The Edinburgh Orthopaedic Trauma Unit collected their experience with this entity. Patients without fractures were more likely to have muscle necrosis at fasciotomy, simply indicative of a delay in diagnosis. Vigilance is the answer to dealing with this situation. As an orthopedic community dealing with the multiply injured patient, significant hypotension must be widely disseminated as a "flashing red light" for persistent assessment and frequent use of intercompartmental pressure measurement.

M. F. Swiontkowski, MD

Symptoms of Posttraumatic Stress Disorder After Orthopaedic Trauma

Starr AJ, Smith WR, Frawley WH, et al (Denver Health Med Ctr; Parkland Mem Hosp, Dallas)

J Bone Joint Surg Am 86-A:1115-1121, 2004 4–4

Background.—Posttraumatic stress disorder was originally described in combat veterans but is being recognized more frequently in civilians who have experienced trauma. Symptoms of posttraumatic stress disorder are divided into 3 categories: intrusion symptoms, such as recurrent recollections of the event, dreams about the event, or feeling that the event is recurring; avoidance symptoms, such as efforts to avoid activities, places, memories, or thoughts associated with the event, and arousal symptoms such as hypervigilance, irritability, outbursts of anger, sleeplessness, or difficulty concentrating. The prevalence of posttraumatic stress disorder among patients who experienced a traumatic orthopedic injury was determined, as was whether injury-related or demographic variables are associated with the disorder.

Methods.—A Revised Civilian Mississippi Scale for Posttraumatic Stress Disorder questionnaire was completed by 580 patients who had experienced orthopedic trauma. Demographic and injury data were collected for analysis of potential variables associated with posttraumatic stress disorder.

Results.—The criteria for diagnosis of posttraumatic stress disorder were met by 295 respondents (51%). Patients with posttraumatic stress disorder had significantly higher Injury Severity Scores, a higher sum of Extremity Abbreviated Injury Scores, and a longer duration since the injury than those without posttraumatic stress disorder. However, none of these variables showed good or excellent capability to discriminate between patients who had posttraumatic stress disorder and those who did not. A response to 1 test item in particular—"The emotional problems caused by the injury have been more difficult than the physical problems"—was significantly associated with the presence of posttraumatic stress disorder and demonstrated a fair capability to identify patients with the disorder.

Conclusions.—Posttraumatic stress disorder seems to be a common occurrence after orthopedic trauma. Patients who indicate that the emotional problems they have experienced after the injury are more difficult than the physical problems may meet the diagnostic criteria for posttraumatic stress disorder and should undergo further evaluation.

▶ The Denver and Parkland orthopedic groups are to be commended for pointing out the phenomenon of posttraumatic stress disorder in patients who sustain musculoskeletal trauma. One shortcoming of this study is that there is not a comparative cohort of patients who sustained blunt trauma but did not sustain fractures or dislocations. Nevertheless, the criteria for diagnosis of this disorder were met in 51% of the patients. Individual orthopedic trauma services should identify resources available in their institutions to manage patients with this phenomenon and provide appropriate referral.

M. F. Swiontkowski, MD

Cigarette Smoking Delays Bone Healing: A Prospective Study of 200 Patients Operated on by the Hemicallotasis Technique

W-Dahl A, Toksvig-Larsen S (Univ Hosp, Lund, Sweden)

Acta Orthop Scand 75:347-351, 2004 4–5

Introduction.—Tibial osteotomy via the hemicallotasis technique (HCO) is based on external fixation. Delayed healing and nonunion prolong treatment and increase the risk of additional complications. The impact of smoking on healing times and complication rates was investigated in 200 patients with knee deformities who underwent HCO.

Methods.—The patients were from 18 to 75 years old (mean age, 53 years) and included 34 smokers and 166 nonsmokers. The HCO technique was performed in the proximal tibia; 186 patients underwent knee arthrosis. Smoking habits were recorded preoperatively, along with postoperative complications and duration of treatment with external fixation.

Results.—Complications occurred in half of the smokers and one fifth of the nonsmokers. The mean duration of external fixation was 96 days. Smokers required an average of 16 additional days in external fixation, compared with that of nonsmokers. Delayed healing and pseudoarthrosis occurred more frequently in smokers than in nonsmokers. The risk ratio for complications to develop in smokers versus nonsmokers was 2.5.

Conclusion.—Smokers who underwent HCO for knee deformities required a longer time in external rotation and had more complications, compared with those of their nonsmoking counterparts. Smoking cessation prior to surgery is recommended for patients undergoing HCO.

► The negative effects of cigarette smoking on fracture healing are well-documented. In this retrospective review, the authors looked at the impact of cigarette smoking on a group of 200 patients treated with hemicallotasis applied to the proximal tibia for unicompartmental arthrosis. The risk ratio for complications increased to 2.5%. Surgeons are well-advised to insist upon discontinuing the use of cigarettes and nicotine products prior to any procedure requiring rapid bone healing.

M. F. Swiontkowski, MD

Early Fracture Fixation

External Fixation as a Bridge to Intramedullary Nailing for Patients With Multiple Injuries and With Femur Fractures: Damage Control Orthopedics

Scalea TM, Boswell SA, Scott JD, et al (Univ of Maryland, Baltimore)

J Orthop Trauma 18:S2-S12, 2004 4–6

Introduction.—Early fracture fixation has many advantages, but patients with multiple injuries and those at risk for complications from major operative procedures may experience poorer outcomes if treatment of musculoskeletal injuries includes prompt surgical intervention. In cases of pelvic fracture, stabilization with external fixation (EF) may reduce the risks associated with early intramedullary nail fixation (IMN). Patients with femur fracture were compared for outcomes after EF versus IMN.

Methods.—The charts and registry data of patients admitted to a level I trauma center with a femur fracture between July 1995 and June 1998 were retrospectively reviewed. During this period, 281 patients treated with IMN and 43 with EF met entry criteria. Outcomes of interest included ICU length of stay, hospital length of stay, mortality, and discharge destination.

Results.—The patient group was predominantly male (71%) and white (63%); the mean age was 30.5 years. Motor vehicle crashes were the cause of 59% of injuries. Five percent of patients were in shock at admission and 40% required an ICU stay (median, 9 days). The EF and IMN groups were similar in patient age, sex, race, and mechanism of injury, but the EF group was more seriously injured, with 83% requiring ICU care.

Twelve EF patients had severe head injuries requiring intracranial pressure monitoring, and half had thoracoabdominal injuries. The median operating room time for EF was 35 minutes; estimated blood loss was 90 mL. In the IMN group, median operating room time was 135 minutes and estimated blood loss was 400 mL. There were 4 deaths in the EF group, 3 from head injuries and 1 from acute organ failure. One patient died before IMN. One complication, bleeding around a pin site, occurred with EF. One patient who underwent IMN after EF had bone infection and another had acute hardware failure.

Overall, approximately half of patients were discharged to home and half to another care setting. Discharge to an acute care facility or a rehabilitation hospital was more common, however, in the EF group (72% vs 49% in the IMN group).

Conclusion.—The timing of fracture fixation requires balancing the risks of operative stress with any benefit of early fixation. In cases of multiple injuries, EF can be performed rapidly with little blood loss, then followed by IMN after the patient is stabilized.

Changes in the Management of Femoral Shaft Fractures in Polytrauma Patients: From Early Total Care to Damage Control Orthopedic Surgery

Pape H-C, Hildebrand F, Pertschy S, et al (Hannover Med School, Germany; Mount Sinai School of Medicine, New York)

J Trauma 53:452-462, 2002 4–7

Introduction.—The immediate and complete definitive operative care for all fractures is often the most beneficial approach for patients with multiple orthopedic injuries. But in those with head and chest trauma or with increased risk for postoperative complications, initial temporary fixation may be preferable. Adult patients who sustained blunt polytrauma including a femoral shaft fracture were retrospectively reviewed to determine the effect of the management of this fracture on outcomes.

Methods.—A total of 514 patients treated at a level I trauma center between January 1981 and December 2000 fulfilled entry criteria. Eligible patients were aged 19 to 65 years and had blunt multiple trauma, an Injury Severity Score of 18 or greater, and a femoral shaft fracture eligible for intramedullary stabilization. They underwent primary surgery within 8 hours of admission.

The protocol for patients treated between 1981 and 1989 was early total care (ETC), with definitive stabilization of the fracture within 24 hours. In the intermediate period (INT) of 1990 through 1992, early temporary fixation was used. Damage control orthopedic surgery (DCO), the protocol followed from 1993 on, consisted of early (less than 24 hours) stabilization with secondary conversion to intramedullary nailing.

Results.—The ETC, INT, and DCO groups were comparable in age, gender distribution, and mechanism of injury. Primary external fixation was performed in only 16.6% of the ETC group, versus 23.9% and 35.6%, respectively, for the INT and DCO groups. Plating of the femur was fairly common in the ETC period (23.4%) but infrequent in the DCO period (6.8%). Reamed nailing was used in most ETC patients (96.1%) and in the majority of INT patients (73.7%) but in few DCO patients (13.5%).

The incidence of local complications did not differ significantly among treatment groups, but there was a significant decrease in multiple organ failure from the ETC to the DCO periods. In the DCO period, the incidence of acute respiratory distress syndrome was significantly higher in an intramedullary nailing subgroup than in an external fixation subgroup.

Conclusion.—The outcomes of polytrauma patients with femoral shaft fractures improved over time. Factors cited were increased frequency of air rescue, a decrease in plate osteosynthesis procedures, a change from reamed to unreamed nailing, and greater awareness of thoracic and abdominal injuries. The DCO protocol is a beneficial alternative for patients at high risk for development of posttraumatic systemic complications.

▶ Since the seminal publication of Bone and Johnson in the late 1980s, the orthopedic trauma community has struggled to define more clearly the place of definitive femoral fracture management in the most severely injured group of patients. The most recent phenomenon is "damage care" orthopedics, in which the most seriously injured are treated with temporary external fixation. In the first study (Abstract 4–6), the outcomes appeared to be more successful with temporary stabilization using external fixation followed by definitive treatment. This is a seriously injured group with a high percentage of patients admitted in shock, with 40% requiring an extended ICU stay. In the second study (Abstract 4–7), the investigators look at their experience and outcomes over a 20-year period. The outcomes of multiply injured patients with femoral shaft fractures have improved over time, and the group cites the increase in the use of temporary external fixation in recent years. The orthopedic community needs to pursue this issue further with a controlled multicenter trial where we can investigate the true impact of damage-care orthopedics in a way that will more clearly answer this question.

M. F. Swiontkowski, MD

Upper Extremity

Percutaneous Closed Reduction of Fracture-Dislocation of the Shoulder

Silver MD, Menezes P, Silver JW (Yale Univ, New Haven, Conn; New York Methodist Hosp, Brooklyn)
Orthopedics 27:713-714, 2004 4–8

Introduction.—Depending on the patient and the fracture type, fracture-dislocations of the shoulder can be treated using closed methods or operative intervention. Whichever treatment approach is chosen, reduction of the humeral head within the glenoid when dealing with a fracture-dislocation of the shoulder can be challenging. A technique for reducing this injury using a small percutaneous incision was described.

> *Surgical Technique.*—Man, 49, injured his left shoulder while holding on to a trapeze. His niece pulled on his shoulder, which produced extreme pain and inability to raise his arm. Radiographs obtained in the emergency department showed a 3-part fracture-dislocation of the shoulder, which was confirmed on CT. Closed reduction was not successful. A small percutaneous incision was made over the anterior aspect of the deltoid. A threaded tip guide pin from the 7.3-mm Synthes cannulated hip screw instruments was positioned using fluoroscopic views into the humeral head, with the en-

try point on the surface of the fractured fragment. The soft tissue was carefully spread to drill through a drill guide to minimize damage to any neurovascular structures, especially the axillary nerve. To achieve better control of the dislocated humeral head, a cannulated tap was advanced over the guide wire into the humeral head under fluoroscopic image. The humeral head was carefully reduced into the glenoid using the cannulated tap as a "joystick." A sling and swathe was used postoperatively. The fracture healed; the patient was lost to follow-up.

Conclusion.—This technique has been used successfully in 3 patients without complications. Greater control of the dislocated humeral head is possible using the cannulated hip tap, particularly in osteoporotic bone, to help reduce the shoulder. This approach also eliminates conversion to open reduction to reduce the humeral head.

▶ This "technical tip" points out the use of closed reduction with a fracture dislocation of the proximal humerus. Percutaneous insertion of a tap was shown to be very useful in reducing the humeral head into the glenoid cavity. This simple maneuver will allow more time for preoperative planning and shared decision making with the patient regarding whether to proceed with internal fixation or hemiarthroplasty.

M. F. Swiontkowski, MD

A Prospective, Randomized Trial Comparing the Limited Contact Dynamic Compression Plate With the Point Contact Fixator for Forearm Fractures

Leung F, Chow S-P (Univ of Hong Kong)
J Bone Joint Surg Am 85-A:2343-2348, 2003 4–9

Background.—Which type of plate fixation for diaphyseal forearm fractures is most effective? The limited contact dynamic compression plate (LC-DCP) decreases the bone-contact area by about 50% compared with conventional plating, which minimizes complications. However, with the LC-DCP device, the screws are still locked into bone. In contrast, the point contact fixator (PC-Fix) does not have surface contact with the bone, and the screws are locked into a plate rather than the bone. To determine if 1 type of device has an advantage over the other, the efficacy and safety of the LC-DCP were compared with those of the PC-Fix for use in diaphyseal forearm fractures.

Methods.—The study included 92 patients (76 males, 16 females; average age, 36 years) with 125 diaphyseal forearm fractures. Patients were selected randomly to receive either an LC-DCP (47 patients, 66 fractures) or a PC-Fix (45 patients, 59 fractures). Operative time, callus formation, and intraoperative complications were recorded. Patients were followed up for an average of 22 months to evaluate pain, function, and bony union.

Results.—Operative time did not differ significantly in the LC-DCP and PC-Fix groups (mean, 92 vs 78 minutes, respectively). Callus formation was also similar in the 2 groups. Deep infection occurred in 1 patient in each group. Most patients in both groups (LC-DCP, 98%; PF-Fix, 86%) were free of pain at the last follow-up, and most (LC-DCP, 98%; PF-Fix, 89%) had full ROM. Time to union did not differ significantly between the 2 groups, nor did the number of delayed unions (5 patients [5 fractures] in the LC-DCP group and 3 patients [4 fractures] in the PC-Fix group). One patient in each group had a refracture; both events occurred at the site of a screw track. At implant removal, the bone under the implants was well vascularized in both groups. However, the bone under the LC-DCP showed an ingrowth of fibrous tissue around the screw holes, an effect that was not seen with the PC-Fix.

Conclusion.—The concepts of fixation differ, but the LC-DCP and the PC-Fix are equally effective and safe for treating diaphyseal forearm fractures.

► In this randomized controlled trial comparing LC-DCP with the PC-Fix, the outcomes were equal in terms of range of motion, time to union, and refracture. To document a real difference between the 2 implants (assuming this report represents a beta error), roughly 1000 patients would be required in each group. This study is likely not possible in today's environment.

M. F. Swiontkowski, MD

Radial Head and Neck Fractures

Fractures of the Radial Head and Neck Treated With Radial Head Excision

Herbertsson P, Josefsson PO, Hasserius R, et al (Malmö Univ, Sweden)

J Bone Joint Surg Am 86-A:1925-1930, 2004 4–10

Introduction.—Fractures of the radial head or neck most often occur after a fall on the outstretched arm. Minimal immobilization is usually effective for undisplaced or slightly displaced fractures, whereas open reduction and fixation or excision of the radial head are frequently the treatment choice for displaced or comminuted fractures. The long-term outcomes of fractures of the radial head and neck were examined in a group of patients treated with radial head excision at a single institution.

Methods.—Sixty-one of 131 patients treated between 1970 and 1990 were available for follow-up. This group included 31 women and 30 men with a mean age of 44 years at the time of injury. Thirty-seven patients had sustained a low-energy injury and 21 a high-energy injury (this information was unknown for 3 patients).

There were 39 Mason type II fractures, 10 Mason type III fractures, and 12 Mason type IV fractures. No patient had any other major fractures or soft tissue trauma of the upper extremity. Forty-three fractures were treated with primary radial head excision and 18 with delayed radial head excision at a median of 5 months after the injury.

Results.—At a mean follow-up of 18 years, 28 patients were symptom free, 27 had occasional elbow pain, and 6 (4 with a Mason type IV fracture) had daily pain. In terms of flexion, extension, and supination, the ROM of the injured upper extremities was only slightly less than that of the uninjured upper extremities. But compared with uninjured elbows, the previously injured elbows had a higher percentage of cysts, sclerosis, and osteophytes (73% vs 7%). Reduced joint space was not noted in any treated fracture, and objective outcomes were similar after primary radial head excision and delayed excision.

Conclusion.—Outcomes in patients with isolated, closed fractures of the radial head and neck appeared to depend more on type of fracture than on whether excision of the radial head was primary or delayed. Mason type IV fractures had the worst results. Radiographic changes had developed in most cases with long-term follow-up, but joint space reduction was not observed.

Uncomplicated Mason Type-II and III Fractures of the Radial Head and Neck in Adults: A Long-term Follow-up Study

Herbertsson P, Josefsson P-O, Hasserius R, et al (Univ Hosp MAS, Malmo, Sweden)

J Bone Joint Surg Am 86-A:569-574, 2004 4–11

Introduction.—Fractures of the radial head or neck are usually caused by a fall on the outstretched arm. The incidence and long-term outcomes of isolated, closed Mason type II and III fractures of the radial head and neck were evaluated in patients who were adults (mean age 47 years) at the time of injury.

Methods.—The registry from a hospital in Malmo, Sweden was searched for individuals who sustained radial head or neck fractures between 1969 and 1979. All those with the fracture type of interest and still living in Malmo were invited to return for re-examination. Of 131 potentially eligible individuals, 100 were older than 16.5 years at the time of the injury and agreed to participate in the study. Patients were 70 women and 30 men; 76 fractures were Mason type II and 24 were Mason type III. Twenty-eight fractures involved the radial neck, and 72 involved the radial head. All patients completed a survey on long-term outcomes, and 75 returned for a clinical and radiographic evaluation.

Results.—The initial treatment consisted of an elastic bandage or a collar and cuff sling with mobilization in 44 cases, cast immobilization in 34, resection of the radial head in 19, open reduction of the radial head in 2, and a collateral ligament repair in 1. With a mean follow-up of 19 years, 77 patients had no symptoms in the injured elbow, 22 had occasional pain, and 2 had daily pain. Compared with the uninjured elbow, the elbows that had radial fractures of the head or neck had a higher prevalence of degenerative changes, a slight flexion deficit, and a small extension deficit.

Conclusion.—The annual incidence of radial head and neck fractures in a population that was 16.5 years or older was 2.9 per 10,000 individuals. Long-term follow-up was largely favorable for isolated Mason type II or III fractures. Ten patients required a secondary operation because of persistent pain, and they were somewhat more likely to have minor complaints in later years than patients who did not undergo a secondary procedure.

► In the first study (Abstract 4–10), the authors retrospectively review the impact of radial head excision over a 20-year period in their institution. Seventy-three percent of patients had radiographic evidence of osteoarthrosis at follow-up. However, 27 of 43 were asymptomatic. Delayed excision did not seem to affect the outcome in a major way.

In the second study (Abstract 4–11), the group took a retrospective look at all patients with fractures of the radial head or neck in their hospital registry. Only 10% of patients required a secondary operation because of persistent pain. The majority had excellent functional outcomes.

M. F. Swiontkowski, MD

Hip

Antibiotic Prophylaxis in Hip Fracture Surgery: A Metaanalysis

Southwell-Keely JP, Russo RR, March L, et al (Univ of Sydney, Australia; Research and Statistics Unit NSW, Sydney, Australia)

Clin Orthop 419:179-184, 2004 4–12

Introduction.—Antibiotic prophylaxis is important in reducing the incidence of wound infection after surgical treatment of fractures of the proximal femur. Wide variability exists, however, in both the type and dosage of antibiotics. The finding that many patients receive multiple IV dosages followed by prolonged oral administration prompted an effort to identify the optimal prophylactic antibiotic regimen for patients who have surgical intervention after hip fractures.

Methods.—Computer searches included MEDLINE for the period from 1966 to December 2000 and EMBASE from 1988 to December 2000. All articles for analysis were cross-referenced, and experts in the field were questioned regarding other trials and unpublished data. Fifteen articles met criteria to be included in the meta-analysis.

Results.—Studies published early in the review period tended to find large differences between patient groups receiving antibiotic treatment and control groups given placebo. Baseline rates of infection have been declining in control subjects, however, with better operating room conditions. Many patients were administered more than the recommended single antibiotic agent and had the treatment continued well beyond the 24-hour postoperative period. Prophylactic antibiotics did reduce the incidence of wound infection after hip surgery, but multiple doses conferred no greater risk reduction than a single dose. The incidence of urinary tract infections was reduced significantly in treated patients, and mortality was nonsignificantly reduced.

Conclusion.—Prophylactic antibiotic administration is a widespread practice in patients undergoing hip fracture surgery. A single dose, usually 1 or 2 g of IV cephalosporin given at induction of anesthesia, appears to be as effective as multiple doses.

▶ This well-done meta-analysis confirms that a single dose of antibiotic prophylaxis (first-generation cephalosporin) appears to be as effective as multiple doses. Clearly no more than 36 hours of prophylaxis is ever necessary.

M. F. Swiontkowski, MD

Association of Timing of Surgery for Hip Fracture and Patient Outcomes

Orosz GM, Magaziner J, Hannan EL, et al (Mount Sinai School of Medicine, New York; Univ of Maryland, Baltimore; State Univ of New York, Albany; et al)

JAMA 291:1738-1743, 2004 4–13

Background.—Hip fractures are becoming more common in the United States among elderly patients. Poor functional outcomes are not uncommon. Surgery is an important part of the management of these patients. Delaying surgery carries the theoretical risk of increasing the complications associated with enforced bed rest, such as thromboembolism, urinary tract infection atelectasis, and pressure ulcers. Perioperative complications may be increased if surgery is done precipitously without stabilizing other medical conditions. The association of timing of hip fracture surgery with mortality, functional outcomes, pain, lengths of stay, and the development of complications was investigated.

Methods.—A prospective cohort design allowed matching cases of early and late surgery to be analyzed with the use of a propensity score. Early surgery was defined as that occurring within 24 hours of hospital arrival, and late surgery was defined as occurring longer than 24 hours after coming for treatment. The 1206 patients analyzed were 50 years or older and had been admitted to 1 of 4 hospitals in the New York City metropolitan area. Outcome measures included function, as determined by the Functional Independence Measure (FIM), survival, pain, and length of stay in the hospital.

Results.—After excluding 28 patients who did not have surgery, 398 patients (33.8%) had surgery within 24 hours of hospital arrival. A total of 780 patients had late surgery. The adjusted mortality at 2 months was 8.2%, and that at 6 months was 17.5%. No improved mortality rate was associated with earlier surgery. Four hundred eighty-seven patients completed an assessment of pain control. Compared with those not assessed for pain, these individuals tended to have better function, tended to be younger, and tended not to have dementia. Those undergoing earlier surgery had lower pain scores (difference, –0.24 points) and fewer days among the first 5 days in the hospital when they experienced severe and very severe pain. The length of stay for those having early surgery was 1.94 days shorter than for those having late surgery. The differences in pain and length of stay were accounted for by the delay in surgery. Improved FIM self-care was linked to early surgery, but fewer complications were not. At 6 months, the FIM locomotion scores were the same, regardless of the timing of surgery.

Conclusions.—The outcomes of hip fracture surgery were essentially the same, regardless of whether it was performed early or late. Survival rates and functioning at 6 months were not improved. However, less pain and a shorter length of stay in the hospital were consistently linked to earlier surgery, along with possibly reduced major complications in patients who were medically stable on admission. Therefore, early surgery seems a reasonable goal for medically stable patients with hip fractures, with the expected results of less pain, a shorter hospital stay, and possibly fewer major complications.

► The optimal timing for surgery for patients with hip fractures has been long debated. In a well-done prospective cohort design, patient survival rate and functional outcomes at 6 months were not different. Improved pain and shorter length of hospital stay are the benefits of surgery within the first 24 hours. This seems to be appropriate for patients who can be medically cleared unless systems problems prevent it.

M. F. Swiontkowski, MD

Patients With Pertrochanteric Hip Fracture May Benefit From Preoperative Intravenous Iron Therapy: A Pilot Study

Cuenca J, García-Erce JA, Muñoz M, et al ("Miguel Servet" Univ Hosp, Zaragoza, Spain; Univ of Málaga, Spain)

Transfusion 44:1447-1452, 2004 4–14

Introduction.—Patients undergoing pertrochanteric hip fracture (PHF) repair surgery frequently undergo perioperative allogeneic blood transfusions (ABTs) to avoid the deleterious effects of anemia. Concerns regarding the adverse effects of ABTs have prompted a review of transfusion practices and the search for a safer treatment of perioperative anemia.

Methods.—The effect of preoperative administration of 200 to 300 mg IV iron sucrose on transfusion requirements and postoperative morbidity and mortality was prospectively evaluated. A prior series of 102 patients with PHF acted as control subjects. All participants were older than 65 years and underwent surgery performed by the same medical team with the same type of implant on the third day after hospital admission.

Results.—Iron sucrose administration was well-tolerated and decreased the transfusion rate in patients with admission hemoglobin levels higher than 120 g/L ($P < .05$); these patients also received fewer units of red blood cells ($P < .05$). Iron sucrose decreased the postoperative infection rate ($P <$ .05) but not the 30-day mortality rate or the mean length of the hospital stay. No differences were found in the transfusion requirements between groups for patients with (stable) PHFs and an AO1 classification. In control subjects, the transfusion rate decreased by 34% when patients with unstable PHFs (AO2 and AO3 classifications) were compared (Table 2).

TABLE 2.—Transfusion Requirements in Patients with PHF, According to the Type of Fracture and to Admission Hb Level

	Number (%) of Transfused Patients*	
	Group 1 (n = 102)	Group 2 (n = 55)
AO classification of PHF		
1 (stable)	17/40 (37.5)	2/6 (33.3)
2-3 (unstable)	42/62 (67.7)	22/49 (44.9)†
Admission Hb level (g/L)		
≤120	31/39 (79.5)	14/17 (82.4)
>120	26/63 (41.3)	10/38 (26.3)†

*Group 1, control; Group 2, iron sucrose 200-300 mg.
†$P < .05$.
Abbreviations: PHF, Pertrochanteric hip fracture; *Hb,* hemoglobin.
(Reprinted with permission from Cuenca J, García-Erce JA, Moñoz M, et al: Patients with pertrochanteric hip fracture may benefit from preoperative intravenous iron therapy: A pilot study. *Transfusion* 44:1447-1452, 2004. Reprinted by permission of Blackwell Publishing.)

Conclusion.—Administration of IV iron sucrose seems to decrease the ABT requirements in patients with PHFs and is associated with lower postoperative morbidity.

► Recently, there has been an increased concern regarding the negative impact of allogenic blood transfusion on patients with hip fractures. Several centers are conducting studies to try to develop methods to limit the use of allogenic blood transfusions. In this cohort study, 102 patients received IV iron, which decreased the transfusion rate by 34%. The institution of this treatment will require significant discussions with the hospital pharmacy, anesthesia, and physicians who manage the medical aspects of hip fracture patient care.

M. F. Swiontkowski, MD

Physical Therapy and Mobility 2 and 6 Months After Hip Fracture

Penrod JD, Boockvar KS, Litke A; et al (Bronx Veterans Affairs Med Ctr, New York; Mount Sinai School of Medicine, New York; Univ of Maryland, Baltimore; et al)

J Am Geriatr Soc 52:1114-1120, 2004 4–15

Introduction.—Physical therapy (PT) after hip fracture is standard in most elderly persons, but a lack of consensus exists concerning the frequency and timing of therapy to maximize functional recovery postoperatively. The association between early PT, later PT, and mobility at 2- and 6 months after hip fracture was assessed in a prospective, multisite, observational investigation.

Methods.—The study included 443 hospitalized older patients discharged after surgery for hip surgery between 1997 and 1998. Data were recorded concerning demographics, fracture type, comorbidities, dementia, number of new impairments at discharge, amount of PT between days of surgery and postoperative day 3 (POD3), and amount of therapy between

POD4 and 8 weeks later. Patient prefracture, 2-, and 6-month mobility were determined via the Functional Independence Measure.

Results.—More PT immediately after hip fracture surgery was linked with significantly better locomotion at 2 months postoperatively. Every additional session from the day of surgery through POD3 was correlated with an increase of 0.4 points (P = .032) on the 14-point locomotion scale; the positive association between early PT and mobility was attenuated by 6 months after fracture. No link was noted between later therapy and 2- or 6-month mobility.

Conclusion.—Patients who undergo PT immediately after hip fracture surgery have greater benefits than those who undergo later therapy. Better mobility was observed at 2 months postoperatively in the immediate PT group. Later therapy (POD4 through 8 weeks) was not associated with mobility at 2 or 6 months after fracture.

▶ Orthopedic surgeons have long questioned the value of PT in improving the functional outcomes after hip fracture surgery. In this prospective, multicenter observational investigation, patients undergoing PT immediately after hip fracture surgery had better functional outcomes. PT instituted later in the hospital course had no impact. Selection bias is a significant concern in this study, and further investigation is warranted.

M. F. Swiontkowski, MD

Effects of Extended Outpatient Rehabilitation After Hip Fracture: A Randomized Controlled Trial

Binder EF, Brown M, Sinacore DR, et al (Washington Univ, St Louis)
JAMA 292:837-846, 2004 4–16

Background.—Hip fractures are common among the elderly and can be very disabling. It was hypothesized that in community-dwelling, frail, elderly patients with hip fracture, 6 months of an extended outpatient rehabilitation program that included whole-body progressive resistance exercise training would result in greater improvements in measures of disability and physical performance than low-intensity home exercise that focused primarily on flexibility.

Study Design.—The study group consisted of 90 frail, elderly, community-dwelling patients who had just completed standard care for hip fracture. Participants completed the Physical Performance Test (PPT), the Functional Status Questionnaire (FSQ), and performed 9 activities of daily living to assess functional status. They were then randomly assigned to receive either standard care at home or 6 months of supervised therapy with progressive resistance training. Participants were reevaluated at 3 and 6 months.

Findings.—PPT and FSQ scores improved significantly more in the therapy group as compared with the standard care group. The physical therapy group also had significantly greater improvements in muscle strength, walking speed, balance, and perceived health, but not in bone mineral density or fat-free mass.

Conclusions.—Extended supervised outpatient physical therapy improved physical function and quality of life in elderly, community-living patients after hip fracture.

▶ In this study, an extended period of outpatient rehabilitation was investigated in a cohort of 90 patients. The physical therapy group had greater improvements in strength, walking, speed, balance, and perceived health. Selection bias and detection bias are concerns in this study. Further research into the use of prolonged physical therapy is warranted.

M. F. Swiontkowski, MD

Predictors of Adherence to the Use of Hip Protectors in Nursing Home Residents

Warnke A, Meyer G, Bender R, et al (Univ of Hamburg, Germany; Johannes-Gutenberg-Univ Mainz, Germany)

J Am Geriatr Soc 52:340-345, 2004 4–17

Introduction.—Hip protectors are effective in decreasing the incidence of hip fractures in nursing homes. Nonetheless, even with free provision of hip protectors and structured education of nursing staff and residents, hip protectors have been worn in only about 60% of falls. Predictors of hip-protector use in nursing home residents under usual-care conditions and after interventions consisting of structured education and provision of free hip protectors were evaluated in 49 nursing homes.

Methods.—In a randomized controlled trial with 18 months' follow-up, nursing home residents with at least 1 fall were evaluated with the use of nested cohort analyses within a cluster. There were 237 participants in an intervention group and 274 in a usual-care group. Regression analyses were conducted for each of the 2 cohorts of patients who had fallen, and the time to the first fall without a hip protector was the dependent variable. Predefined nursing home cluster-related variables (ie, center, staffing ratio, proportion of registered nurses in nursing staff, and hip-protector use before initiation of the trial) and resident-related variables (ie, sex, history of falls and fractures, fear of falling, urinary incontinence, use of a walking aid, and extent of disablement) acted as explanatory variables.

Results.—Ninety-seven percent of the usual-care group (266 residents) versus 62% of the intervention group (148 residents) experienced at least 1 fall without hip protection. Predictors of hip-protector use in the intervention group were use of a walking aid (hazard ratio [HR], 1.53; 95% CI, 0.98-2.39) and no urinary incontinence (HR, 1.47; 95% CI, 1.03-2.09); predictors for the usual-care group were nursing staff per 10 residents (HR, 0.78; 95% CI, 0.63-0.96), a high degree of disablement (HR, 1.38; 95% CI, 1.06-1.80), and a strong fear of falling (HR, 0.78; 95% CI, 0.60-1.02). For control subjects, the nursing home cluster was a significant predictor ($P = .029$); this was not true for the intervention group ($P = .100$).

Conclusion.—Only a few weak predictors of hip-protector use were identified in both the intervention and usual-care groups and were of questionable relevance.

▶ Variable results have been reported in the literature regarding the use of hip protectors in preventing hip fractures in nursing homes. In this cluster randomized controlled trial with 18-month follow-up, the use of these hip protectors was investigated in 49 nursing homes. The devices designed to date have been relatively poorly accepted because of bulkiness, difficulty in application, and patient complaints. No strong predictors of hip protector use could be identified. The individual nursing home and its individual characteristics, such as staffing ratio, appear to have the greatest impact on the use of these devices.

M. F. Swiontkowski, MD

Delayed Internal Fixation of Fractures of the Neck of the Femur in Young Adults: A Prospective, Randomised Study Comparing Closed and Open Reduction

Upadhyay A, Jain P, Mishra P, et al (Maulana Azad Med College, New Delhi, India)

J Bone Joint Surg Br 86-B:1035-1040, 2004 4–18

Introduction.—An intracapsular fracture of the neck of the femur in young adults is a management challenge. The results and complications after closed and open reduction with internal fixation were compared in young adults with displaced intracapsular fractures (Garden grades III and IV) of the neck of the femur. Risk factors that influenced nonunion and the development of AVN were determined.

Methods.—A total of 102 patients (ages 15-50 years) with displaced intracapsular fractures of the neck of the femur were randomly assigned to receive either closed or open reduction. Groups were compared for age, sex, time to surgery, posterior comminution, union, and complications. Univariate and multivariate analyses were used to evaluate the factors influencing nonunion and AVN.

Results.—Of 102 patients treated between January 1997 and June 2000, 92 were available for review. No significant difference was found between groups for union ($P = .93$) and AVN at 2 years ($P = .85$). Posterior comminution, poor reduction, and improper placement of the screws were the most important factors contributing to nonunion. The overall rate of AVN was 16.3% (15/92 patients); it was not influenced by these factors. A delay of more than 48 hours before surgery did not affect the rate of union or the development of AVN compared with surgery within 48 hours of the injury.

Conclusion.—No significant difference in results was obtained for closed versus open reduction with internal fixation. The extent of posterior comminution influences the chances of union. It is possible that injuries with severe posterior comminution need to be managed via a posterior approach with additional bone grafting. Injuries likely to result in nonunion should be determined so that primary arthroplasty can be considered.

► This is a retrospective review of patients younger than 50 years with displaced femoral neck fractures. The overall rate of AVN was 16.3%, and this did not appear to be affected by a delay to surgery, even beyond 48 hours. This is in contrast to other retrospective cohort studies. Here again, a multicenter, prospective trial where each site simply collects the variables of injury time, time to surgery, quality of reduction, stability of fracture fixation, and other risk factors, would answer the questions posed by conflicting cohort studies. Because of the low incidence of this injury, a randomized controlled trial will be difficult, if not impossible.

M. F. Swiontkowski, MD

Femur

Factors Affecting Rates of Infection and Nonunion in Intramedullary Nailing

Malik MHA, Harwood P, Diggle P, et al (Royal Preston Hosp, England)
J Bone Joint Surg Br 86-B:556-560, 2004 4–19

Background.—Intramedullary nailing has become a standard procedure for the treatment of fractures of the long bones. This procedure is associated with an excellent healing potential and a low complication rate. However, controversy exists as to whether to ream the medullary canal before insertion of the nail and the optimal location of nailing in open fractures. The advantage of reaming is that it allows the insertion of a tighter fitting nail across the isthmus of a long bone, which provides greater stability and a lower rate of implant failure than do unreamed nails. This provides an internal bone graft, which acts locally to stimulate union of the fracture. There are concerns that reaming destroys the endosteal blood supply and may delay union. However, the published data on this subject are equivocal. The incidence of infection and nonunion after intramedullary nailing of a fracture of a long bone was determined.

Methods.—A retrospective study was conducted over 5 years to determine the incidence of infection and nonunion after intramedullary nailing in fractures of 214 long bones: 122 femoral, 75 tibial, and 17 humeral. The indications for nailing were trauma in 161 patients, pathologic fractures in 30 patients, and nonunion in 23 patients (Table 2). There were 30 open fractures. The overall rates of deep infection and nonunion were 3.8% and 14.2%, respectively.

Results.—Multiple logistic regression analysis was used to determine the relationships between deep infection and nonunion and the preoperative and perioperative factors of age, American Society of Anesthesiologists (ASA) score, indication for nailing, the use of reaming, the use of antibiotics, whether the fracture was open, and the operating time. A significant associa-

TABLE 2.—The Number of Cases for Each Indication That Were Reamed or Unreamed, Open at Presentation or at Surgery, Deeply or Superficially Infected, and Those That Developed Nonunion

Site	Indication	Reamed	Unreamed	Open Fracture	Open at Surgery	Deep Infection	Wound Infection	Nonunion
Femur	Trauma (n = 91)	59	32	10	8	3	16	10
	Revision (n = 9)	9	0	0	5	1	3	2
	Pathological (n = 22)	21	1	0	3	1	3	6
Tibia	Trauma (n = 58)	22	36	18	3	3	9	4
	Revision (n = 14)	14	0	0	7	0	5	3
	Pathological (n = 0)	0	0	0	0	0	0	0
Humerus	Trauma (n = 12)	8	4	2	2	0	3	3
	Revision (n = 0)	0	0	0	0	0	0	0
	Pathological (n = 5)	5	0	0	2	0	0	2

(Courtesy of Malik MHA, Harwood P, Diggle P, et al: Factors affecting rates of infection and nonunion in intramedullary nailing. *J Bone Joint Surg Br* 86-B:556-560, 2004.)

tion was observed between open fractures and deep infection. The outcome may also be affected by the length of the operation. Opening of the fracture at the time of surgery and the ASA score were found to be significantly associated with the development of nonunion after intramedullary nailing. These findings were compared with findings from previously published data from the large teaching hospital units.

Conclusions.—Opening the site of the fracture should be avoided if possible. This study was a retrospective analysis and was, therefore, limited, but the results suggest that strategies for risk management to avoid the complications of intramedullary nailing can be developed. A randomized controlled prospective trial is presently under way to gather such data.

▶ In a retrospective analysis of 214 long bone fractures, the variables associated with nonunion were investigated. Release of the fracture hematoma with opening of the fracture site must be avoided wherever possible. This is an issue that will only be answered by a prospective trial. It is unlikely that this will ever be performed, however, since the use of closed interlocking nailing has been broadly accepted for the femur and the tibia and is really only an option in the humerus.

M. F. Swiontkowski, MD

Femoral Nail Removal Should Be Restricted in Asymptomatic Patients

Gösling T, Hufner T, Hankemeier S, et al (Hannover Med School, Germany)
Clin Orthop 423:222-226, 2004 4–20

Background.—The preferred treatment for most femoral shaft fractures is intramedullary nailing. However, it is unclear whether the implant should be removed after fracture consolidation. In the past, hardware removal was considered to be a routine procedure after fracture healing. Patients with persisting pain after femoral nailing might improve after hardware removal.

The recommended interval for nail removal after implantation is 24 months. However, complications, such as wound healing problems, have been reported after nail removal, and these reports have recommended removal of femoral nails only for symptomatic patients. Whether asymptomatic patients have long-term complaints after femoral nail removal was determined.

Methods.—A retrospective review was conducted of 149 patients who had removal of 164 femoral nails after fracture consolidation. The patients' charts and radiographs were reviewed.

Results.—The operation time was not influenced by either the interval between nail implantation and removal or the use of an end cap. The qualifications of the surgeon and the depth of the nail were the only variables that influenced operation time. The operation time, nail depth, surgeon's qualifications, and grade of heterotropic ossification had a significant influence on the incidence of wound healing problems. Of the patients for whom data were collected, 109 (73%) were available for a follow-up interview. Local complaints were reported preoperatively by 58 (53%) of these patients, of whom 78% reported improvement and 7% reported an aggravation of their local complaints. Among the 51 patients who were asymptomatic before surgery, 20% reported long-term complaints at follow-up.

Conclusions.—Only symptomatic patients should be considered for removal of femoral nails.

► Implant removal is a common procedure in the United States, usually ranking fourth among the most common CPT codes used in orthopedic surgery. Clinical research into the impact of this procedure is lacking. In this retrospective review of 149 patients who had 164 femoral nails removed, 78% reported improvement in their symptoms. Of the 51 patients who were asymptomatic before the surgery, 20% reported long-term complaints. It seems logical, based on the limited amount of data that we have today, to leave intermedullary nails in place in asymptomatic patients and only consider the removal in patients who are having significant symptoms around the hip. This is an area that is ripe for well-done prospective randomized clinical research.

M. F. Swiontkowski, MD

Tibia and Fibula Fractures

Complications Associated With Internal Fixation of High-Energy Bicondylar Tibial Plateau Fractures Utilizing a Two-Incision Technique

Barei DP, Nork SE, Mills WJ, et al (Harborview Med Ctr, Seattle, Wash)
J Orthop Trauma 18:649-657, 2004 4–21

Introduction.—Single incision open reduction and double plate fixation of complex tibial plateau fractures has been linked with high rates of wound complications. Minimally invasive methods have been recommended to reduce the wound complication rate compared with open techniques. Laterally applied fixed-angle devices seem to diminish late varus deformities without the need for additional medial stabilization. Accurate reduction of comminuted lateral and/or medial articular surfaces often necessitates visualization through an open reduction. Reported are the complications, infection rates, and radiographic evaluation of reductions linked with double plating of complex AO/OTA 41-C3 tibial plateau fractures with the use of 2 incisions.

Methods.—During a 77-month period, the 2-incision technique was used to treat 83 patients with complex bicondylar tibial plateau fractures. Dual plating was performed with the use of anterolateral and posteromedial incisions. The primary outcome measures were the type and incidence of septic and nonseptic complications and the radiographic evaluation of articular reduction and axial alignment.

Results.—Eleven fractures were open (13.3%). Twelve patients had compartment syndrome that was treated with fasciotomies (14.5%). The average time from injury to definitive surgical treatment was 9 days. During the evaluation period, an increasing percentage of fractures were temporarily spanned. Seven patients had deep wound infections develop (8.4%). Three patients had associated septic arthritis (3.6%). Clinical resolution of infections occurred at an average of 3.3 additional procedures. The presence of a dysvascular limb needing vascular reconstruction was statistically correlated with a deep wound infection ($P = .006$). Secondary procedures for complications were needed by 13 patients who required removal of implants secondary to local discomfort, by 5 who needed knee manipulation, by 2 managed with excision of heterotopic ossification to improve knee motion, by 1 who needed an equinus contraction release, and by 1 who was treated for a metadiaphyseal nonunion. Sixteen patients (19.3%) experienced deep venous thromboses. Satisfactory articular reductions, coronal alignment, sagittal alignment, and condylar width were observed in 62%, 91%, 72%, and 98% of procedures, respectively.

Conclusion.—Lateral fixed-angle implants have largely replaced the need for medial metadiaphyseal plating, but the 2-incision technique continues to be useful in high-energy bicondylar tibial plateau fractures, especially when reduction and stabilization of a medial articular injury is needed.

▶ Operative management of bicondylar tibial plateau fractures is fraught with significant complications. In this retrospective review, the 2-incision approach was utilized. Satisfactory articular reduction and alignment were achieved in the vast majority of these cases, with a deep infection rate of 8.4%. Management of these injuries takes significant skill and clinical judgment. A full armamentarium of limited internal fixation, with and without arthroscopic guidance and with and without external fixation, must be utilized.

M. F. Swiontkowski, MD

Functional Recovery in Patients With Nonunion Treated With the Ilizarov Technique

Barker KL, Lamb SE, Simpson AHRW (Nuffield Orthopaedic Centre NHS Trust, Oxford, England; Coventry Univ, England; New Royal Infirmary, Edinburgh, Scotland)

J Bone Joint Surg Br 86-B:81-85, 2004 4–22

Introduction.—The Ilizarov technique for limb salvage has yielded good results in the treatment of nonunion, osteomyelitis, and malunion, but few studies have objectively measured recovery in terms of functional outcome and quality of life. Forty consecutive patients undergoing correction of nonunion of a lower limb fracture with the use of the Ilizarov technique were studied prospectively for functional and subjective outcomes.

Methods.—Patients were evaluated for at least 30 months after completion of the surgery. All had previously had 1 or more surgical procedures fail. Treatment consisted of excision of nonviable bone and soft tissue, when required, and removal of any fixation device. An Ilizarov fixator with distraction osteogenic techniques was used for stabilization and reconstruction. Functional capability was measured on the day before surgery and at 6, 12, 24, and 30 months after removal of the external fixator. Patients completed the Toronto Extremity Salvage Score (TESS) survey at the same preoperative and postoperative periods.

Results.—Of 40 patients (32 men and 8 women; mean age, 33 years), 18 had active infections at the time of surgery. None of the performance tests for walking speed, sit-to-stand ability, and stair climbing showed any significant improvement at the first follow-up 6 months after the frame was removed. However, by 1 year, overall walking speed had increased by 0.15 m/s over baseline, 4.4 more stand-to-sit repetitions could be completed, 12 more steps could be climbed in 60 seconds, and the TESS score improved by 19 points. Improvements were statistically significant up to 2 years of follow-up but not beyond this period. Functional recovery did not differ between cases of femoral and tibial nonunion.

Conclusion.—All 4 tests showed a similar pattern of recovery, and little change was seen in the first 6 months or after 2 years. This finding has important implications for rehabilitation program follow-up, prediction of patient status for legal claims, and the design of future studies. The sit-to-stand test, which is easy to complete and sensitive to change, is recommended if a single physical measure is required. The TESS is also recommended for the usefulness of its data.

► The Ilizarov technique continues to be a useful tool for management of patients with nonunion. This prospective evaluation for functional and subjective improvement reveals continued improvement after removal of the external fixation up to 2 years, but not beyond. The findings of this study correlate nicely with those from the lower extremity fracture study, from which multiple peer-reviewed publications have been written. In general, patients with severe lower extremity trauma experience functional improvement up to 2 years, but not after.

M. F. Swiontkowski, MD

Intermedullary Nailing of Tibial Diaphyseal Fractures

Should Insertion of Intramedullary Nails for Tibial Fractures Be With or Without Reaming? A Prospective, Randomized Study With 3.8 Years' Follow-up

Larsen LB, Madsen JE, Høiness PR, et al (Ullevål Univ Hosp, Oslo, Norway)
J Orthop Trauma 18:144-149, 2004 4–23

Introduction.—Solid, small-diameter unreamed nails were introduced to improve outcomes in patients undergoing surgery for tibial fractures. The previously used reamed nails appeared to be associated with a number of adverse effects, relative to unreamed nails, including a slower return to normal cortical blood flow and a higher infection rate. Patients who underwent reamed or unreamed nailing of tibial fractures were compared for fracture healing and major complications.

Methods.—Forty-eight patients met inclusion criteria and were prospectively randomly assigned to either a reamed Grosse-Kempf tibial nail or an unreamed AO tibial nail as their primary treatment. All had displaced closed and open Gustilo type I-IIIA fractures of the central two thirds of the tibia and were treated in a standardized manner at the same hospital. Three patients were lost to follow-up, which left 22 in the reamed group and 23 in the unreamed group. The mean follow-up time was 3.8 years.

Results.—The study groups were comparable in age, sex, fracture type, and trauma score, but the unreamed group had more open fractures. The mean time to union was 16.7 weeks for reamed nails and 25.7 weeks for unreamed nails, which was a significant difference. Thirteen unreamed and 3 reamed nails were dynamized, and the dynamized unreamed nails required a mean time of 28.1 weeks for union. All 3 nonunions occurred in the unreamed group, which also had 4 malunions; 1 of the nonunions failed to heal after further treatments. Two malunions occurred in the reamed group.

Discussion.—Unreamed nailing of tibial fractures resulted in a significantly longer time to union when compared with reamed nailing. In addition, unreamed nailing was associated with more malunions and a greater need for secondary operations. Reamed nailing is, thus, recommended as the treatment of choice for displaced, closed, and open type I-IIIA central two thirds tibial shaft fractures.

► In this prospective randomized study comparing reaming and unreaming, the time to union was more rapid with reamed nailing and the malunion, and need for secondary operation was higher with unreamed nailing. The SPRINT study has features not utilized in this study, such as blinded assessment of union, and is in a cohort more than 25 times this size. It will be interesting to compare the results of this larger trial with this smaller study.

M. F. Swiontkowski, MD

Rotational Malalignment of the Tibia Following Reamed Intramedullary Nail Fixation

Puloski S, Romano C, Buckley R, et al (Univ of Calgary, Alta, Canada)
J Orthop Trauma 18:397-402, 2004 4–24

Introduction.—Reamed intramedullary nail fixation of fractures of the tibial diaphysis provides superior functional results when compared with other treatment options, but rotational malreduction is a potentially serious complication. Twenty-five consecutive patients with 25 tibial shaft fractures were prospectively studied for the incidence of this complication and the accuracy of CT as a measurement tool.

Methods.—Four different surgeons treated the patients at a level I trauma center over a 4-month period in 2001. Fracture data recorded included AO fracture pattern, fracture location, soft tissue and wound status, mechanism of injury, and degree of postoperative displacement. In addition to CT scans of both tibiae, patients had preoperative and postoperative standard plain x-ray studies. A single staff radiologist and a second investigator read scans without knowledge of the patients' identity. Readings were averaged to determine the overall degree of tibial malrotation for each patient.

Results.—Complete data were available for 22 patients (18 men and 4 women) with a mean age of 34 years. Nine fractures were in the distal third of the diaphysis, 12 in the middle third, and 1 in the proximal third. There were 13 AO type A fractures, 7 AO type B, and 2 AO type C. Four fractures were open. Preoperative displacement was classified as minor in 12 cases, moderate in 6, and severe in 4. Acceptable angular reduction was present postoperatively in 20 of 22 fractures.

Axial CT images of the normal and fractured limb revealed a mean absolute rotational difference of 6.7°. Rotational malreduction ranged from 15° of internal rotation to 22° of external rotation. Five (22%) tibia were malrotated greater than 10° and 3 were malrotated 15° or greater.

Conclusion.—The signs of tibial malrotation are subtle, and lesser degrees of malrotation may be fairly common. In this series, more than 20% of patients showed CT evidence of rotational malreduction greater than 10°. High energy, greater prereduction displacement, and distal third fractures appear to be more prone to malreduction. A CT comparison of fractured and normal limbs yields accurate information on rotational malalignment.

► The complication of rotational malreduction is significant with reamed and unreamed nailing. CT assessment was used to assess this phenomenon in 22 patients. It is surprising that only 20% of patients showed a rotational malreduction of greater than 10°. Patients need to be counseled that this is a possibility because of the closed management of these fractures. In general, rotational malunion of greater than 20° is not functionally significant.

M. F. Swiontkowski, MD

Comparison of Intramedullary Nailing of Distal Third Tibial Shaft Fractures: Before and After Traumatologists

Obremskey WT, Medina M (Vanderbilt Univ, Nashville, Tenn; Univ of North Carolina, Chapel Hill)

Orthopedics 27:1180-1184, 2004 4–25

Introduction.—Intramedullary nailing techniques have advanced during the past 10 years, yet obtaining an acceptable closed reduction using an intramedullary nail can be challenging. A comparison and evaluation of the time to union, alignment, return to function, and complications of intramedullary nailing of distal-third tibia fractures were retrospectively undertaken in a level II trauma center before and after implementation of orthopedic trauma surgeons.

Methods.—The medical records and radiographs of all patients with tibial shaft fractures treated with intramedullary nails between 1992 and 2000 were examined. All fractures were isolated, closed, and occurred in adult patients (closed physes). In 1996, orthopedic trauma surgeons were introduced, and between 1996 and 2000, patients were treated by either a community surgeon or a trauma surgeon. Patients were followed up until radiographic union or established nonunion occurred. Patients were contacted to ascertain their ability to return to work and activities (sports and recreational). Functional outcomes were determined with the use of the MODEMS lower limb module.

Results.—Fifty-seven fractures of the distal third of the tibia were treated during the evaluation period with intramedullary nail fixation. Patients were grouped according to whether they were treated by a community orthopedic surgeon or an orthopedic trauma surgeon (39 and 18 patients, respectively). Nine (23%) of the patients treated by a community orthopedic surgeon exhibited more than 5° of angulation in at least 1 direction; 5 (13%) displayed angulation in more than 1 direction, and 3 had more than 10° of angulation. One (5%) of the patients treated by an orthopedic trauma surgeon had more than a 5° angulation in any plane ($p < .05$). No between-group differences were observed in time to union, nonunion, delayed union, hardware failure, or infections. A between-group comparison in patients with less than a 5° angulation and average scores in physical functioning, physical limitation, and bodily pain did not differ significantly.

Conclusion.—This small patient series indicates that orthopedic surgeons who regularly perform intramedullary nailing of long bone fractures are more likely to obtain good results (ie, less incidence of malalignment) when fixing a distal-third tibia fracture.

► In this retrospective review, the management of distal third tibial shaft fractures by closed interlocking nailing by general orthopedic surgeons is compared with those obtained by specialists in orthopedic trauma. Malalignment was significantly less in patients managed by experienced surgeons. This is consistent with the volume of literature looking at technical procedures. In almost every instance, outcomes are improved by surgeons performing specific procedures more frequently.

M. F. Swiontkowski, MD

---

450 Closed Fractures of the Distal Third of the Tibia Treated With a Functional Brace

Sarmiento A, Latta LL (Coral Gables, Fla; Plantation, Fla)

Clin Orthop 428:261-271, 2004 4–26

Introduction.—Closed intramedullary nailing has gained wide acceptance in the treatment of tibial fractures and is the preferred treatment for many surgeons. It is, however, associated with several complications. Some trials that have found unsatisfactory results with functional fracture bracing did not meet well-established criteria. A total of 450 closed fractures of the distal third of the tibial diaphysis treated with a functional brace were evaluated.

Methods.—Fractures were evaluated in 126 females (28%) and 324 males (72%). Their ages ranged from 16 to 82 years (average, 33.5 ± 12.0 years).

Findings.—Nonunion occurred in 4 fractures (0.9%). The average healing time was 16.6 weeks (range, 10-40 weeks). The average final shortening was 5.1 mm (range, 0.25 mm). A total of 424 fractures (94.2%) healed with less than 12 mm of shortening. The initial shortening at the time of the injury was nearly unchanged (from 4.4 ± 4.5 mm to 4.4 ± 3.9 mm final shortening). Axially unstable closed tibial fractures did not shorten beyond the initial shortening. A total of 405 fractures (90.0%) healed with less than 8° of angular deformity in either the frontal or sagittal planes; 302 (67.1%) healed with less than 5° of deformity in any plane. A total of 391 fractures (87%) healed with less than 12 mm of shortening and less than 8° of angulation in any plane.

Conclusion.—The degrees of angular deformity and shortening in this cohort seem to compare favorably with those reported by other investigators who used intramedullary nails. Functional bracing seems to be an effective treatment method for a select group of patients with tibial fractures.

► Functional bracing remains an effective technique for the closed management of a tibial shaft fracture, particularly in the distal third. In this retrospective review, 90% of 405 fractures healed with less than 8° of deformity. The technique requires experienced judgment, and attention to detail, and is clearly an option that should be offered to patients with isolated closed tibial fractures.

M. F. Swiontkowski, MD

Foot and Ankle Fractures

The Efficacy of the A-V Impulse System in the Treatment of Posttraumatic Swelling Following Ankle Fracture: A Prospective Randomized Controlled Study

Caschman J, Blagg S, Bishay M (Royal United Hosp, Bath, England; Nuffield Orthopaedic Centre, Oxford, England)

J Orthop Trauma 18:596-601, 2004 4–27

Introduction.—Patients with ankle fractures may experience soft tissue injuries at the time of the fracture severe enough to preclude planned early surgical intervention. Immediate surgery may not be possible because of a delay in patient presentation or the unavailability of an operating time. Soft tissue swelling may increase during the delay, compromising optimal treatment. The clinical benefit of the A-V Impulse "in-cast" system in the treatment of posttraumatic swelling after an ankle fracture was evaluated in a prospective, randomized investigation that compared the effectiveness of the A-V Impulse "in-cast" system with that of elevation and plaster in the treatment of preoperative swelling.

Methods.—Sixty-four adults with closed unilateral ankle fractures necessitating internal fixation for whom immediate surgery was not possible were evaluated. All fractured ankles were treated with the use of an initial application of a plaster back-slab splint. Patients were randomly assigned to either a control group of limb elevation or a study group in which an A-V Impulse bladder was fitted under the arch of the foot within the plaster back-slab and intermittent pneumatic pedal compression was provided until surgery. Participants underwent daily circumferential ankle girth measurements. The time taken for swelling to resolve adequately to allow surgery, the development of skin complications, and the duration of hospitalization were documented.

Results.—Twenty-seven patients in each treatment group were followed up until discharge from outpatient care. A significant decrease in the time taken for ankle swelling to settle before surgery ($P = .01$) was observed in the A-V Impulse System group, along with a decrease in wound and skin complications ($P < .01$) and final preoperative ankle swelling ($P = .03$).

Conclusion.—The A-V Impulse "in-cast" system provided a significant benefit in the management of adults with isolated ankle fractures who could not undergo immediate open reduction and internal fixation.

► The impact of sequential compression devices within the cast and the management of posttraumatic swelling after ankle fracture fixation were evaluated. The AV impulse system provided a decrease in wound and skin complications and in final swelling. This was a randomized open-label study, with a significant potential for detection bias. With caution, the use of this device can be recommended. The use of the device should be investigated further to see if it results in earlier return to function.

M. F. Swiontkowski, MD

Stress Examination of Supination External Rotation-Type Fibular Fractures

McConnell T, Creevy W, Tornetta P III (Boston Univ)

J Bone Joint Surg Am 86-A:2171-2178, 2004 4–28

Introduction.—There is a large volume of literature that promotes both operative and nonoperative treatment of indirect ankle fractures. The outcomes of these injuries correlate closely with alignment of the ankle mortise at the time of union. Tenderness over the deltoid, swelling, or ecchymosis has been assumed to indicate a deltoid rupture and concomitant ankle instability. This concept has yet to be verified; it is possible that these findings have led to surgery in patients with stable ankle fractures that could have been effectively treated with functional bracing. Stress radiography was evaluated for its capability to determine ankle stability in patients with a reduced ankle mortise, a Lauge-Hansen type-suppination–external rotation (SE)/Weber type-B lateral malleolar fracture, and no medial malleolar fracture and was compared with the value of medial joint-line tenderness, swelling, and ecchymosis in predicting instability of the ankle to differentiate between SE2 and SE4 fractures.

Methods.—During a 32-month period, 138 patients were seen emergently for a Weber type-B SE fibular fracture and were evaluated for tenderness in 9 locations, ecchymosis, and swelling. Patients with an apparently isolated fibular fracture and an intact ankle mortise (with a medial clear space of 4 mm or less and no talar subluxation) were assessed with the use of stress radiography to ascertain deltoid competence. Patients were grouped according to their fractures: SE2 fracture (stable ankle on stress radiograph), stress (+) SE4 fracture (unstable ankle on stress radiograph), SE4 fracture (presentation with a wide medial clear space), and bimalleolar fracture. At presentation, the 4 groups underwent measurement of tenderness, swelling, and ecchymosis, and these variables were then compared among the 4 groups. Patients with SE2 fractures were permitted immediate weight-bearing.

Results.—Sixty-one of 97 patients with isolated fractures and intact mortises had stable SE2 injuries, and 36 had unstable stress (+) SE4 injuries. Every stable SE2 injury healed with an intact mortise. Findings of medial tenderness, ecchymosis, and swelling were not predictive of deltoid incompetence (instability).

Conclusion.—Stress radiographs permit the accurate diagnosis of deltoid incompetence in patients with Weber type-B fibular fractures and no other osseous injuries. Soft tissue indicators should not be considered accurate predictors of instability.

► The issue of deltoid tenderness swelling or ecchymosis as it relates to ankle stability after lateral malleolus fracture was investigated in 138 patients. These indicators did not prove to be predictive of instability. Stress radiographs are strongly recommended in the group where this is a consideration. Practically speaking, an early trial of weight bearing with 7 to 10 days' follow-up seems to be a cost-effective stress test. Regardless of which venue is chosen, careful follow-up of these patients is required.

M. F. Swiontkowski, MD

Ankle Stress Test for Predicting the Need for Surgical Fixation of Isolated Fibular Fractures

Egol KA, Amirtharage M, Tejwani NC, et al (Jamaica Hosp, New York)
J Bone Joint Surg Am 86-A:2393-2398, 2004 4–29

Introduction.—Differentiation between stage II and stage IV supination-external rotation fractures of the ankle is clinically important in determining the need for surgical intervention. The usefulness of stress radiographs as a method for distinguishing supination-external rotation stage II from stage IV ankle fractures was examined, along with functional outcomes in patients treated nonoperatively, despite a diagnosis of a supination-external rotation stage IV injury on stress radiography.

Methods.—A total of 101 patients with evidence of an isolated fibular fracture and an intact mortise were assessed with stress radiographs. A positive test finding was considered to be 4 mm or more of widening of the medial clear space. Patients with a negative stress test finding were treated nonsurgically; those with a positive stress test finding and clinical signs of a medial injury were treated surgically; those with a positive stress test finding and no signs of a medial injury were treated according to surgeon and patient preferences. Participants were followed up prospectively with radiographs and ankle outcome scores.

Results.—Sixty-six patients(65%) had positive stress radiograph findings. Of these, 36 had signs of a medial injury, and 30 had no medial injury. For the prediction of a positive finding on a stress radiograph, medial tenderness had a sensitivity of 56% and a specificity of 80%; these rates for swelling were 55% and 71%, respectively; for ecchymosis, the rates were 26% and 91%, respectively. In the subset without signs of a medial injury, 20 were treated nonoperatively, and 10 were treated operatively. Two of the 20 patients treated nonoperatively had evidence of persistent widening of the medial clear space at the latest follow-up (mean, 7.4 months); 1 was symptomatic. The average American Orthopedic Foot and Ankle Society score was 94 for patients treated nonoperatively and 93 for those treated operatively.

Conclusion.—A high rate of positive findings on stress radiographs was seen for patients with isolated fibular fractures and intact ankle mortises. Median tenderness, swelling, and ecchymosis were not sensitive for predicting a widening of the medial clear space on radiographs. All patients with positive signs and no clinical symptoms who were treated nonsurgically had good or excellent results.

► In this study, stress radiographs were used to investigate instability in supination–external rotation (SER) II fractures by differentiating SER II from SER IV ankle fractures. Here again, medial tenderness had a sensitivity of 56%

and a specificity of 80%, and swelling had 55% for sensitivity and 71% for specificity. The authors suggest that patients with instability detected on stress radiographs without clinical signs can be treated nonoperatively. However, 2 patients had persistent widening of the medial clear space out of the total of 20. As with the prior study (Abstract 4–28), the wise course would seem to be operative stabilization of the fibula and examination of the syndesmosis under direct supervision where widening of the clear space is detected within the first 2 weeks.

M. F. Swiontkowski, MD

Combined Conservative and Orthotic Management of Acute Ruptures of the Achilles Tendon

Wallace RGH, Traynor IER, Kernohan WG, et al (Musgrave Park Hosp, Belfast, Northern Ireland; Univ of Ulster, Northern Ireland)

J Bone Joint Surg Am 86-A:1198-1202, 2004 4–30

Introduction.—Considerable debate exists concerning the optimal treatment for acute rupture of the Achilles tendon. Trials addressing treatment of Achilles tendon ruptures have usually dealt with small numbers of patients; results of surgical management were reported more often than nonoperative measures. A well-documented and structured program of nonsurgical management of Achilles tendon rupture that uses casts and a removable orthosis was described.

Methods.—The program included 140 consecutive patients with complete rupture of the Achilles tendon who had been treated nonsurgically between 1992 and 1998 who were evaluated on the basis of subjective results and clinical findings with physiologic testing.

Results.—Overall, 56% of the cohort had excellent results, 30% had good results, 12% had fair results, and 2% had poor results. The overall incidence of complications was 8%. Three complete and 5 partial tendon reruptures, 2 deep vein thromboses, and 1 temporary dropfoot occurred.

Conclusion.—The results of nonoperative treatment in this cohort were better than those of published results of operative repair of acute Achilles tendon rupture. Patient satisfaction was high with nonoperative treatment.

► The use of a removable orthosis for the conservative management of Achilles tendon rupture was investigated in 140 consecutive patients. There were 3 complete and 5 partial tendon reruptures, which the authors state is better than the results reported with operative management. Based on the peer-reviewed literature that we have today, patients should be provided with the options and should select the treatment that best meets their needs in a discussion with the managing surgeon.

M. F. Swiontkowski, MD

Calcaneus Fractures

Fracture of the Calcaneus Associated With Talocalcaneal Coalition

Kim DH, Berkowitz MJ (Univ of Colorado, Denver; Tripler Army Med Ctr, Honolulu, Hawaii)

Foot Ankle Int 25:426-428, 2004 4–31

Introduction.—Calcaneal fractures rarely occur in children. Most patients have good outcomes with nonsurgical treatment. In the presence of a significantly displaced fracture, surgical treatment may be the optimal approach. A case of a fracture of the calcaneous associated with talocalcaneal coalition was described.

> *Case Report.*—Boy, 15 years, cross-country runner, fell and sustained an axial load to his heel. His uninjured side had absent subtalar motion. Plain radiograph showed the presence of an intra-articular calcaneous fracture with reduced Bohler's angle and widened heel; the coalition was not clearly observed. CT was performed to verify suspicion of a coalition. Middle facet coalition, likely fibrous, was probable bilaterally. An open reduction and internal fixation was performed to treat the fracture displacement using the modified Letournel lateral approach on 14 days postinjury. Intraoperatively, the middle facet coalition was verified. The fracture healed, and he had equal ROM; the hardware was not symptomatic. He returned to full activity, including cross-country running and surfing at 4-year follow-up. Follow-up radiographs at 4 years showed maintenance of the reduction.

Conclusion.—Open reduction and internal fixation was performed without excision of the intact coalition in a 15-year-old patient with a previously asymptomatic middle facet talocalcaneal coalition who experienced a displaced intra-articular calcaneous fracture after falling from a height. The patient was completely asymptomatic and returned to competitive cross-country running at 4-year follow-up. The literature was totally void of any clinical guidance in this setting. Surgery was performed in this case because of the depressed Bohler's angle and widened heel.

▶ This is an unusual case of a fracture of the calcaneus associated with a talocalcaneal coalition. Three percent of the population will have these coalitions. Management of the fracture by the usual treatment principles and techniques provided a good result.

M. F. Swiontkowski, MD

Functional Outcome (SF-36) of Patients With Displaced Calcaneal Fractures Compared to SF-36 Normative Data

van Tetering EAA, Buckley RE (Univ of Maastricht, The Netherlands; Foothills Med Ctr, Calgary, Alberta, Canada)

Foot Ankle Int 25:733-738, 2004 4–32

Introduction.—Physical functioning is usually the most important determinant of a patient's general health during hospitalization. After discharge, patients need to deal with all aspects of general health. The general health status of patients with displaced intra-articular calcaneal fractures was evaluated with the use of the Short Form 36 Health Status Survey (SF-36) and was compared with that of normative control subjects.

Methods.—A total of 312 patients between 25 and 64 years of age were treated for displaced intra-articular calcaneal fractures at a level I trauma center. Participants were followed up for 2 to 8 years. The primary outcome measure was the SF-36 score.

Results.—The scores in 8 SF-36 categories in the patient group differed by more than 5 points from population norms (Fig 1), which indicates that this injury has both clinical and social relevance. Outcomes in patients with displaced intra-articular calcaneal fractures were not as good across most SF-36 categories as were outcomes of patients with other orthopedic conditions. The outcomes of patients with intra-articular calcaneal fractures were worse across most categories than were the outcomes of patients who underwent organ transplants or who had myocardial infarction.

Conclusion.—When the treatment for displaced intra-articular calcaneal fractures is compared with the treatment for other orthopedic problems or

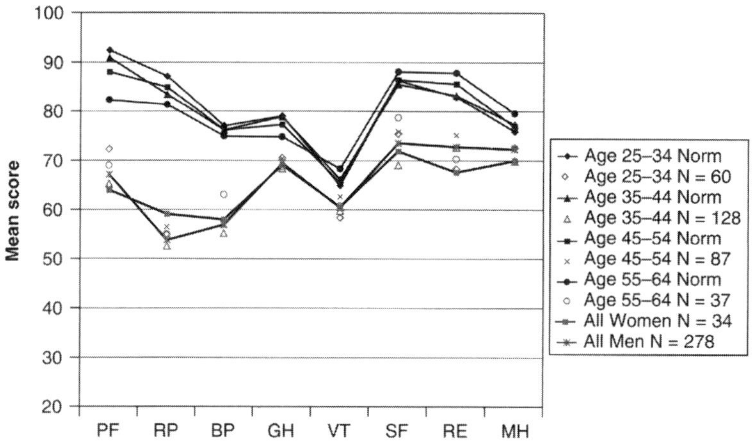

FIGURE 1.—Normative data compared to all patients with a displaced intra-articular calcaneal fracture subdivided by age. *Abbreviations:* PF, Physical functioning; *RP*, role physical; *BP*, bodily pain; *GH*, general health; *VT*, vitality; *SF*, social functioning; *RE*, role emotional; *MH*, mental health. (Courtesy of van Tetering EAA, Buckley RE: Functional outcome (SF-36) of patients with displaced calcaneal fractures compared to SF-36 normative data. *Foot Ankle Int* 25(10):733-738, 2004. Copyright 2004 by the American Orthopaedic Foot and Ankle Society. Reproduced with permission.)

other disease processes, it seems that intra-articular calcaneal fractures are serious life-changing events.

▶ In this subreport from the Canadian Orthopaedic Trauma Association Study Group, the functional results using the SF-36 in patients sustaining calcaneus fractures were compared with normative control subjects. Not surprisingly, patients with these fractures had significant functional disability. These results were reported earlier in the LEF study with multiple peer-reviewed publications.

M. F. Swiontkowski, MD

Results of Isolated Lisfranc Injuries and the Effect of Compensation Claims

Calder JDF, Whitehouse SL, Saxby TS (Brisbane Private Hosp, Australia; Prince Charles Hosp, Brisbane, Australia)

J Bone Joint Surg Br 86-B:527-530, 2004 4–33

Background.—Lisfranc injuries are dislocations and fracture dislocations through the tarsometatarsal joints. The outcome for these injuries is improved after anatomical open reduction and internal fixation; however, up to 20% may be misdiagnosed or overlooked. Several studies have reported a high incidence of unsatisfactory results after treatment. However, most articles include patients with associated injuries, which may affect the outcome of these studies. The long-term outcome of isolated, displaced Lisfranc injuries that required operative intervention was determined, as was whether the results of treatment are influenced by compensation claims.

Methods.—A retrospective study was conducted to identify patients who underwent surgery for Lisfranc injuries and who were operated on by the senior author. The presence of a compensation claim arising as a direct result of the injury was recorded, and where appropriate, workers' compensation records were examined to identify the financial implications of these injuries. The study group was composed of 46 patients with isolated Lisfranc injuries at a minimum of 2 years after surgery.

Results.—Of the 46 patients evaluated, 13 had poor outcomes and had to change employment or were unable to find work as a result of their injuries. The presence of a compensation claim and a delay in diagnosis of more than 6 months were associated with poor outcomes. No association was observed between a poor functional outcome and age, sex, mechanism of injury, or previous occupation.

Conclusions.—Patients who are pursuing compensation claims after surgery for displaced Lisfranc injuries have poor prognoses, independent of other factors. These findings may have medicolegal implications for reporting the prognosis of such injuries. In addition, the findings highlight the importance of a prompt diagnosis and treatment.

▶ Midfoot fracture dislocations result in significant functional disability in the short and the long term. In this retrospective cohort, patients with worker's compensation claims for which a delay in diagnosis occurred had a marked negative impact on the functional outcome. This is likely related to educational level and employment opportunity. Patients who have high functional demands of manual labor types of positions will not be able to function normally. With limited education, their employment options are limited, thereby increasing the stress on the worker's compensation system.

M. F. Swiontkowski, MD

Surgical Amputation Issues

Influence of Transmetatarsal Amputation in Patients Requiring Lower Extremity Distal Revascularization

Glass H, Rowe VL, Hood DB, et al (LAC +USC Med Ctr, Los Angeles)
Am Surg 70:845-849, 2004 4–34

Introduction.—Patients with symptomatic peripheral vascular disease who require extensive tissue resections and arterial bypass are sometimes deemed inappropriate candidates for limb salvage and instead undergo transtibial or transfemoral amputations. The influence of transmetatarsal amputation (TMA) on limb salvage in patients undergoing lower extremity revascularization was evaluated.

Methods.—The medical records of all patients with symptomatic peripheral vascular disease requiring lower extremity revascularization to the tibial vessels between 1986 and 2002 were reviewed. Limb salvage was assessed with the use of life-table analysis.

Results.—The average age of 15 men and 9 women (29 limbs) was 64.2 years. Gangrene was the indication for bypass and TMA in 25 cases (86.5%). The outcomes of 7 limbs were lost to follow-up. Nine of 22 remaining limbs needed below-knee (8) or above-knee (1) amputations. Of 7 limbs that underwent major amputations within the first 3 months, graft thrombosis was the cause of leg amputation in 6 cases (85.7%). No significant predictors of early major amputation were observed. Limb salvage was 62% at 1 year in the TMA cohort. Among historical control subjects needing distal revascularization and no adjunctive toe or foot amputations, limb salvage was 76.5% (P = NS).

Conclusion.—Long-term salvage depends on successful lower extremity revascularization. The need for TMA should not affect the decision for limb salvage.

▶ The result of disvascular patients requiring amputation has been a focus of concern for the last 4 decades. In this retrospective cohort over a 16-year period, limb salvage was noted to be dependent on successful lower extremity revascularization.

M. F. Swiontkowski, MD

Mortality in Diabetic and Nondiabetic Patients After Amputations Performed From 1990 to 1995: A 5-Year Follow-up Study

Tentolouris N, Al-Sabbagh S, Walker MG, et al (Univ of Manchester, England)

Diabetes Care 27:1598-1604, 2004 4–35

Introduction.—Diabetes is the cause of nearly 50% of all nontraumatic lower extremity amputations worldwide. The lifetime risk for amputation in patients with diabetes is 10% to 15%, which is 10 to 30 times higher than the general population. The outcome of amputees was examined and compared between patients with and without diabetes to ascertain whether there are any modifiable risk factors for increased mortality in patients with diabetes.

Methods.—All amputations performed at a single center between 1990 and 1995 (100 cases without and 151 with diabetes) were reviewed retrospectively. Survival status was evaluated from the first amputation until December 31, 2001.

Results.—A total of 61% of patients with and 54.3% of patients without diabetes died a mean of 5.2 years (4.5-5.8 years) and 5.3 years (4.7-5.9 years) after their first amputation, respectively ($P = .80$). The survival duration among patients with and without diabetes was not significantly different after adjustment was made for the level (major vs minor) ($P = .67$) and the cause (ischemia vs infection) of amputation ($P = .72$). No sex differences were observed for survival in either group. Independent predictors of mortality for the diabetic group were the duration of diabetes ($P = .05$), a history of a stroke ($P = .02$), and serum creatinine level ($P < .0001$). In the nondiabetic group, the independent predictors were a history of a stroke ($P = .04$), serum creatinine level ($P < .005$), and higher white blood count ($P = .02$). The peak incidence of amputations occurred between the ages of 67 and 76 years for both groups. Major amputations occurred more often in patients without diabetes in all age groups. The median hospital stay and postoperative complications were similar for both groups.

Conclusion.—The all-cause mortality rate is high after nontraumatic amputations for patients with and without diabetes. Both groups have similar mortality rates, hospital lengths of stay, and postoperative complications. No modifiable factors, except nephropathy, improved the survival duration in patients who had undergone amputation. Peripheral vascular disease and neuropathy are the most important causes of amputations; therefore, they must be prevented to avoid amputations and the subsequent high rates of mortality.

▶ The impact of diabetes on the long-term outcome of patients requiring amputation was evaluated in a single-site study over a 5-year period. Major, more proximal amputations occurred more often than in the nondiabetic group, which had a high incidence of associated comorbidity. Median hospital stay and postoperative complications were similar. Peripheral vascular disease and neuropathy seemed to be the most pertinent factors.

M. F. Swiontkowski, MD

Trial of Amitriptyline for Relief of Pain in Amputees: Results of a Randomized Controlled Study

Robinson LR, Czerniecki JM, Ehde DM, et al (Univ of Washington, Seattle; Good Samaritan Hosp, Puyallup, Wash)

Arch Phys Med Rehabil 85:1-6, 2004 4–36

Introduction.—Tricyclic antidepressants (TCAs) are commonly used to treat phantom limb pain (PLP). Trials assessing the efficacy of TCAs for PLP are almost nonexistent. Whether amitriptyline is more effective than placebo in improving PLP or residual limb pain was determined in a randomized controlled trial.

Methods.—The study included 39 participants with amputation-associated pain persisting more than 6 months who underwent a 6-week trial of amitriptyline (titrated up to 125 mg/d) or an active placebo (benztropine mesylate). The primary outcome measure was average pain intensity, and the secondary outcome measures were disability, satisfaction with life, and degree of handicap.

Results.—No significant differences were seen between the treatment group in outcome variables when controlling for initial pain scores.

Conclusion.—These findings do not support the use of amitriptyline for treatment of postamputation pain syndrome.

▶ Pain relief for patients experiencing phantom limb pain is an important area of study. In a group of 39 participants, the TCA amitriptyline was investigated. The drug did not have any impact whatsoever on the outcome measures assessed, which included disability, handicap, pain intensity, and satisfaction with life. Its use cannot be recommended in patients with this diagnosis.

M. F. Swiontkowski, MD

Explaining Racial Variation in Lower Extremity Amputation: A 5-Year Retrospective Claims Data and Medical Record Review at an Urban Teaching Hospital

Rucker-Whitaker C, Feinglass J, Pearce WH (Northwestern Univ, Chicago; Rush-Presbyterian-St Luke's Med Ctr, Chicago)

Arch Surg 138:1347-1351, 2003 4–37

Introduction.—Population-based hospital data show that African American patients undergo major lower-extremity (LE) amputations 2- to 3-times more than do Caucasian patients. Concern has been expressed that this finding is caused by a lack of access to LE revascular procedures by African Americans. A 2-step retrospective investigation was performed to determine (1) the likelihood that racial disparities in amputation rates are linked to treatment choice; (2) the incidence of primary amputation (major amputation without any previous attempt at revascularization); and (3) the incidence of repeat amputation.

Methods.—Administrative discharge data for all 1127 patients undergoing LE arterial bypass graft, angioplasty, or major amputation between January 1, 1995, and February 1, 2000, were reviewed to evaluate racial differences in the risk of admission for major amputation in comparison with that for revascularization. Medical records were reviewed for an approximately full sample of 60 African American major amputees and a random sample of 60 (two thirds of the total) white major amputees. Racial disparities in the incidence of primary and repeat amputation were analyzed, controlling for age, sex, and diabetes mellitus status. African Americans and white people were evaluated for the odds of amputation versus revascularization and the odds of primary versus repeat major amputation.

Results.—African Americans were significantly younger ($P < .05$), more often female ($P < .01$), and more likely to undergo major amputation (odds ratio [OR], 1.68; $P = .005$), compared to white people. After adjusting for age, sex, and diabetes mellitus prevalence, an equal likelihood of primary amputation was seen among African Americans and white people. Repeat amputees were 2.5 times more likely to be African American than white ($P = .04$).

Conclusion.—The racial disparity observed in this cohort was primarily due to African American patients undergoing repeat major amputation at a significantly higher rate, compared with that of white patients.

► The investigation of racial disparities is an important area of research in the musculoskeletal community. Compared with whites, African Americans were significantly more likely to become repeat amputees. The causes of this discrepancy needs to be carefully investigated in a prospective cohort study, again requiring a multicenter cooperative design.

M. F. Swiontkowski, MD

Functional Outcomes Following Trauma-Related Lower-Extremity Amputation

MacKenzie EJ, Bosse MJ, Castillo RC, et al (Johns Hopkins Bloomberg School of Public Health, Baltimore, Md; Carolinas Med Ctr, Charlotte, NC; Harborview Med Ctr, Seattle; et al)

J Bone Joint Surg Am 86-A:1636-1645, 2004 4–38

Introduction.—Trauma-related lower-limb amputations are often performed in or near the zone of injury to preserve limb length. This practice can result in atypical wound closures, use of skin grafts or flaps, and a residual limb that is less than ideal. Patients who had undergone above-the-ankle amputation at a trauma center were assessed for functional outcome according to amputation level and other factors.

Methods.—The study group included 161 patients who had undergone amputation within 3 months of injury and were followed up prospectively at 3, 6, 12, and 24 months after the injury. The principal measure of outcome was the Sickness Impact Profile (SIP). Additional outcomes of interest included pain, degree of independence, and the physician's satisfaction with clinical, functional, and cosmetic recovery of the limb.

Results.—The average hospital stay for initial acute care was 17.7 days, and 29.8% of patients were rehospitalized at least once because of a complication. Scores on the SIP did not differ significantly between patients treated with above-the-knee and those treated with below-the-knee amputation, but the below-the-knee subgroup performed better on the timed test for walking speed. Compared with both below- and above-the-knee subgroups, patients with through-the-knee-amputation had worse regression-adjusted SIP scores and slower self-selected walking speeds. Overall, differences in physical function were most affected by the level of amputation.

Physicians were less satisfied with the outcome, particularly in terms of clinical and cosmetic recovery, of patients with through-the-knee amputations. Factors other than level of amputation that significantly predicted a poor overall SIP score included a pre-existing medical condition, smoking, an ipsilateral limb injury, less than a college education, low self efficacy, and nonwhite race. These predictors were the same for all levels of amputation.

Conclusion.—Major lower-limb amputation caused by trauma is most often performed in adolescents and young adults. In this study, functional outcomes at 24 months were poor, particularly after through-the-knee amputations. High self-efficacy was a more important determinant of better outcome than the technological sophistication of the prosthetic device.

► Non-injury-related factors seem to be the most cogent predictors of poor outcomes after trauma-related lower limb amputation in this prospective cohort. Preexisting medical conditions, ipsilateral limb injury, low education, smoking, low self-advocacy, and nonwhite race are the important predictors. Preventive strategies to enhance the quality of function after these devastating injuries must be investigated as the cause for poor outcomes, which clearly do not seem to be related to surgical technique or amputation level.

M. F. Swiontkowski, MD

Prosthetic Related Amputation Issues

Houghton Scale of Prosthetic Use in People With Lower-Extremity Amputations: Reliability, Validity, and Responsiveness to Change

Devlin M, Pauley T, Head K, et al (Univ of Toronto; West Park Healthcare Centre, Toronto; Village Square Physiotherapy, Calgary, Alta, Canada, et al)

Arch Phys Med Rehabil 85:1339-1344, 2004 4–39

Introduction.—The Houghton Scale is an instrument that evaluates a patient's perception of prosthetic use in cases of lower-extremity amputation. Compared with other tools that measure prosthetic use, the 4-question Houghton Scale is quickly administered and easy to score. A prospective single-center study was designed to evaluate the scale's responsiveness to change in patient status and its test-retest reliability.

Methods.—Participants were 125 individuals who were receiving prostheses because of unilateral or bilateral lower-extremity amputation. All were medically stable, and none had problems related to the prosthesis. The group was divided into sample 1 (49 participants, 26 men and 23 women with a mean age of 60.9 years) and sample 2 (76 participants, 58 men and 18 women with a mean age of 65.5 years).

Data from sample 1 were used to establish the test-retest reliability of the Houghton Scale. Sample 2 data were used to evaluate its responsiveness to change, internal consistency, and validity. Houghton Scale results were reported as a total score out of 12, with higher scores indicating greater performance and greater comfort.

Results.—Most amputations in both samples had been performed for diabetes mellitus and peripheral vascular disease. Evaluation of responsiveness to change after rehabilitation showed that the total Houghton Scale score increased from a mean of 6.14 at discharge to a mean of 7.70 at 3-month follow-up. Floor and ceiling effects were observed for the individual subscales but not for the overall score.

Internal consistency was judged moderate at both discharge and follow-up. There was a moderate, yet significant correlation between the Houghton Scale and the physical composite score of the Medical Outcomes Study 36-Item Short-Form Health Survey and the 2-minute walk test at admission and discharge. Reliability of the scale was high (the intra-class correlation coefficient for total score test-retest was 0.96).

Conclusion.—The Houghton Scale proved responsive to change in prosthetic use in patients with lower-limb amputation after rehabilitation. Changes over time for the first 3 items that make up the scale were significant. The authors recommend that item 4, which assesses comfort at negotiating different outdoor surfaces, be omitted.

▶ The Houghton Scale is proven in this study to be a responsive and internally consistent questionnaire to evaluate amputation outcomes. Its use can be recommended to evaluate patient perception of prosthetic use in lower extremity amputation.

M. F. Swiontkowski, MD

The Effects of Added Prosthetic Mass on Physiologic Responses and Stride Frequency During Multiple Speeds of Walking in Persons With Transtibial Amputation

Lin-Chan S-J, Nielsen DH, Yack HJ, et al (Texas Woman's Univ, Dallas; Univ of Iowa, Iowa City; Natl Yang Ming Univ, Taipei, Taiwan)

Arch Phys Med Rehabil 84:1865-1871, 2003 4–40

Background.—People with transtibial amputation use up to 55% more energy during walking than people with 2 normal legs. To enhance motor performance in these patients, prosthesis manufacturers have reduced prosthetic mass and improved the dynamic capabilities of the prosthetic foot. However, the new, lightweight prosthetic materials, such as titanium, are more expensive than traditional stainless-steel devices; in addition, many patients prefer a heavier foot mass. The extent to which prosthetic mass could be increased without significantly affecting physiologic responses during walking was investigated.

Methods.—The study included 8 ambulatory men, 20 to 64 years old, (mean age, 36 years) with unilateral traumatic transtibial amputation. Three prosthetic masses (60%, 80%, and 100% of the estimated intact shank and foot mass) were tested at 5 speeds during treadmill walking (4 minutes each at 54, 67, 80, 94, and 107 m/min, without resting between accelerations). Patients were allowed to acclimate to each mass for 3 hours before testing. Oxygen consumption, gait efficiency, relative exercise intensity (ie, percentage of age-predicted maximum heart rate), and stride frequency were assessed during each condition.

Results.—Oxygen consumption and gait efficiency increased with increasing walking speed, yet neither parameter differed significantly according to mass percentage. However, as the mass of the prosthesis increased from 60% to 100%, and as walking speed increased, the relative exercise intensity increased significantly, and stride frequency decreased significantly.

Conclusion.—A prosthesis even up to 100% of the estimated intact below-knee mass did not increase oxygen consumption or gait efficiency during accelerated walking for these patients with transtibial amputation. However, increased prosthesis mass did increase relative exercise intensity and decreased stride frequency during accelerated walking. The possibility of providing more prosthetic options at lower cost for these patients deserves further study.

▶ The weight of the prosthesis is a significant concern for patients with transtibial amputation. Increasing the prosthetic mass decreases the stride frequency as well as the relative exercise intensity, which makes good sense. The tradeoff of the cost of the prosthesis versus these fractures is a difficult one and requires thoughtful consideration from patients, prosthetists, and the groups responsible for funding medical care.

M. F. Swiontkowski, MD

Residual Function in Peripheral Nerve Stumps of Amputees: Implications for Neural Control of Artificial Limbs

Dhillon GS, Lawrence SM, Hutchinson DT, et al (Univ of Utah, Salt Lake City)
J Hand Surg [Am] 29A:605-615, 2004 4–41

Introduction.—Potential impediments to interfacing artificial limbs to the peripheral system of long-term (>3 months) amputated stumps include axotomy-induced loss of central connections, questionable viability of the proximal nerve stump, and reorganization of CNS areas related to the missing limb regions. It is not known if the motor and sensory patterns that are associated with a missing or denervated limb remain functionally intact during periods of several months or years after amputation or chronic peripheral nerve transection injury. The degree to which activity on chronically severed motor nerve fibers could be controlled by human amputees and whether distally referred tactile and proprioceptive sensations could be induced by stimulation of sensory axons in the nerve were investigated.

Methods.—Eight amputee research subjects undergoing stump revision surgery had longitudinal intrafascicular electrodes threaded percutaneously and implanted in severed nerves. The electrodes were interfaced to an amplifier and a stimulator system that was controlled by a laptop computer. Electrophysiologic testing was performed for 2 consecutive days after recovery from surgery.

Results.—It was possible to record volitional motor nerve activity uniquely associated with missing limb movement. Electrical stimulation through the implanted electrodes produced discrete, unitary, graded sensations of touch, joint movement, and position, referring to the missing limb.

Conclusion.—Both central and peripheral motor and somatosensory pathways retain significant residual connectivity and function for several years after limb amputation, suggesting that peripheral nerve interfaces could be used to provide amputees with prosthetic limbs with more natural feel and control than is possible using current myoelectric and body-powered control systems.

▶ In this investigational study, the authors investigate the potential for amputated nerve stumps to provide a viable interface for functional electrical stimulation. They found that the peripheral nerve interfaces were intact enough to allow motor and somatosensory pathways to be communicated with. The potential for designing limbs with a more natural feel and control seems real.

M. F. Swiontkowski, MD

Effects of a Simple Functional Electric System and/or a Hinged Ankle-Foot Orthosis on Walking in Persons With Incomplete Spinal Cord Injury

Kim CM, Eng JJ, Whittaker MW (Univ of British Columbia, Vancouver, Cana)

Arch Phys Med Rehabil 85:1718-1723, 2004 4–42

Introduction.—The traditional way to augment foot clearance during the swing portion of the gait is to use an ankle–foot orthosis (AFO). An alternative approach that aids in foot clearance is electric stimulation of the peroneal nerve to induce ankle dorsiflexion during the swing. The effect of functional electric stimulation (FES) was compared with that of a hinged AFO for assisting foot clearance, walking speed, and endurance and to ascertain whether added benefits exist for the use of FES in conjunction with AFO in patients with incomplete spinal cord injuries (SCIs).

Methods.—A within-subject comparison of walking under 4 conditions was performed in 19 participants with incomplete SCIs: AFO, FES, AFO and FES, and no orthosis. A plastic hinged AFO was used in all AFO conditions. The primary outcome measures were self-selected walking speed, 6-minute walk distance, and foot clearance values; these were compared for all conditions.

Results.—The walking speed increased with FES ($P < .05$) and with an AFO ($P = .06$); the 6-minute walk distance increased with the an AFO ($P < .05$). No significant differences were observed between the 2 forms of orthoses in either walking speed or endurance. The greatest increase in walking speed and endurance for the no-orthosis condition was observed with the combined AFO and FES condition. Foot clearance improved with FES but not with an AFO. Participants whose walking speed increased with FES had weaker hip flexors, knee flexors, and ankle dorsiflexion compared with those who did not benefit from FES.

Conclusion.—Both FES and the hinged AFO promote walking; FES was only superior to the AFO in increasing foot-clearance values. The hinged AFO and FES together may provide advantages over either device alone.

▶ The use of FES to improve function with the use of an AFO was investigated for patients with incomplete SCI. It proved to be advantageous for increasing foot clearance values. Combining FES with a hinged AFO seems to have promise for this small group of patients with very high functional demand needs.

M. F. Swiontkowski, MD

5 Total Hip Arthroplasty

Introduction

The literature continues to reflect tremendous interest in joint replacement arthroplasty. As applied to the hip, a blend of long-term outcome studies using established systems with information regarding newer articular surfaces is included. The use of navigation and limited invasive surgery are hot topics, but only a trickle of peer review literature is available on these topics of growing interest. The effectiveness of revision surgery is also highlighted in this year's selections, which hopefully will offer insight with regard to the tried and true as well as innovative thoughts that are in the process of evolution and assessment.

Bernard F. Morrey, MD

Thirty-Day Mortality Following Hip Arthroplasty for Acute Fracture

Parvizi J, Ereth MH, Lewallen DG (Mayo Clinic and Mayo Found, Rochester, Minn)

J Bone Joint Surg Am 86-A:1983-1988, 2004 5–1

Introduction.—Hip fractures are linked with increased mortality. Earlier reports addressing perioperative mortality associated with hip arthroplasty in the treatment of acute fracture have not documented demographic and surgical characteristics that increase the possibility of death. The prevalence of and associate risk factors for perioperative death after hip arthroplasty was examined in patients treated for acute fracture.

Methods.—Data were compiled from the computerized joint registry at a single institution to ascertain the mortality rate after hip arthroplasty according to age, gender, diagnosis, implant type, and fixation mode. Database review showed that 7774 consecutive patients had undergone hip arthroplasty for treatment of an acute fracture between 1969 and 1997. The medical records of all patients who had died within 30 days after hip arthroplasty were examined retrospectively.

Results.—The overall incidence of mortality within 30 days after hip arthroplasty for treatment of an acute fracture was 2.4% (186/7774). Marked variations were observed within clinical subgroups. The 30-day incidence of mortality was significantly higher among patients who had received a cemented implant, female patients, elderly patients, those with cardiorespiratory comorbidities, and patients with intertrochanteric fractures. No significant difference was observed in mortality between patients managed with THA and those managed with hemiarthroplasty.

Conclusion.—Hip arthroplasty for the diagnosis of acute fracture is associated with a nearly 10-fold higher incidence of perioperative mortality compared to elective hip arthroplasty. Medical optimization, an appropriate choice of implants, and vigilant intraoperative management are crucial for these patients.

► Significant strides have been made with regard to anesthetic and surgical technique allowing improved management of displaced femoral neck fractures in the elderly. Nonetheless, this is a sobering report, indicating a 10-fold increase in mortality in this patient population compared with elective surgery at our institution. Attempts to rehydrate the patient before surgery, as well as a rapid and efficient procedure, are within the control of the surgeon and are demonstrated to be important to minimize this disastrous complication.

B. F. Morrey, MD

Closed Suction Drainage for Hip and Knee Arthroplasty: A Meta-analysis

Parker MJ, Roberts CP, Hay D (Peterborough District Hosp, England)

J Bone Joint Surg Am 86-A:1146-1152, 2004 5–2

Introduction.—Closed-suction drainage systems are commonly used after total joint replacement. The theoretical advantages for using drains are decreases in the incidence of wound hematomas and infection. A meta-analysis was performed to ascertain the advantages and adverse effects of surgical drains, based on evidence from randomized controlled trials.

Methods.—Hand searches of journals and computer-aided searches of MEDLINE, EMBASE, CINAHL, CENTRAL, the Cochrane Collaboration, and Current Contents were performed to identify all randomized trials involving elective hip and knee arthroplasty. There were no restrictions on languages or source. Methods of all identified trials were examined.

Results.—Eighteen trials involving 3495 patients with 3689 wounds were included. Pooled results indicated that there was no significant difference between wounds treated with and those treated without a drain in the occurrence of wound infection (relative risk [RR], 0.73; 95% confidence interval [CI], 0.47-1.14) wound hematoma (RR, 1.73; 95% CI, 0.74-4.07), or reoperation for wound complications (RR, 95% CI, 0.13-1.99). A drained wound was linked with a significantly higher need for transfusion (RR, 1.43; 95% CI, 1.19-1.72).

Reinforcement of the wound dressing was necessary more frequently in the group managed without drains. No between-group differences were observed in limb swelling, venous thrombosis, or hospital stay.

Conclusion.—Meta-analyses revealed that closed suction drainage increases the transfusion requirements after elective hip and knee arthroplasty and provides no major benefit. More data are needed before the outcome of wound infection can be linked to closed suction drainage.

► The editor discontinued the use of closed suction drains for hips and knees approximately 15 years ago. This was based on our interpretation of the emerging literature that, in my judgment, is very clearly confirmed by this meta-analysis. Specifically, retaining the use of suction drainage does not decrease the infection rate or the complication of hematoma. It does add an unnecessary cost, and the data presented here clearly demonstrate the additional disadvantages of increasing the transfusion requirements. It would be hoped that data such as these will provoke the elimination of this unnecessary ritual which does add, albeit small, some cost to the procedure.

B. F. Morrey, MD

Patient-Reported Outcome in Total Hip Replacement: A Comparison of Five Instruments of Health Status

Ostendorf M, van Stel HF, Buskens E, et al (Univ Med Ctr, Utrecht, The Netherlands)

J Bone Joint Surg Br 86-B:801-808, 2004 5–3

Introduction.—Health status questionnaires are especially important when comparing the cost-to-benefit ratio of medical interventions. The minimum set of patient-reported outcome measures necessary to evaluate health status after total hip replacement (THR) was examined in 114 patients.

Methods.—The preoperative characteristics and sensitivity to change of the Oxford hip score (OHS), the Western Ontario and McMaster Universities osteoarthritis index (WOMAC), the short-form-36 (SF-36), the SF-12 (derived from the SF-36), and the Euroqol questionnaire (EQ-5D) were evaluated.

Results.—At 1 year postoperatively, very large effect sizes were seen for the disease-specific measures, the physical domains of the SF-12, SF-36, and the $\text{EQ-5D}_{\text{index}}$ (1.3-3.0). Patients in Charnley class A experienced more change in the OHS, the WOMAC pain and function, the physical domains of the SF-36, and the $\text{EQ-5D}_{\text{vas}}$ ($P < .05$) compared with those in the Charnley class B and C groups. In the Charnley class A group, the effect size for the OHS more than doubled the size effect of the WOMAC pain and physical function.

High correlations and correlations of change were observed between the OHS, the WOMAC, the physical domains for the SF-12, the SF-36, and EQ-5D scores at 1 year postoperatively. They approached scores for the general population. A binomial distribution of the preoperative $\text{EQ-5D}_{\text{index}}$ score and a preoperative discrepancy and postoperative agreement between the $\text{EQ-5D}_{\text{vas}}$ and $\text{EQ-5D}_{\text{index}}$ were observed.

Conclusion.—The OHS and SF-12 are recommended for evaluation of THR. The SF-36 may be used when smaller changes in the health status are evaluated (ie, follow-up of THR). The EQ-5D is helpful in situations in which utility values are necessary to calculate cost effectiveness or quality-adjusted life years, including the evaluation of new techniques in THR.

▶ This is a detailed assessment of the relative values and effectiveness of several different patient-reported outcome measurement tools. As the need to demonstrate cost effectiveness continues, measurements such as these will be important to record and have available to demonstrate improvement in quality of life as well as cost effectiveness of the hip and knee replacement procedures.

B. F. Morrey, MD

Results of Charnley Total Hip Arthroplasty at a Minimum of Thirty Years: A Concise Follow-up of a Previous Report

Callaghan JJ, Templeton JE, Liu SS, et al (Univ of Iowa, Iowa City; Iowa Methodist Med Ctr, Des Moines)

J Bone Joint Surg Am 86-A:690-695, 2004 5–4

Introduction.—The results of a prospective investigation in a single-surgeon series of primary Charnley THAs, which were previously published after 2, 10, 15, and 25 years of follow-up, were now extended to a minimum follow-up of 30 years.

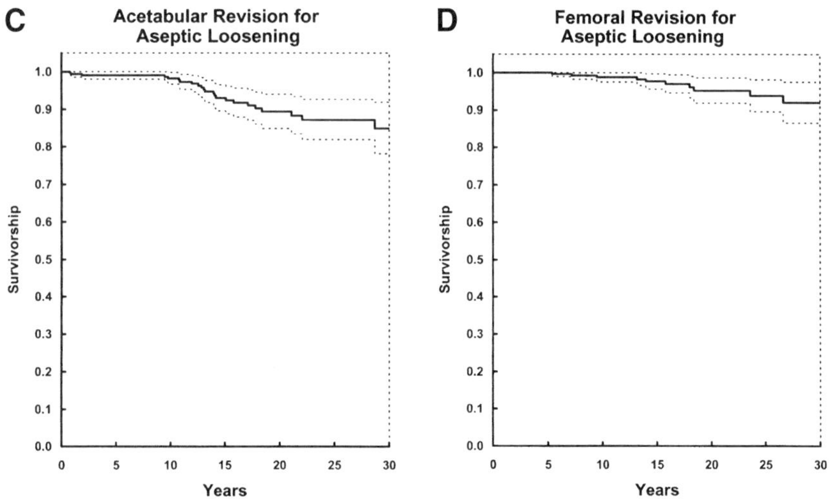

FIGURE 1.—C Survivorship curve with revision because of acetabular loosening as the end point. D Survivorship curve with revision because of femoral loosening as the end point. (Republished with permission of the Journal of Bone and Joint Surgery, Inc, from Callaghan JJ, Templeton JE, Liu SS, et al: Results of Charnley total hip arthroplasty at a minimum of thirty years: A concise follow-up of a previous report. *J Bone Joint Surg Am* 86-A:690-695, 2004. Reproduced by permission of the publisher Copyright Clearance Center, Inc.)

Findings.—The original series included 134 women and 128 men whose average age was 65.1 years (range, 29-86 years) at the time of surgery. Twenty-seven patients (34 hips [10.3%] in the initial group) were alive at a minimum of 30 years postoperatively and serve as the basis of the present investigation. Revisions because of aseptic loosening of the acetabular component were performed in 23 (7.3%) hips from the original cohort (excluding those revised because of infection or dislocation) and in 8 (26%) hips in the living cohort. Revisions necessary because of aseptic loosening of the femoral component were performed in 10 (3.2%) hips of the original cohort (excluding those caused by infection or dislocation) and in 3 (10%) hips in living patients. Since the 25-year review, 3 hips underwent revision (1 for acetabular loosening, 1 for femoral loosening, and 1 for instability) (Fig 1).

Conclusion.—The remarkable durability of cemented Charnley total hip replacements were demonstrated during a span of 3 decades; 88% of the original prostheses were intact at the time of final follow-up or at the time of patient's death.

► Although the numbers are of necessity relatively small, there is merit in documenting the long-term outcome of this patient population. The long-term Kaplan-Meier survival curve for acetabular and femoral revision rates after a cemented Charnley hip replacement is clearly impressive. The editor continues to emphasize the distinction between patients in whom a revision occurred and those who had radiographic evidence of implant loosening. The absence of a revision procedure does not necessarily imply a successfully functioning implant. On the other hand, radiographic evidence of loosening does not necessarily indicate functional failure. Regardless, the long-term outcome of the cemented implant continues to serve as the standard against which the newer systems must be considered.

B. F. Morrey, MD

Cementless Acetabular Fixation at Fifteen Years: A Comparison With the Same Surgeon's Results Following Acetabular Fixation With Cement

Gaffey JL, Callaghan JJ, Pedersen DR, et al (Univ of Iowa, Iowa City; Iowa Methodist Med Ctr, Des Moines)

J Bone Joint Surg Am 86-A:257-261, 2004 5–5

Introduction.—Loosening of the acetabular component is an important long-term problem linked with THA with cement. The minimum 13-year results of cementless acetabular components inserted by a single surgeon were evaluated and compared with results of cemented acetabular components inserted by the same surgeon.

Methods.—The study included 120 consecutive, nonselected primary total hip replacements that were performed in 108 patients using a Harris-Galante-I cementless acetabular component and a cemented femoral component with a 28-mm head. Patients were examined clinically using a standard terminology questionnaire. They underwent radiographic examination to identify loosening, component migration, wear, and osteolysis. The revision rates for aseptic loosening and radiographic evidence of loosening for this cohort were compared with the rates for 4 previously reviewed consecutive series of hips in which the acetabular component was inserted with cement. All patients were managed by the same surgeon, were followed up for 13 to 15 years, and were assessed using the same 2 criteria (revision and loosening) as end points for Kaplan-Meier analysis.

Results.—Sixty-two patients, (72 hips) were alive, and 42 patients (48 hips) had died at the time of analysis. No acetabular component had been revised because of aseptic loosening, and none had migrated. With revision of the acetabular component for any reason as the end point, the 15-year survival rate was 81%. With revision of the acetabular component for clinical failure (osteolysis, wear, loosening, or dislocation) as the end point, the 15-year survival rate was 94%. Among 70 hips with a minimum of 13 years of radiographic follow-up, 5 had pelvic osteolysis and 3 had revision of a well-fixed acetabular component because of pelvic osteolysis secondary to polyethylene wear. The average linear wear rate was 0.15 mm/y and was higher for hips that needed revision of the femoral component (0.28 mm/y). The average linear wear rate was 0.12 mm/y when the outlier was not included.

Conclusion.—The Harris-Galante-I cementless components performed better, compared to the cemented 22-mm–inner-diameter Charnley acetabular components, along with the 28-mm–inner-diameter all-polyethylene and metal-backed acetabular components that were inserted by the same surgeon. The wear rate was greater in Harris-Galante-I cementless components than in the Charnley cemented all-polyethylene components.

► This article is worthwhile in that it provides useful information on expectations referable to the outcome of a specific design acetabular lining from the perspective of implant loosening. Fortunately, implant loosening is no longer a real issue with any of the current available metal shells. The issue is wear of the acetabular liner.

Unfortunately, this article does not address this subject in sufficient detail to allow the orthopedic surgeon to select an appropriate design as a function of the age of the patient. There is a great deal of information to indicate cemented cups in patients older than 70 or 75 years have as long, if not longer, survival as do uncemented acetabular components. Additional studies addressing these important issues continue to be needed and are awaited in order that the most cost-effective implant selection can be made.

B. F. Morrey, MD

Clinical and Radiographic Results Associated With a Modern, Cementless Modular Cup Design in Total Hip Arthroplasty

González Della Valle A, Zoppi A, Peterson MGE, et al (Hosp for Special Surgery, New York)

J Bone Joint Surg Am 86-A:1998-2004, 2004 5–6

Introduction.—The second generation of cementless cups designed for use in THA reduced the number of complications and the rate of failure associated with first-generation cementless modular cups. Advances in the newer cups include fewer screw-holes (or no holes), improved locking mechanisms, and maximized shell-liner conformity. A consecutive group of patients who received a modern modular acetabular cup was followed up for 4 to 7 years for evaluation of fixation, wear, and the rate of periprosthetic osteolysis.

Methods.—The 271 patients (136 women and 135 men) available for study had 308 primary hybrid total hip replacements between October 1996 and January 1998. The average age of the patient cohort was 64 years. In all hips, a Trilogy cementless acetabular cup (Zimmer, Warsaw, Indiana) was implanted through a posterolateral approach. A single orthopedic surgeon performed all procedures. Patients were evaluated according to the Hospital for Special Surgery hip-scoring system.

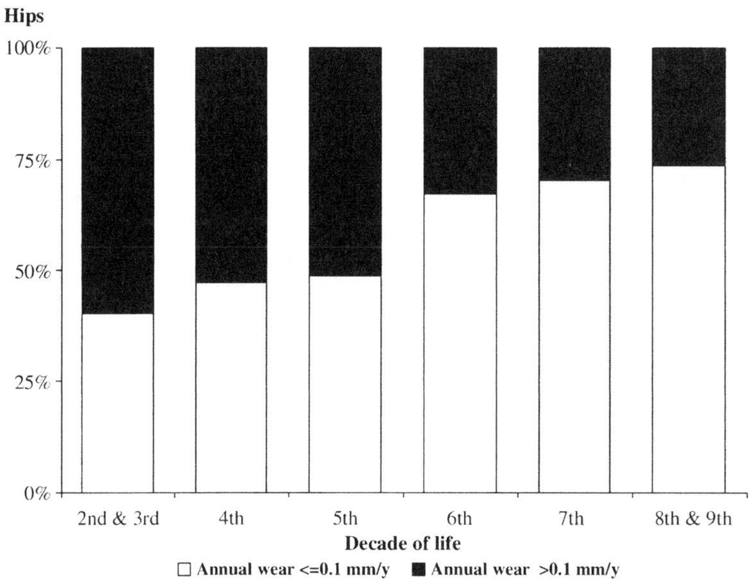

FIGURE 2.—Annual wear rates of 0.01 mm or less or more than 0.01 mm according to the decade of life at the time of surgery. (Courtesy of González Della Valle A, Zoppi A, Peterson MGE, et al: Clinical and radiographic results associated with a modern, cementless modular cup design in total hip arthroplasty. *J Bone Joint Surg Am* 86-A:1998-2004, 2004. Republished by permission of the Journal of Bone and Joint Surgery, Inc. Reproduced by permission of the publisher via Copyright Clearance Center, Inc.)

Results.—At the latest follow-up, 288 of 303 unrevised hips in 267 living patients were rated as excellent, 14 as good, and 1 (in a patient with amyloidosis) as fair. Hip scores for pain, walking ability, motion, and function averaged 4.05, 4.02, 3.08, and 4.02, respectively, preoperatively; postoperatively, the scores increased to 9.08, 9.6, 8.5, and 9.3, respectively. There were 8 revisions (6 for aseptic loosening and 2 for infection).

In the group of 229 patients (262 hips) with complete radiographic follow-up, 259 cups were well fixed. The average wear rate for 246 hips was 0.09 mm/y. Annual wear rates varied according to the decade of life at the time of surgery (Fig 2). Osteolysis, detected in 12 (5%) hips, was associated with the annual wear rate and male gender. No calcar resorption was noted in 138 hips. In hips with calcar resorption, the average extent was 5.9 mm. There was a significant correlation between extent of calcar resorption and the annual wear rate.

Conclusion.—The rates of revision for aseptic loosening (0.3%) and of periprosthetic osteolysis (5%) were both quite low in this series of patients who received total hip replacement with a cementless, second-generation acetabular component. At the last follow-up, 97% of the 271 patients who were still alive had good or excellent clinical results.

► This is a complementary article to that of Parvizi et al (Abstract 5–7) and portrays a second generation cementless modular cup. The outcome of this second generation design does show less osteolysis and comparable mechanical fixation to the earlier designs. It should be emphasized that the ultimate problem is absolutely a function of the duration of follow-up. Further, several different designs are used in this report, and the surveillance is significantly shorter than the prior study of Parvizi et al. Simply stated, the single most important factor that relates to wear is the duration of follow-up, thus defining a significant difference between these 2 reports.

B. F. Morrey, MD

Fifteen-Year Clinical Survivorship of Harris-Galante Total Hip Arthroplasty

Parvizi J, Sullivan T, Duffy G, et al (Mayo Clinic and Mayo Found, Rochester, Minn)

J Arthroplasty 19:672-677, 2004 5–7

Introduction.—After 3 decades of use, it is not clear whether uncemented THA has achieved the objective of minimizing aseptic failure. Some femoral components have had suboptimal long-term performance, while others have exhibited excellent survivorship. The long-term outcome of uncemented THA using Harris-Galante Porous I acetabular and femoral components was evaluated in 90 hips (80 patients) submitted to primary surgery between 1984 and 1986.

Methods.—The average age of the 35 women and 45 men was 57.5 years (range, 23-80 years). The average patient follow-up was 14.9 years; none were lost to follow-up. The Harris Hip Score for THAs was used to evaluate clinical outcome. Serial AP and lateral radiographs were reviewed to determine the position of the prosthesis and loosening and wear. The average radiographic follow-up was 12.6 years.

Results.—The preoperative Harris Hip Scores improved significantly from 52.1 (range, 30-71) to 89.2 (range, 72-95) at the latest follow-up ($P < .001$). Review of the latest radiographs showed nonprogressive radiolucent lines around 11 femoral components. The femoral component was positioned in slight varus in 6 hips and in slight valgus in 3 hips. The position of the acetabular component was optimal and acceptable on the first postoperative radiographs in 83 hips. The acetabular components were not within the optimal range for placement in 7 hips.

At the latest follow-up, 3 femoral components were loose; all were radiographically stable. None were revised for aseptic loosening. Circumferential radiolucency was observed around 1 cup, and another cup had evidence of mild polyethylene wear. Revision surgery was probably going to be needed for both components in the near future.

Three patients experienced dislocation, despite well-positioned acetabular and femoral components. Two patients underwent reoperation: 1 for psoas tendon release and 1 for excision of heterotopic ossification. There were 11 revisions: 8 for failure of the femoral component, 3 for failure of the acetabular component, and 1 for deep infection. Survivorships free of revision and free of mechanical failure for the acetabular component at 15 years were 95.7% (95% confidence interval [CI], 0.89-1.0) and 91.9% (95% CI, 0.83-0.98), respectively. For the femoral component, survivorship was 86.8% (95% CI, 0.78-0.95) for freedom from revision and 82.0% (95% CI, 0.71-0.92) for freedom from mechanical failure (Fig 1). During follow-up, there were 3 deaths unrelated to hip surgery.

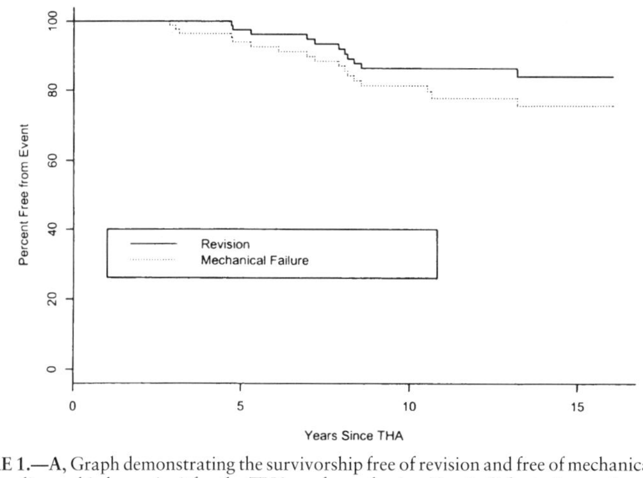

FIGURE 1.—A, Graph demonstrating the survivorship free of revision and free of mechanical failure (revision and radiographic loosening) for the THA performed using Harris-Galante Porous I acetabular and femoral components at 14.9 years' clinical and 12.6 years' radiographic follow-up. (Courtesy of Parvizi J, Sullivan T, Duffy G, et al: Fifteen-year clinical survivorship of Harris-Galante total hip arthroplasty. *J Arthroplasty* 19:672-677, 2004.)

Conclusion.—The uncemented Harris-Galante Porous I acetabular component had outstanding durability at long-term follow-up. It continues to be an attractive uncemented component for THA.

▶ This is an important contribution since it is one of the longest, if not the longest, surveillance studies for an uncemented cup. It is also important to recognize that the Harris-Galante Porous I used a type of polyethylene that previous studies have suggested fared well with regard to wear characterisitics.

This perception is reflected in the data, which show an outstanding 15-year survival free of mechanical loosening and quite acceptable outcome referable to osteolysis. It should be noted that the long-term survival of the metal-back cups does shift the burden to one of wear and osteolysis rather than fixation, as is reflected in these results.

B. F. Morrey, MD

A Comparison of Polyethylene Wear Rates Between Cemented and Cementless Cups: A Prospective, Randomised Trial

McCombe P, Williams SA (Frankston Hosp, Melbourne, Australia; Geelong Hosp, Australia)

J Bone Joint Surg Br 86-B:344-349, 2004 5–8

Introduction.—The long-term success of hip replacement relies on avoiding early complications and attaining lasting fixation of the components, with avoidance of aseptic loosening and osteolysis. There is sufficient evidence that high rates of wear of polyethylene and high rates of osteolysis are linked with higher rates of failure from aseptic loosening. The linear rates of penetration and rates of osteolysis of a typical hybrid hip replacement were compared with those of a typical cemented hip replacement using an all-polyethylene cup in a randomized controlled trial.

Methods.—A consecutive series of 162 patients needing primary hip replacement surgery for 1 hip between mid 1993 and 1995 were randomly as-

TABLE 1.—Patient Demographics and Results

	Duraloc	Exeter
Patients randomized	78	84
Exclusions	26	21
Patients studied	52	63
Age (yrs)	68.2 (41 to 83)	66.6 (48 to 82)
Follow-up (yrs)	6.51 (5.1 to 9.1)	6.43 (5.0 to 8.03)
Polyethylene thickness (mm)	10.44 (7 to 13.2)	10.87 (9 to 15)
Acetabular inclination (degrees)	41.6 (28 to 56)	42.6 (30 to 52)
Pelvic osteolysis	2	0
Calcar osteolysis	13	3
Wear rate (mm/yr)	0.15 (0 to 0.4)	0.07 (0 to 0.22)

(Courtesy of McCombe P, Williams SA: A comparison of polyethylene wear rates between cemented and cementless cups. *J Bone Joint Surg Br* 86-B:344-349, 2004.)

signed to receive either a cementless, hemispheric, modular titanium acetabular cup or a cemented, all-polyethylene cup. All replacements were performed by 2 surgeons at 4 general hospitals. The same technique and a 26-mm metal-head femoral component were used in every patient.

Results.—After exclusions, 115 hips were evaluated for differences in rates of wear and osteolysis. The mean clinical and radiologic follow-ups were 8 and 6.5 years, respectively. The cementless and cemented cups wore at a mean rate of 0.15 mm/y and 0.07 mm/y, respectively ($P < .0001$) (Table 1).

Conclusion.—It appears that the cemented all-polyethylene cup may function better in the longer term, compared to the evaluated uncemented cup. Caution is recommended concerning the widespread use of modular uncemented cups in total hip replacement.

▶ These investigators provide a scientific basis for that which has been long known; specifically: modular acetabular components are associated with a greater tendency for wear than are the monoblock cemented acetabular components. (See comment regarding acetabular revision, Abstract 5–23). Specifically, these investigators have provided the objective difference, at least in their experience, that the modular cup wears at twice the rate as does a monoblock cemented cup, a difference that is highly significant ($P < .0001$). It is precisely this reality that prompts the editor to cement acetabular components in patients over the age of 70 since the data clearly demonstrate that at this age group, the cups tend to remain in situ for the duration of the person's life time in over 95% of instances.

B. F. Morrey, MD

Wear of the Cup in the Charnley LFA in the Young Patient

Wroblewski BM, Siney PD, Fleming PA (Wrightington Hosp, Wigan, England)

J Bone Joint Surg Br 86-B:498-503, 2004 5–9

Introduction.—Some of the factors impacting the rate of wear of the cup after arthroplasty are damage to the head of the femoral component by ingress of cement and the patient's activity level. Reported were the long-term results in a series of young patients who underwent a Charnley low-friction torque arthroplasty using the ultra high molecular weight polyethylene cup.

Methods.—A total of 1092 patients under the age of 51 years at the time of surgery underwent 1434 low-friction torque arthroplasties performed between November 1962 and December 1990. Factors associated with either low wear (0.02 mm/y or less) or high wear (0.2 mm/y or more) were assessed.

Results.—A total of 190 patients (13.2%) experienced low wear and 149 (10.4%) had high wear. Significant factors in the low-wear group were female gender ($P = .042$), rheumatoid arthritis ($P = .014$), Charnley grade C ($P = .03$), and varus position of the stem ($P = .003$). The use of the acetabular cement pressurization ($P = .07$) and medialization of the cup ($P = .07$) approached significance.

TABLE 2.—Details of the Statistical Analysis in Both Groups (*P* Value)

Low-wear group	
Female gender	0.042
Rheumatoid arthritis	0.014
Charnley category 'C' post-op	0.03
Varus position of stem	0.003
No revision for aseptic loosening of the cup	<0.0001
High-wear group	
Male gender	0.042
Primary osteoarthritis	0.006
Valgus position of stem	0.023
Charnley category 'C' post-op	0.01
Revision for aseptic loosening of the cup	<0.0001
Approaching significance to the low-wear group	
Acetabular pressuriser used	0.07
Medialised cup position	0.07
Approaching significance to the high-wear group	
Support of the cup by the rim of the acetabulum	0.07
Not significant	
Revision for aseptic loosening of the stem/stem fracture	0.49
Cup flange	0.14

(Courtesy of Wroblewski BM, Siney PD, Fleming PA: Wear of cup in the Charnley LFA in the young patient. *J Bone Joint Surg Br* 86-A:498-503, 2004.)

There was a predominance of men in the high-wear group ($P = .042$), with osteoarthritis ($P = .006$) as the underlying pathology, and the stem in the valgus position ($P = .023$). Support of the cup by the rim of the acetabulum approached significance ($P = .07$). There were no significant between-group differences in revision for aseptic loosening of the stem or fracture of the stem ($P = .49$) (Table 2). A highly significant difference ($P = .0001$) was observed between the 2 groups for revision for wear and aseptic loosening of the cup (5.3% vs 39%).

Conclusion.—Changes in cup geometry are probably adequate in explaining the increasing incidence of loosening and revisions with the increasing depth of penetration of the cup. There is much to be gained from the use of a low-wearing, ceramic, ultra high molecular weight combination. Tissue reaction to polyethylene particles is not the cause of aseptic loosening of the stem.

► The factors associated with variable wear rates of the same implant design is quite a valuable contribution to the understanding of this problem. Clearly, "batch differences" of the polyethylene account for some of the variation reported in this study. The authors point out the underlying diagnosis, such as rheumatoid arthritis, and the male gender as being additional risk factors. With the high incidence of osteoarthritis in males, the correlation of this complication in males with osteoarthritis should be noted particularly in the younger age groups.

B. F. Morrey, MD

Factors Influencing the Longer-term Survival of Uncemented Acetabular Components Used in Total Hip Revisions

Jones CP, Lachiewicz PF (Univ of North Carolina, Chapel Hill)

J Bone Joint Surg Am 86-A:342-347, 2004 5–10

Introduction.—Revision of the acetabular component with a cementless porous-coated component and concomitant bone-grafting provides the possibility of long-term mechanical stability and reconstitution of deficient acetabular bone structure. Fixation with multiple screws offers the rigid fixation that is needed for initial stability and bone ingrowth. The longer-term survivability after 211 revision hip arthroplasties performed by a single surgeon using a hemispherical titanium-fiber metallic–porous-coated acetabular component fixed with multiple screws was assessed using prospectively gathered data to ascertain factors that could influence failure and determine the results and complications of isolated acetabular revisions.

Methods.—The same surgical technique was used in all patients: the component was impacted and fixed with multiple screws. Bone deficiencies were augmented using supplemental bone graft. Both the acetabular and femoral components were revised in 142 hips; an isolated acetabular revision was performed in 69 hips. All 211 revisions were entered into a survivorship analysis to 12 years. Prospectively evaluated clinical results in 135 hips and radiographic results in 131 hips were analyzed at a minimum of 5 years postoperatively.

Results.—Of 7 acetabular components that were removed, 3 were due to infection, 1 was for recurrent dislocation, and 3 for mechanical loosening. A symptomatic radiologic loosening was detected in 1 additional acetabular component (total rate of aseptic loosening, 2%). The 12-year prosthetic survival rate was 95% (95% confidence interval [CI], 91%-99%); failure was considered component removal for any reason. No significant difference was noted in the survival rate of the cup or femoral component between the 69 hips treated with isolated acetabular revision and the 142 hips in which both components underwent revision. A significant difference was observed in the rate of dislocation between hips treated with isolated acetabular revision (dislocation, 14 [20%] hips) versus those in which both components were revised (dislocation, 11 [8%] hips; $P = .03$); no difference was seen in component survival when a dislocation occurred. A significant correlation was seen between patient weight of more than 82 kg and acetabular failure ($P = .04$).

Conclusion.—The titanium fiber metal-coated hemispheric component fixed with multiple screws had a 12-year survival rate of 95%, with a dislocation rate that was significantly higher in patients treated with isolated acetabular revision; routine postoperative bracing is now recommended for these patients.

► This article provides insight with regard to the function of an uncemented acetabular component in revision hip surgery. The 95% survival rate is indeed comforting. Yet the study would seem more homogeneous if the revisions for sepsis were excluded, since this diagnosis introduces yet additional variables. Further, the 20% instability rate of isolated acetabular component revision is of concern, and although the recommendation is to brace patients with this procedure, we are left without a clear understanding as to the reason for its occurrence. Our experience does demonstrate that at the time of revision, retaining a 22-mm femoral head is statistically more unstable than a larger femoral head. In addition, the revision acetabular component generally is of larger size than the original one, thus, adversely altering the head and neck ratio and increasing the chance of dislocation. Data have revealed that the use of an elevated liner would be appropriate, or use of a captive acetabular liner as alternate strategies to avoid this complication should be considered.

B. F. Morrey, MD

Comparison of Primary Total Hip Replacements Performed With a Standard Incision or a Mini-Incision

Woolson ST, Mow CS, Syquia JF, et al (Stanford Univ, Calif)

J Bone Joint Surg Am 86-A:1353-1358, 2004 5–11

Introduction.—Advantages claimed by the proponents of mini-incision techniques for primary total hip replacement include decreases in blood loss, transfusion requirements, postoperative pain, and soft-tissue trauma, compared to standard techniques through a longer incision. There are no known well-designed comparison investigations that support these claims. A retrospective controlled investigation was performed that used the in-hospital data and initial radiographic results for a series of patients who underwent total hip replacement with the mini-incision technique.

Methods.—Of 135 primary unilateral total hip replacements, 50 were performed for selected patients using a mini-incision (ó10 cm) and 85 were performed using a standard incision. A posterior approach was used in all surgeries. In-hospital data were gathered retrospectively. Initial postoperative radiographs were evaluated. Due to the selection process, patients who had a mini-incision had both a significantly lower average body-mass index ($P = .008$) and a lower average score on the American Society of Anesthesiologists rating ($P = .006$), suggesting that they were thinner and healthier than patients with a standard incision.

Results.—No significant differences were observed between groups in measurements of average surgical time, intraoperative blood loss, in-hospital transfusion rate, length of hospital stay, or patient disposition after hospital discharge. The mini-incision group had a significantly higher risk of wound complication ($P = .02$), a higher percentage of acetabular component malposition ($P = .04$), and poor fit and fill of femoral components inserted without cement ($P = .0036$).

Conclusion.—There was no evidence that the mini-incision technique was associated with less bleeding or less trauma to the soft tissues of the hip, factors that would have produced a quicker recovery and a shorter hospital stay. Further analysis of the mini-incision technique is necessary before it can be recommended for general use.

► With the exploding interest in the mini-incision technique, any valid data regarding the efficacy of this approach is of great value. Although this is a retrospective cohort study, it does provide very important insight with regard to the value of the mini-incision technique used by these surgeons. In their experience, there was a statistically significant higher complication rate, with no lasting advantages that could be measured. The orthopedic community must view the increasing acceptance of mini-incision with significant skepticism, and objective data of the value of such an approach must be provided. It would be anticipated and hoped that the increased complication rate, which is known to be associated with the mini incision technique, might be decreased as the greater familiarity with this technique is realized.

B. F. Morrey, MD

Failure Rates for 4762 Revision Total Hip Arthroplasties in the Norwegian Arthroplasty Register

Lie SA, Havelin LI, Furnes ON, et al (Univ of Bergen, Norway; Haukeland Univ, Bergen, Norway)

J Bone Joint Surg Br 86-B:504-509, 2004 5–12

Introduction.—During a 10-year period, 11% of all primary prostheses in the Norwegian Arthroplasty Register failed. The results of total hip revision surgeries were reviewed using data from the Norwegian Arthroplasty Register.

Methods.—A total of 4762 revision THAs with no prior infection in the hip were reported to the Norwegian Arthroplasty Register between 1987 and 2003. Separate revision surgeries were performed for acetabular and femoral components. Fixation of the components was classified as either uncemented or cemented with antibiotic-containing cement.

Results.—In acetabular components, significantly decreased risk of failure for uncemented revision was observed both with (relative risk [RR], 0.66; 95% confidence interval [CI], 0.43-0.99) and without (RR, 0.37; 95% CI, 0.22-0.61) allograft. In femoral components, a significantly decreased risk of failure for uncemented revisions was observed both with (RR, 0.27; 95% CI, 0.16-0.46) and without (RR, 0.22; 95% CI, 0.11-0.46) unimpacted allograft.

This decreased risk of failure also applied to cemented revision components with allograft (RR, 0.53; 95% CI, 0.33-0.84) and with impaction bone grafting (RR, 0.34; 95% CI, 0.19-0.62). Adjusted for gender and age, a significantly decreased risk of re-revision was seen for uncemented revision components with (RR, 0.66; 95% CI, 0.43-0.9) and without (RR, 0.37; 95% CI, 0.22-0.61) bone grafting (Fig 1).

Conclusion.—Revision prostheses are usually inferior, compared to primary prostheses. Recementation without allograft, and uncemented revi-

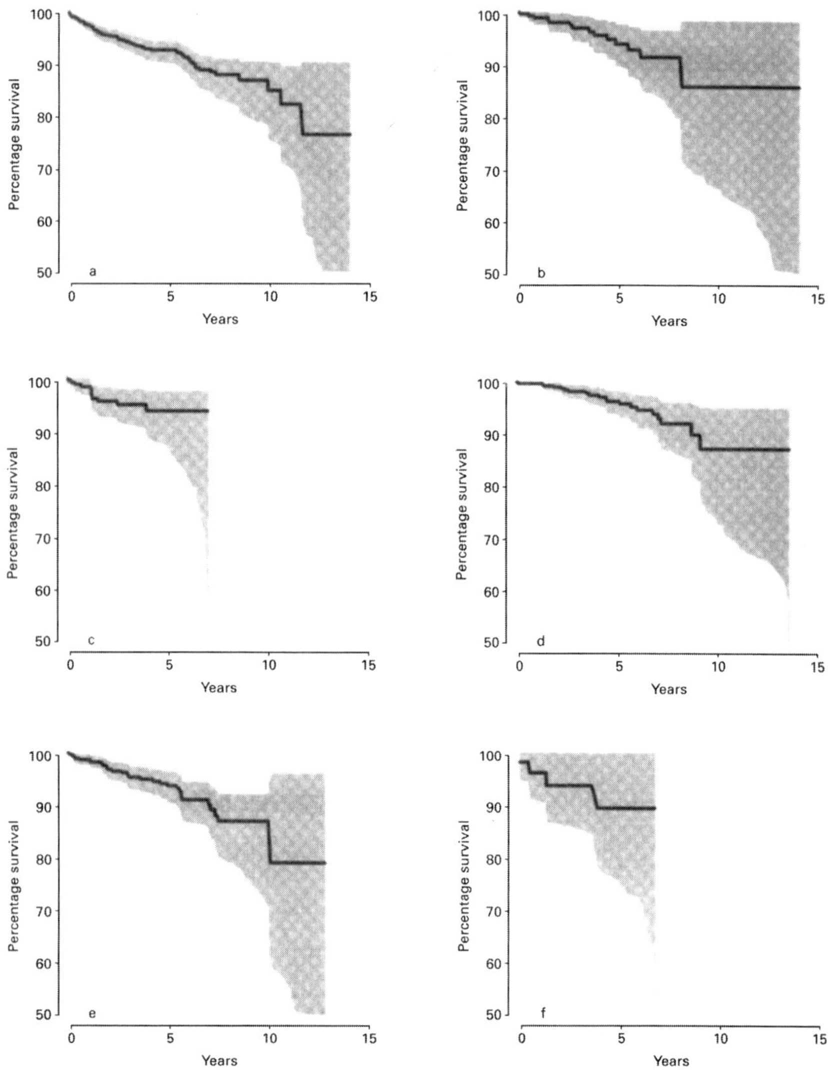

FIGURE 1.—Survival curves for the acetabular revision prostheses, categorized by both bone transplantation and fixation techniques. **a**, cemented without allograft; **b**, cemented with allograft; **c**, cemented with impaction bone grafting; **d**, uncemented without allograft; **e**, uncemented without allograft; and **f**, uncemented with impaction bone grafting. (Courtesy of Lie SA, Havelin LI, Furnes ON, et al: Failure rates for 4762 revision total hip arthroplasties in the Norwegian Arthroplasty Register. *J Bone Joint Surg Br* 86-B:504-509, 2004.)

sion with bone impaction, were linked with worse results, compared to other revision techniques.

▶ This study emphasizes the value of national registries to at least provide a general insight as to success and failure of implant types and surgical strategy.

The message of this report is very straightforward and does not require too much interpretation. Hence, recementation without the use of allograft or uncemented revision with bone impaction appear to be inferior options and associated with an increase in revision failure.

B. F. Morrey, MD

The Cumulative Long-term Risk of Dislocation After Primary Charnley Total Hip Arthroplasty

Berry DJ, von Knoch M, Schleck CD, et al (Mayo Clinic, Rochester, Minn)

J Bone Joint Surg Am 86-A:9-14, 2004 5–13

Background.—Different series have reported widely varying prevalence figures for dislocation after THA. The prevalence of dislocation after THA is affected by many factors, including patient-related factors, surgical technique, and implant design. However, another, less-studied factor is that varying durations of follow-up have been used in these reports. The effect of demographic factors on the long-term risk of dislocation as a function of time after THA has not been well studied. The risk of dislocation as a function of time after Charnley total hip arthroplasty was investigated, and the demographic factors that affect the cumulative risk of dislocation were identified.

Methods.—Included in this study were 6623 consecutive primary Charnley THAs performed for 5459 patients at a single institution between 1969 and 1984. The mean age of these patients (2869 women and 2590 men) was 63 years. All procedures were performed with a 22-mm femoral head, and all femoral and acetabular components were fixed with cement. The patients were followed up at routine intervals and specifically asked about dislocation. Kaplan-Meier analysis was used to determine the cumulative risk of dislocation.

Results.—There were 320 dislocations (4.8%). The cumulative risk of a first-time dislocation was 1% at 1 month and 1.9% at 1 year. After the first postoperative year, this risk increased at a constant rate of approximately 1% every 5 years to 7% at 25 years for patients who were alive and had not had a revision by that time (Fig 2).

The relative risk for dislocation for women compared with men was 2.1, and the relative risk for patients who were age 70 years or older—as compared with younger patients —was 1.3. Patients with an underlying diagnosis of osteonecrosis of the femoral head, acute fracture or nonunion of the proximal part of the femur, and inflammatory arthritis has a significantly greater risk of dislocation than did patients with osteoarthritis.

Conclusion.—There is a significantly greater cumulative long-term risk of dislocation after THS than has been reported in short-term studies. The highest incidence of dislocation is in the first year after arthroplasty, and the risk will increase at a relatively constant rate for the life of the arthroplasty. The patients at greatest risk are women and those with a diagnosis of osteo-

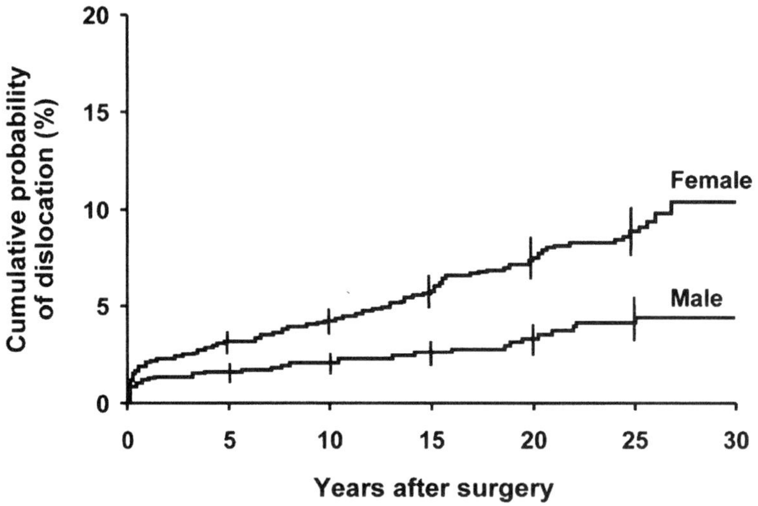

FIGURE 2.—Cumulative probability of a first-time hip dislocation for patients less than 70 years of age and those 70 years of age or older at the time of arthroplasty. (Reproduced with permission of the Journal of Bone and Joint Surgery, Inc, from Berry DJ, von Knoch M, Schleck CD, et al: The cumulative long-term risk of dislocation after primary Charnley total hip arthroplasty. *J Bone Joint Surg Am* 86-A:9-14, 2004. Reproduced by permission of the publisher via Copyright Clearance Center, Inc.)

necrosis of the femoral head or an acute fracture or nonunion of the proximal part of the femur.

► The value of this particular study is that it includes over 6000 patients assessed over a 15-year period to determine the implications of long-term hip dislocation. The findings, therefore, are particularly relevant. The observation that almost 5% of patients will experience instability at some point in time is approximately twice the 2.5% to 3% risk usually quoted to our patients. Multivariate analysis confirms the increased incidence with females and aging.

B. F. Morrey, MD

Efficacy of Abduction Bracing in the Management of Total Hip Arthroplasty Dislocation

DeWal H, Maurer SL, Tsai P, et al (New York Univ)

J Arthroplasty 19:733-738, 2004 5–14

Introduction.—Many surgeons use bracing or casting for 6 to 12 weeks for patients treated for dislocation after THA. Few studies, however, have assessed the need for immobilization or restriction of motion in this setting. A large series of patients who underwent successful closed reduction for total hip dislocation was retrospectively reviewed to determine the effectiveness of an abduction brace.

Methods.—The 149 patients included in the study had undergone THA between 1993 and 2000. Patients were classified as having a primary THA or a revision THA, and dislocations were categorized as first time or recurrent. Osteoarthritis was the most common preoperative diagnosis in both first-time and recurrent groups. Use of an abduction brace was based on the attending surgeon's usual practice, and braces were individually fitted to each patient. Redislocation constituted failure of treatment.

Results.—Braced and nonbraced patients did not differ significantly in age, sex, operative side, previous surgery, surgical approach, component head size, or head/neck ratio. Ninety-one patients had a first-time dislocation and 58 had a recurrent dislocation. The mean follow-up was 4.0 years for the first-time group and 3.7 years for the recurrent group. Among patients in the first-time group, 61% redislocated with a brace and 64% redislocated without a brace. The outcome was similar for the recurrent dislocation group: 55% redislocated with a brace and 56 redislocated without a brace.

Conclusion.—Bracing—a routine practice of many surgeons for patients who have undergone closed treatment of dislocation after THA—is associated with considerable expense and discomfort. Redislocation rates were similar in braced and nonbraced groups, and outcomes were similar for first-time and recurrent dislocation groups. With little proven benefit in preventing redislocation, the use of an abduction brace is difficult to justify.

▶ This is a very interesting article since it questions an accepted practice. Demonstrating the value of hip braces is probably more ritualistic than real. Virtually all surgeons immobilize first-time dislocators in order to allow the hip to "scar in." These investigators provide compelling evidence that use of an abduction brace as a means of stabilizing the hip in order to allow the soft tissue healing has no clinical value. I am not sure this article will provide sufficient confidence for most orthopedic surgeons to change the methods of caring for the first-time dislocator, but based on this study, at least, this practice should be further questioned and investigated.

B. F. Morrey, MD

Mini-incision Anterior Approach Does Not Increase Dislocation Rate: A Study of 1037 Total Hip Replacements

Siguier T, Siguier M, Brumpt B (Clinique Jouvenet, Paris)

Clin Orthop 426:164-173, 2004 5–15

Introduction.—Correct positioning of the prosthetic components in total hip replacements is important to prevent dislocations. Correct positioning is made easier by extensive approaches, but it also is possible using the mini-incision approach. The mini-incision used to facilitate early rehabilitation should not produce a higher dislocation rate than that of the more conventional approaches. The anterior surgical approach we describe allows for good exposure, despite the reduced size of the skin incision. Its length is 5-10 cm and usually 6-8 cm for patients with normal corpulence. Our mini-incision anterior approach using intermuscular planes allows a surgical approach to the hip and implantation of a total prosthesis with no muscle, tendon, or trochanteric section, even partially. This is not possible with any other surgical approach. A series of 1037 primary total hip replacements done between June 1993 and June 2000 was studied retrospectively. The dislocation rate was 0.96% (10 of 1037 hips). The mini-incision approach allows for adequate positioning of the two prosthetic components. Preserving the muscular potential also may contribute to dynamic stabilization of the hip.

▶ There is an increasing number of contributions demonstrating the technique and early outcome of minimally invasive surgery for hip joint replacement. This article was of interest since it attempted to address one of the common concerns regarding limited invasive surgery, specifically an increase in complication rate. With this particular technique, which is rather popular in Europe, and one in which the editor is also investigating, it is encouraging to note that the instability rate is no greater and, in fact, less than what is generally quoted for conventional hip joint replacement. While this broad subject continues to evolve rapidly, there is little question that surgical approaches such as the one demonstrated here will eventually be adopted for at least a select number of patients and will be associated with an acceptable complicate rate. The question continues as to the length of the learning curve and the ultimate risk-to-benefit ratio.

B. F. Morrey, MD

The Use of a Constrained Acetabular Component to Treat Instability After Total Hip Arthroplasty

Shrader MW, Parvizi J, Lewallen DG (Mayo Clinic and Mayo Found, Rochester, Minn)

J Bone Joint Surg Am 85-A:2179-2183, 2003 5–16

Background.—One of the most common complications of THA is dislocation, which can cause major distress for the patient and frustration for the treating surgeon. Recurrent dislocation after THA is a disabling complication that can be difficult to treat and may not be amenable to nonoperative management. Extensive soft tissue deficiency may be an important contributing cause of the instability in these patients. Revision arthroplasty with the use of a constrained cup has been proposed for the treatment of these patients. The clinical and radiographic outcomes associated with the use of a constrained acetabular component as a salvage treatment for instability after hip arthroplasty were evaluated.

Methods.—A retrospective review was conducted of the clinical and radiographic outcomes of 110 THAs for 109 patients. All of these procedures were performed with the use of a single design of constrained acetabular component. In 79 hips, the constrained component was implanted for the treatment of recurrent instability; in 31 hips, it was implanted because of ab-

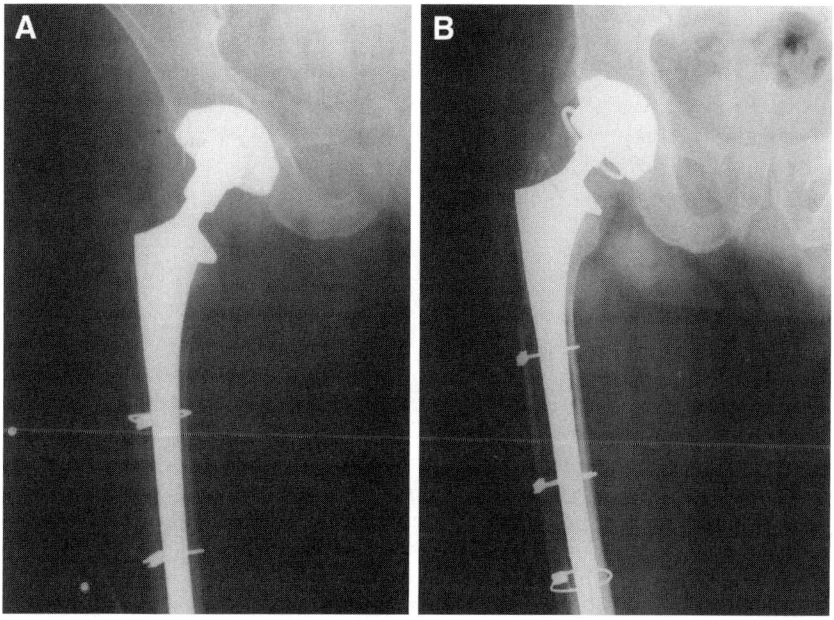

FIGURE 1.—A, Anteroposterior radiograph of a 76-year-old man who had undergone multiple failed previous stabilization procedures for recurrent instability. B, The instability, which was related mostly to soft tissue deficiency, was fully addressed by the insertion of a constrained liner into the well-fixed cup with cement. (Republished with permission of the Journal of Bone and Joint Surgery, Inc, from Shrader MW, Parvizi J, Lewallen DG: The use of a constrained acetabular component to treat instability after total hip arthroplasty. *J Bone Joint Surg Am* 85-A:2179-2183, 2003. Reproduced by permission of the publisher via Copyright Clearance Center, Inc.)

sent or grossly deficient soft tissue attachments that were believed to be associated with a high risk for subsequent instability.

Results.—The constrained acetabular device was successful in eliminating or preventing hip instability in all but 2 patients, who continued to have sensations of subluxation (Fig 1). The mean Harris hip score was significantly improved, from 62.7 points preoperatively to 76.4 points at the time of the latest follow-up. There were no instances of dislocation or disassembly of the hip components. Radiographic analysis demonstrated radiolucent lines around the cup in 15 hips (14%). There were 9 revisions performed, 6 for deep infection, 2 for acetabular loosening, and 1 for a periprosthetic fracture of the femur.

Conclusion.—A constrained acetabular component can reliably restore and maintain hip stability in patients with recalcitrant recurrent instability and can reliably prevent dislocation in patients who are at high risk because of absent or deficient soft tissues about the hip. However, the use of these devices should be reserved for situations in which other methods are inadequate or have failed.

▶ This large experience from the Mayo Clinic confirms and reinforces earlier reports of the short-term effectiveness of the constrained acetabular component for the purpose of treating hip instability. While this report demonstrates excellent short- to intermediate-term results, we are aware of an increasing number of mechanical failures with this and other designs that attain stability through a captive head in the acetabular construct. The editor emphasizes that the selection of this implant, in most instances, should be one of a salvage procedure and not the first-line choice for routine THA.

B. F. Morrey, MD

Persistent Infection Associated With Residual Cement After Resection Arthroplasty of the Hip

Buttaro M, Valentini R, Piccaluga F (Italian Hosp, Buenos Aires, Argentina)

Acta Orthop Scand 75:427-429, 2004 5–17

Background.—Removal of all implants, cement, and devitalized and necrotic tissue is an important aspect of surgical debridement of an infected hip arthroplasty. However, this is a technically demanding process that carries a risk of bone stock deficiency. There is disagreement as to the danger of residual unremoved polymethylmethacrylate (PMMA) after resection of infected prosthetic components. Evaluated were the outcomes in a group of patients with infected hip arthroplasty who continued to have persistent infection with residual cement after previous treatment with resection arthroplasty and antibiotic treatment.

Methods.—An analysis was conducted of 10 patients with infected total hip prosthesis who had been treated previously with resection arthroplasty and antibiotics and who had persistent infection with residual cement. Surgical debridement with resection of all the PMMA was performed in 9 patients, and adequate antibiotics were administered. Surgical treatment was refused by 1 patient; however, this patient accepted antibiotics.

Results.—The average duration of follow-up was 4 years (range, 1-18 years). In 8 patients, there were no signs or symptoms of recurrent infection. One severely immunodeficient patient died 2 years after removal of the residual cement, but this death was attributable to reasons other than the hip arthroplasty. The patient who refused surgical treatment continued to have an active sinus 4 years after the first consultation.

Conclusion.—Chronic infection after resection of an infected total hip prosthesis may be attributable to the presence of residual cement. All devitalized tissue and foreign material must be removed as part of the treatment of an infected hip arthroplasty.

► We have all been taught to remove all cement at the time of debridement for infection. However, this is not always accomplished due to the difficulty of removing well fixed cement or of lack of recognition of its presence. The findings of this study should prompt us to redouble our efforts to remove all cement when managing the patient with the infected total joint.

B. F. Morrey, MD

► The importance of complete debridement in the management of an infected failed implant is again emphasized by this article. This is a lesson we learned long ago that residual cement and foreign material increases the risk of persistent infection following resection. It is critically important that all of the foreign material is removed and that routine intraoperative radiographic evaluation of a debridement be performed in the course of treatment of a patient with an infected failed implant.

C. P. Beauchamp, MD

Metal-on-Metal Hybrid Surface Arthroplasty: Two to Six-Year Follow-up Study

Amstutz HC, Beaulé PE, Dorey FJ, et al (Orthopaedic Hosp, Los Angeles)

J Bone Joint Surg Am 86-A:28-39, 2004 5–18

Background.—The rates of revision THA are higher in young and active patients than in older patients, and these rates are increased in the setting of osteonecrosis. After reintroduction of metal-on-metal bearings in THA in Europe in the late 1980s, the potential utility of metal-on-metal surface arthroplasty in young and active patients was first investigated in the United States in the early 1990s.

It was believed that there was no satisfactory biological or prosthetic solution for the treatment of advanced arthritis in these patients. The clinical and radiographic results of the first 400 hips treated with metal-on-metal hybrid surface arthroplasties at an average follow-up of 3½ years was described.

Methods.—The 400 metal-on-metal hybrid surface arthroplasties included in this review were performed between November 1996 and November 2000 for 355 patients. All of the femoral head components were cemented, but only 59 of the short metaphyseal systems were cemented. The average age of the patients was 48 years; 73% of patients were men, and 66% had a diagnosis of osteoarthritis. Clinical and radiographic follow-up were performed at 3 months postoperatively and then yearly.

Results.—Most of the patients were able to return to a high level of activity, including athletic activity, and 54% had activity scores of more than 7 on the University of California at Los Angeles activity assessment system. The Kaplan-Meier survivorship showed that the rate of survival of the components at 4 years was 94.4%.

Patients with a surface arthroplasty had a risk score of greater than 3; the rate of survival of the components at 4 years in these patients was 89% compared with a rate of 97% for patients with a score of 3 or less. Patients with a higher risk index were 4.2 times more likely to undergo revision to a total hip replacement at 4 years. Revision to a total hip replacement was performed in 12 hips (3%). Of these 12 hips, 7 were revised because of loosening of the femoral component, and 3 were revised because of fracture of the femoral neck.

Substantial radiolucencies were observed around 16 uncemented metaphyseal femoral stems. No femoral radiolucencies were observed among the hips in which the metaphyseal stem was cemented. The most important risk factors for loosening of the femoral component and the presence of substantial stem radiolucencies were large femoral head cysts, patient height, female gender, and smaller component size in male patients.

Conclusions.—The early outcomes for metal-on-metal hybrid surface arthroplasty are encouraging. Optimal femoral bone preparation and component fixation are crucial to improving the durability of these arthroplasties. If necessary, the metal-on-metal hybrid surface arthroplasty can easily be revised to a standard femoral component.

► This article is the largest United States experience of a growing trend of metal-on-metal surfacing type implant, a technique becoming increasingly popular in Europe. The favorable clinical outcome of this experience is consistent with other reports that are beginning to appear in the literature. The major remaining concern that cannot be answered by this study or any other without a significantly longer follow-up is the potential adverse effect of the increased metallic ion concentration in serum and in cells.

B. F. Morrey, MD

Computer-Assisted Cup Placement Techniques in Total Hip Arthroplasty Improve Accuracy of Placement

Jolles BM, Genoud P, Hoffmeyer P (Univ Hosp of Lausanne, Switzerland; Univ Hosp of Geneva)

Clin Orthop 426:174-179, 2004 5–19

Introduction.—Malposition of the acetabular component during hip arthroplasty increases the occurrence of impingement, reduces range of motion, and increases the risk of dislocation and long-term wear. To prevent malpositioned hip implants, an increasing number of computer-assisted orthopaedic systems have been described, but their accuracy is not well established. The purpose of this study was to determine the reproducibility and accuracy of conventional versus computer-assisted techniques for positioning the acetabular component in total hip arthroplasty. Using a lateral approach, 150 cups were placed by 10 surgeons in 10 identical plastic pelvis models (freehand, with a mechanical guide, using computer assistance). Conditions for cup implantations were made to mimic the operating room situation. Preoperative planning was done from a computed tomography scan. The accuracy of cup abduction and anteversion was assessed with an electromagnetic system. Freehand placement revealed a mean accuracy of cup anteversion and abduction of 10° and 3.5°, respectively (maximum error, 35°). With the cup positioner, these angles measured 8° and 4° (maximum error, 29.8°), respectively, and using computer assistance, 1.5° and 2.5° (maximum error, 8°), respectively. Computer-assisted cup placement was an accurate and reproducible technique for total hip arthroplasty. It was more accurate than traditional methods of cup positioning.

► This contribution is included as a sample of several that have appeared in the literature this last year documenting the accuracy of navigation in the placement of the acetabular component for hip joint replacement. As with the knee, the theoretic value of computer-assisted placement continues to be attractive. There is little question that in time, the technology will allow a wider spread use of its application to the clinical practice. The increasing interest in minimally invasive surgery should accelerate the development of more user-friendly systems and their adaptation to the clinical practice. A noninvasive means of demonstrating inertial skeletal landmarks will be a key in the development of more efficient systems which, once developed, should be of value for the accurate placement of the acetabular component, especially if a limited incision has been used.

B. F. Morrey, MD

Rapid Bone and Blood Flow Formation in Impacted Morselized Allografts: Positron Emission Tomography (PET) Studies on Allografts in 5 Femoral Component Revisions of Total Hip Arthroplasty

Sörensen J, Ullmark G, Långström B, et al (Uppsala Univ, Sweden; Univ Hosp, Uppsala, Sweden)

Acta Orthop Scand 74:633-643, 2003 5–20

Introduction.—Despite the widespread clinical use of impaction bone allografts, little is known regarding the physiologic events that occur in the graft bed during the first year. The dynamics of bone blood flow and the rate of mineralization were investigated using positron emission tomography (PET) in patients who underwent revision THA to better understand the biological response of morselized bone allografts.

Methods.—Five patients underwent revision with impaction of morselized frozen allograft and a cemented THA because of loosening and osteolysis of a primary hip arthroplasty. Plain film radiographs of the stems revealed stable implants at 15 to 24 months postoperatively. Clinical results were good in all patients. Patients underwent 4 studies as follows: (1) PET to assess vascularization and new bone formation in the allograft; (2) kinetic (^{18}F)-fluoride PET to produce quantitative images that were interpreted as new bone formation in the allograft surrounding the femur stem; (3) (^{15}O)-water PET to quantify bone blood flow; and (4) {^{15}O)-carbon monoxide to ascertain blood flow. Patients were evaluated twice postoperatively: at 1 to 8 days and at 12 months; 3 patients were also evaluated at 4 months.

Results.—As early as 8 days postoperatively, blood flow and bone formation had increased greatly adjacent to the allograft. At 4 months, blood flow and bone formation were nearly the same; activity was highest in the graft material. At 1 year postoperatively, blood flow had diminished to the level of the contralateral femur diaphysis in most of the graft bed.

Conclusion.—Angiogenesis and new bone formation occurred early after impaction of morselized bone allografts around the femur component in patients who underwent revision THA. It appears that PET is sensitive in the evaluation of neovascularization and bone formation in the graft beds.

▶ By using noninvasive PET, these investigators documented the very rapid revascularization of the cancellous impaction allograft. This is an important insight and would seem to help explain the low incidence of mechanical failure of impaction grafting. As such, it provides an explanation for the continued favorable reports that have appeared in the literature regarding impaction cancellous grafting for bone deficiency at the time of hip revision.

B. F. Morrey, MD

Impacted Cancellous Graft Plus Cement in Hip Revision

Cabanela ME, Trousdale RT, Berry DJ (Mayo Clinic, Rochester, Minn)
Clin Orthop 417:175-182, 2003 5–21

Introduction.—Revision of the femoral component is challenging when large cavitary defects of the femur are present. Impaction cancellous grafting used in conjunction with a cemented prosthesis has been recommended for restoring bone stock, along with providing excellent and durable clinical results. Between 1993 and 1997, impaction grafting with particulate fresh-frozen cancellous allograft and a collarless, tapered, polished stem was performed in 57 femoral component revisions. Strut allografts were used for femoral reinforcement in 40 hips. In 1999, the outcomes of this early experience with a consecutive group of patients who underwent impaction cancellous allograft with a cemented prosthesis were reported. The outcomes of the same group of patients after a longer follow-up were again discussed.

Results.—None of the patients were lost to follow-up; 3 died of causes not associated with the hip. One patient experienced an infection and underwent resection arthroplasty. At 6.3 years of follow-up, clinical results were excellent. Radiographic assessment revealed no evidence of loosening in any of the 53 surviving hips. Subsidence of 1 to 3 mm was identified in 40 hips, and subsidence of 4 to 6 mm was detected in 2 hips. Cancellous remodeling was seen in 42 hips. The most frequently occurring complications were postoperative femoral fractures. All 6 fractures occurred at the distal end of the prosthesis. They were not linked with prosthetic loosening and were successfully treated via open reduction and internal fixation without prosthetic revision.

Conclusion.—These satisfactory results and limited subsidence observed in radiographs could be explained by the careful attention to the technical details of the procedure. Even with the generous use of strut graft augmentation, postoperative femoral fractures continue to be the most serious complication.

▶ This is an impressive series indicating that in the selected patient with large cavitary defects, impaction grafting is a reliable and effective means of providing a stable hip as well as augmenting the bone lost from osteolysis. It should be observed that approximately 80% of these patients had a supplemental strut graft to help reinforce the integrity of the proximal femur. Although subsidence does occur, it is limited and does not seem to affect the clinical outcome. An explanation for the satisfactory results is provided in the interesting contribution by Sorensen et al (Abstract 5–20).

B. F. Morrey, MD

Acetabular Revision With Impacted Morsellised Cancellous Bone Grafting and a Cemented Cup: A 15- to 20-Year Follow-up

Schreurs BW, Bolder SBT, Gardeniers JWM, et al (Univ Med Centre Nijmegen, The Netherlands)

J Bone Joint Surg Br 86-B:492-497, 2004 5–22

Introduction.—The long-term results of most techniques of acetabular revision are not clear. Few reports are available concerning outcome beyond 10 years. The 15- to 20-year outcome of patients who underwent acetabular revision was reported.

Methods.—Between January 1979 and March 1986, 62 acetabular revisions were performed in 58 patients with the use of impacted morselized bone grafts and a cemented cup. The mean patient age was 59.1 years (23-82 years). At the time of review in April 2001, 17 patients (18 hips) had died within 15 years of the revision surgery. The clinical and radiologic results were examined at a mean follow-up of 16.5 years (range, 15-20 years). The Harris Hip Score was used for clinical assessment. One patient was lost to follow-up.

Results.—Three additional patients (3 hips) died after the minimum follow-up (15, 15, and 17 years post revision, respectively). The mean Harris Hip Score of the remaining 28 patients (30 hips) with acetabular reconstructions alive at a mean of 16 years and 5 months (5-2 years) postoperatively was 86 (range, 50-100). Of the original 61 hips, 11 underwent further revision. Two were for culture-confirmed septic loosening at 3 and 6 years postoperatively; 7 were for aseptic loosening between 6 and 14 years; 1 well-fixed cup was changed at 12 years in the course of femoral revision for aseptic loosening; and 1 was revised again at 17 years due to wear, even though it was well fixed.

Most hips had a stable radiographic appearance with uniform radiodensity of both graft and host bone, even after 20 years of follow-up. The Kaplan-Meier survivorship for the cup with end-point revisions for any reason was 79% at 15 years postoperatively (95% confidence interval [CI], 67-91). Excluding 2 revisions for septic loosening at 3 and 6 years and 1 revision of a well-fixed cup after 12 years, survivorship was 84% at 15 years (95% CI, 73-95). At last review, there were no further cases of loosening, although 7 acetabular reconstructions had radiolucent lines in 1 or 2 zones.

Conclusion.—Acetabular revision with impacted large morselized bone chips (0.7 cm to 1.0 cm) and a cemented cup is a reliable technique of reconstruction, as observed at 15-year follow-up.

► This is a definitive study from Dr Slooff, the originator of this technique, and his group documenting the long-term outcome of this valuable technique. The use of morsellised cancellous bone grafting has become particularly important as osteolysis continues to emerge as a major long-term problem of hip joint replacement. We have used this technique for the revision of acetabular components and found it to be relatively easy and quite effective, as this study clearly demonstrates.

B. F. Morrey, MD

Cementless Acetabular Revision With the Harris-Galante Porous Prosthesis: Results After a Minimum of Ten Years of Follow-up

Hallstrom BR, Golladay GJ, Vittetoe DA, et al (Harvard Med School, Boston)

J Bone Joint Surg Am 86-A:1007-1011, 2004 5–23

Introduction.—Revisions of the acetabular component of a total hip arthroplasty have a higher incidence of complications, especially loosening and dislocation, compared to primary procedures. The results of a consecutive series of revisions performed by a single surgeon using the Harris-Galante Porous acetabular component were evaluated at an average of 12 years. The purpose was to quantify the complications and outcomes of acetabular revision.

Methods.—Clinical and radiographic results were investigated to determine the incidence of loosening, lysis, radiolucencies, and trochanteric union in 188 hips (170 patients) treated between 1984 and 1990. A total of 122 hips in 110 patients were followed up for a minimum of 10 years, a requirement for inclusion. Thirty-one patients (36 hips) died before 10-year postoperative follow-up; 29 (30 hips) patients were lost to follow-up or refused to return for follow-up.

Results.—The average Harris hip score was 78 points at an average of 12.5 years post revision. This was a 29-point improvement compared to the preoperative score. The incidence of repeat revision due to aseptic loosening of the acetabular shell was 4% (5/122). The incidence of repeat revision of the shell for any reason was 15% (18/122). Eight unrevised sockets were loose radiographically. The total incidence of aseptic loosening was 11% (13/122).

Conclusion.—Most acetabular revisions with the cementless hemispheric socket were successful. Few structural grafts and no cages were used for revision.

► An alternative acetabular revision technique is the use of a porous coated prosthesis, the effect of which is well documented by this study. It should be noted that the mean 12-year surveillance of the second report may not be adequate to demonstrate its true long-term effectiveness. Many of the problems seen in acetabular reconstruction become evident only after 10 years of use. This is of particular relevance since the uncemented acetabular component requires a modular insert which is known to be associated with increased incidences of wear and osteolysis, especially after 10 years!

B. F. Morrey, MD

Cementing a Liner Into a Stable Cementless Acetabular Shell: The Double-Socket Technique

Beaulé PE, Ebramzadeh E, LeDuff M, et al (Orthopaedic Hosp, Los Angeles)
J Bone Joint Surg Am 86-A:929-934, 2004 5–24

Introduction.—The advent of cementless fixation of acetabular components and the introduction of modularity have made it possible to perform revision in cases of excessive polyethylene wear or osteolysis by exchanging the liner without removing a stable acetabular shell. In cases of a defective locking mechanism or incompatibility of the liner with the implanted acetabular shell, the extraction of a well-fitted cementless acetabular shell can be challenging.

Cementing a new liner into the existing acetabular shell (the double-socket technique) may be a simple solution. The initial clinical results and potential limitations of this technique were discussed.

Methods.—Thirty-two hips with a preexisting well-fixed acetabular socket that had been in situ for an average of 8.6 years underwent insertion of a new polyethylene liner (17 hips) or a metal liner (15 hips) using cement. The indication for this approach was a deficient locking mechanism and the unavailability of a matching liner in 22 and 10 hips, respectively. AP radiographs of all hips were examined by a single independent reviewer.

Results.—The mean follow-up was 5.1 years. Six hips underwent reoperation at a mean of 29.7 months. Reasons included aseptic failure of the acetabular construct (4 hips), instability (1 hip), and sepsis (1 hip). Significant improvement was observed in the University of California at Los Angeles hip scores ($P < .001$), compared with preoperative values. The mean score improved from 6.2 to 9.1 for pain, from 6.3 to 8.3 for walking, from 6.2 to 7.8 for function, and from 4.7 to 5.8 for activity. The incidence of dislocation was 22%. Kaplan-Meier analysis with revision as the end point showed at 5-year survival rate of 78% (95% confidence interval, 55%-91%).

Conclusion.—The double-socket technique is a reasonable alternative to acetabular socket removal for suitable candidates who have a well-fixed cementless socket with an inner diameter that is larger than the outer diameter of the cemented liner. This approach preserves acetabular bone stock and allows conversion to alternative bearing surfaces. The removal of a well-fixed acetabular shell or the use of a constrained liner should be strongly considered in the presence of a history of hip instability.

▶ This contribution is very relevant since the failure of modular polyethylene liners poses the important question of whether or not the metal shell must be removed or the technique described here—which is relatively easy and straightforward—might be considered an effective alternative. The documentation is substantiated by other similar studies which reveal that simply cementing a polyethylene liner within the shell in instances in which the locking mechanism is no longer reliable is an effective revision option under this particular circumstance.

This is the treatment of choice in this type of patient by the editor and at our institution. The limiting factor of the use of this technique is the presence of significant osteolysis, which requires prompt removal of the uncemented shell even if it is well fixed.

B. F. Morrey, MD

6 Total Knee Arthroplasty

Introduction

The most significant evolution regarding knee replacement continues to be the value of computer-based navigation systems and limited invasive surgery with hemi-joint replacement. The peer review literature on these topics is just now emerging, and the long-term effectiveness of these interventions awaits corroboratory clinical finding as practical and usable navigation systems. The impressive long-term effectiveness of knee joint replacement is also reflected in several studies in which large cohorts of patients are followed for long periods of time. A global perspective has been followed in the selection of this group of patients as we have selected articles from several countries. Finally, the effectiveness of various functional assessments and the necessity to accurately document functional outcome to better aid the orthopedic surgeon in decision making, particularly with regard to implant and technique selection, are reviewed in this selection.

Bernard F. Morrey, MD

The Fate of Patients Not Returning for Follow-up Five Years After Total Knee Arthroplasty

King PJ, Malin AS, Scott RD, et al (Brigham and Women's Hosp, Boston; New England Baptist Hosp, Boston)
J Bone Joint Surg Am 86-A:897-901, 2004 6–1

Introduction.—Patients who undergo TKA are advised to undergo annual or biannual radiographic follow-up examinations. Those who do not return for follow-up after TKA are frequently presumed to have had a worse outcome. With the use of patient records and Internet search techniques, an attempt was made to locate all patients in a consecutive series who were treated by a single surgeon. Outcomes were compared between patients who did and did not attend prescribed postoperative appointments.

Methods.—The outcomes of 161 patients (200 knees) were retrospectively examined at a minimum of 5 years after TKA. All patients who had had no contact of any kind with their surgeon beyond 6 months postopera-

TABLE 2.—Reasons Given for Not Returning for Follow-up Appointments

	Primary Reason	Secondary Reason	Total Responses
Not having any problems with knees	1	10	11
Forgot/did not know follow-up was recommended	8	1	9
Difficult/long trip for follow-up appointment	5	2	7
Patient died	7	0	7
Too busy/preoccupied with other health issues	4	0	4
Seeing another surgeon for convenience	3	0	3
Unhappy with provided care	2	0	2
Delaying the inevitable replacement of other knee	0	1	1

tively were categorized as having not returned for follow-up. When patients could not be located after use of all available information in their medical records, a standardized Internet search algorithm was utilized and made use of readily available free search engines.

Results.—Thirty patients (35 treated knees) met the criteria for not returning for follow-up. Thirteen patients could not be located from the contact information they provided at their last visit. All 13 were located by means of the Internet. No patients had had knee surgery elsewhere. The reasons for not adhering to recommended follow-up were identified (Table 2). This subgroup had improved Knee Society pain and function scores, compared to preoperative values. There were no significant differences between patients who did and did not return for follow-up.

Conclusion.—Patients who did not attend follow-up appointments had not undergone additional knee surgery and did not have significant differences in pain and function scores compared to those who complied with recommended follow-up protocol. The Internet was valuable in locating patients who had not returned for follow-up postoperatively.

▶ The methodology of this article is important since it demonstrates that the use of the Internet can be an effective means of identifying patients otherwise not returning for follow-up. This is also the editor's experience. The outcome of those patients who do not return for follow-up is an ongoing topic of controversy, with some reports indicating these patients selectively do poorer. However, there is a growing body of evidence that indicates that reasons other than outcome account for not complying with follow-up visits, thus indicating that "lost to follow-up" does not necessarily imply poor outcome.

B. F. Morrey, MD

Responses Bias: Effect on Outcomes Evaluation by Mail Surveys After Total Knee Arthroplasty

Kim J, Lonner JH, Nelson CL, et al (Univ of Pennsylvania, Philadelphia)

J Bone Joint Surg Am 86-A:15-21, 2004 6–2

Background.—Postal questionnaires are being used increasingly to follow up patient satisfaction and performance after total joint arthroplasty. However, survey responses are subject to a variety of possible biases. Response behavior in a mail survey of patients undergoing TKA was assessed in this study.

Methods.—Four hundred seventy-two patients who had had primary TKAs between 1996 and 1998 were mailed a questionnaire. The 10-item survey elicited information of patient satisfaction, general health, and Knee Society knee function and clinical scores. The response rate was 83% after a repeat mailing. All nonresponders were eventually contacted, and the 2 groups were compared.

Findings.—Patients responding earliest to the mail survey gave the highest ratings of satisfaction, and the nonresponders gave the lowest ratings. The mean Knee Society knee score was also significantly higher for the early responders than for the nonresponders. In addition, mean function and pain scores were significantly higher in the early responders. Changes in Knee Society knee scores, mean function scores, and mean pain scores from preoperative levels were significantly higher among the early responders than among nonresponders.

Conclusions.—Patients who do not respond to mail surveys for follow-up appear to report significantly worse outcomes than patients who respond to such surveys. Follow-up analyses using postal questionnaire should consider this potential response bias. Assessing patients lost to follow-up is an essential part of accurately analyzing arthroplasty outcomes.

▶ As patients are more and more reluctant to return for postoperative visits, the orthopedic community faces the challenge of documenting intermediate to long-term outcomes. The investigators here provide us a service by documenting that patients for whom follow-up is not available or assessed are not representative of the entire sample. The good results are return data and are recorded, the bad results are embedded in the nonresponders. This is an important issue that must be addressed. We continue to struggle with defining improved methods of long-term surveillance in the face of reluctance by both the patient and payers to afford the opportunity for the patient to return to the clinic for assessment.

B. F. Morrey, MD

Predicting Total Knee Replacement Pain: A Prospective, Observational Study

Brander VA, Stulberg SD, Adams AD, et al (Northwestern Univ, Chicago)

Clin Orthop 416:27-36, 2003 6–3

Background.—Studies describing normal pain patterns after total knee arthroplasty (TKA) or identifying patients at risk for unusual pain after TKA are lacking. This prospective, observational study reported the natural history of pain after TKA and determined predictors of excessive postoperative pain.

Methods.—Clinical and radiographic data on 116 patients were obtained preoperatively and at 1, 3, 6, and 12 months after TKA. A total of 149 knees were treated. The mean patient age was 66 years. Assessments included the visual analog pain scale and other measures of patient health, psychological state, and component reliability.

Findings.—Significant pain was reported by 72.3% preoperatively, 44.4% at 1 months, 22.6% at 3 months, 18.4% at 6 months, and 13.1% at 12 months. Greater preoperative pain was associated with a higher degree of postoperative pain, the use of more home therapy, and postoperative manipulations. Preoperative depression and anxiety correlated with greater pain at 1 year.

Conclusions.—Pain after TKA appears to resolve quickly, decreasing to approximately half within 3 months. However, 1 in 8 patients continues to have moderate to severe pain 1 year postoperatively, despite an absence of clinical or radiographic abnormalities. Office-based preoperative screening tools and interventions for patients at increased risk of persistent pain may improve outcomes.

▶ This is an interesting prospective randomized study with a very relevant clinical question. The major value is quantifying the fact that almost 50% of the patients still had significant pain at 3 months after knee replacement. The information contained herein, in my judgment, does not affect our selection factors or even our technique but rather what we tell patients in terms of expectations.

B. F. Morrey, MD

Effectiveness of Intensive Rehabilitation on Functional Ability and Quality of Life After First Total Knee Arthroplasty: A Single-blind Randomized Controlled Trial

Moffet H, Collet J-P, Shapiro SH, et al (Laval Univ, Quebec City, Canada; Quebec Rehabilitation Inst, Canada; McGill Univ, Montreal; et al)

Arch Phys Med Rehabil 85:546-556, 2004 6–4

Background.—Rehabilitation follow-up after TKA is often limited to a few supervised sessions during a short in-hospital stay. This is typically followed by an unsupervised home exercise program or by a few home physio-

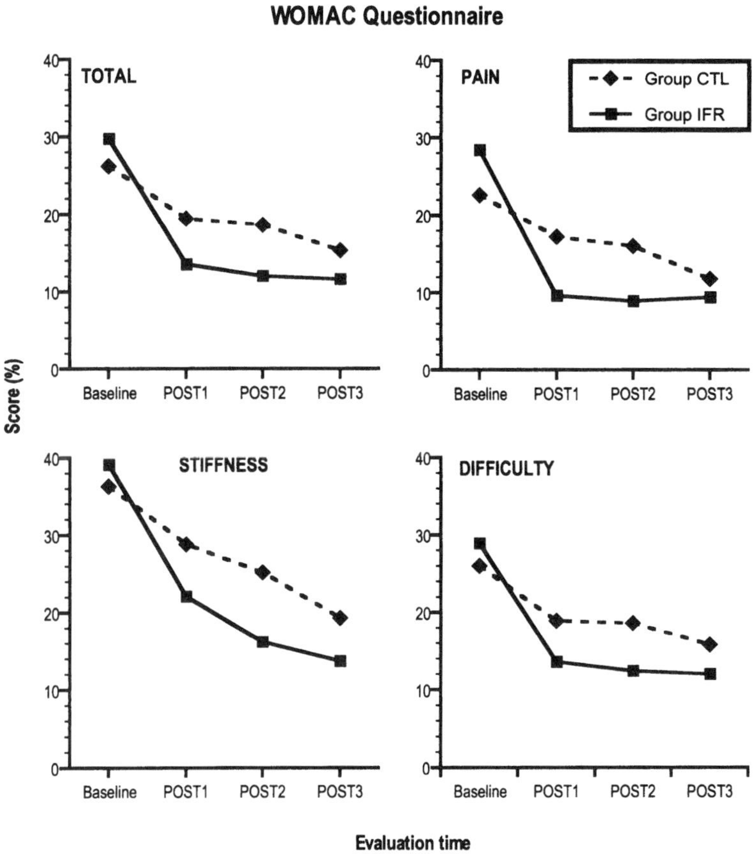

FIGURE 3.—WOMAC questionnaire total and subscale (pain, stiffness, difficulty) scores for both groups of subjects, at baseline and at follow-up evaluations. A decrease in scores represents an improvement in knee pain, stiffness, and/or functional ability. (Reprinted from Moffet H, Collet J-P, Shapiro SH, et al: Effectiveness of intensive rehabilitation on functional ability and quality of life after first total knee arthroplasty: A single-blind randomized controlled trial. *Arch Phys Med Rehabil* 85:546-556, 2004. Copyright 2004 with permission from The American Congress of Rehabilitation Medicine and the American Academy of Physical Medicine and Rehabilitation.)

therapy (PT) visits in the first 2 months after surgery. The efficacy of a new, intensive functional rehabilitation (IFR) program on functional ability and quality of life (QOL) in patients undergoing a first TKA was investigated.

Methods.—Seventy-seven patients with knee osteoarthritis were enrolled in a randomized, controlled study in an ambulatory care setting. By random assignment 2 months after TKA, patients received IFR or standard care. The IFR group underwent 12 supervised rehabilitation sessions combined with exercises at home between 2 and 4 months after TKA. Patients were assessed blindly at baseline (2 months after TKA), immediately after IFR (4 months after TKA), and 2 and 8 months after that.

Findings.—Compared with the control group, patients in the IFR group walked longer distances on the 60-minute walk test at the third postoperative assessment. At the first and second follow-up assessments, IFR recipients had less pain, stiffness, and difficulty performing daily activities (Fig 3). Positive changed in QOL favored IFR only at the second postoperative assessment.

Conclusions.—Intensive functional rehabilitation improves short- and mid-term functional ability after uncomplicated primary TKA. More intensive rehabilitation in the subacute recovery period after TKA is advocated to optimize functional outcomes in the first postoperative year.

▶ We included this article for a somewhat unusual reason. The authors conclude that intensive postoperative physical therapy is of value. However, our interpretation of the data is contrary to that of the authors. The intensive program of 12 visits following surgery while providing measurable improvement is, in our judgment, of very questionable clinical value. The major concern we have is the cost benefit of this approach based on the relatively minimal incremental improvement of the supervised therapy. I do not think the time and financial expenditure is worth the relatively mild improvement. The most important parameter is whether or not the long-term outcome is altered. The literature is replete demonstrating supervised therapy does not influence this parameter, hence, the major value would be in the short-term and this value appears to be limited.

B. F. Morrey, MD

Effect of Tibial Slope or Posterior Cruciate Ligament Release on Knee Kinematics

Jojima H, Whiteside LA, Ogata K (Fukuoka Univ, Japan; Missouri Bone and Joint Ctr, St Louis)

Clin Orthop 426:194-198, 2004 6–5

Introduction.—Correcting the kinematics of a knee that is too tight in flexion is frequently encountered in posterior cruciate ligament (PCL)-sparing TKA. Partial PCL release and increasing the posterior tibial slope have been shown to diminish tension of the PCL. An experimental trial using fresh human cadaver knees was designed to assess the effect of partial PCL release or posterior tibial slope on knee kinematics after TKA.

Methods.—Varus and valgus laxity, rotational laxity, AP laxity, femoral rollback, and maximum flexion angle were assessed in a normal knee, an ideal TKA, and a TKA in which the ligaments were too tight in flexion. The TKA specimens underwent either partial PCL release or increased tibial slope. Posterior tibial slope increased varus and valgus laxity, AP laxity, and rotational laxity in the knee with flexion tightness.

Results.—The PCL release corrected only AP tightness; it had no influence on the abnormal collateral ligament tightness. Increased posterior tibial slope significantly improved varus and valgus laxity and rotational laxity in the knee that was tight in flexion more than with release of the PCL. Thus, increasing posterior tibial slope is preferable in a knee that is tight in flexion during TKA.

► This simple experiment provides great insight with regard to subtle techniques of TKA. The simple observation that the posterior slope of a specific tibial design is more important than PCL release for overall balancing of the knee is of great practical value. With tight collateral ligaments, PCL release improves only the AP tightness. This is an important observation but is design specific. Nonetheless, this is useful information that may be of value in the patient with tight collateral contractures and concurrent limited flexion and extension arc.

B. F. Morrey, MD

Long-term Changes of the Nonresurfaced Patella After Total Knee Arthroplasty

Shih H-N, Shih L-Y, Wong Y-C, et al (Chang Gung Univ, Taoyuan, Taiwan)
J Bone Joint Surg Am 86-A:935-939, 2004 6–6

Introduction.—The most frequently observed complications of TKA involve the patellofemoral joint. The long-term outcome of the nonresurfaced patella after TKA has rarely been reported and was therefore retrospectively examined.

Methods.—Between 1992 and 1993, 227 knees of 181 patients underwent TKA without patellar resurfacing for treatment of osteoarthritis. Follow-up averaged 8.5 years after TKA. The functional results were correlated with radiographic changes. The risk factors leading to abnormal changes of the patella were assessed.

Results.—Before surgery, 186 (82%) of the patellae tracked centrally, 39 (17%) displaced or tilted laterally, and 2 (1%) subluxed laterally. At the latest postoperative follow-up, 133 (59%) patellae still tracked centrally with preservation of the cartilage thickness, 15 (7%) demonstrated early lateral tilt, 68 (30%) had progressive loss of lateral cartilage thickness with lateral tilt or displacement, 7 (3%) had progressed to lateral subluxation, and 4 (2%) tilted medially.

An abnormal patellofemoral joint did not impact the knee and function scores (P = .90 and 0.89, respectively). Yet, symptoms including difficulty rising from a chair or reluctance to use the involved lower limb while climbing stairs were observed. Preoperative patellar maltracking was seen as the only risk factor leading to postoperative patellar abnormalities (relative risk, 2.7; 95% confidence interval, 2.21-3.30; P = .003).

Conclusion.—At an average follow-up of 8.5 years, patellar tracking and the patellofemoral joint remained normal in about 60% of TKAs performed without resurfacing of the patella. Progressive degenerative changes of the nonresurfaced patella (primarily on the lateral facet) and patellar maltracking were the most frequently observed abnormal radiographic changes. Patellar maltracking increases the risk for development of these changes and clinical symptoms. Resurfacing of the patella during TKA may be beneficial for these patients.

▶ These authors address the ongoing and interesting question of whether the patella needs to be replaced at the time of total knee replacement. The key is the frequency of reoperation and the functional impairment when leaving the patella, compared to the frequency of revision and the outcome of a failed patellar resurfacing. These authors do not document the frequency of revision but do clearly demonstrate a high percentage of patients with abnormal kinematics that directly relate to abnormal function. Carefully studied, in the editor's view, this article supports the use of resurfacing the patella as a routine when performing TKA.

B. F. Morrey, MD

The Outcome of Total Knee Arthroplasty in Obese Patients

Foran JRH, Mont MA, Etienne G, et al (Good Samaritan Hosp, Baltimore, Md)

J Bone Joint Surg Am 86-A:1609-1615, 2004 6–7

Introduction.—There is strong evidence for an association between excessive body weight and degenerative joint disease of the knee. A large proportion of patients who undergo TKA are obese or morbidly obese. Several trials have implicated excessive weight as a negative predictor of the success of TKA. The clinical and radiographic results of TKAs performed in obese patients were compared with those performed with the use of the same prosthesis in nonobese individuals.

Methods.—Clinical and radiographic data regarding 78 TKAs in 68 obese patients were compared with data for a matched group of nonobese patients. Analyses were also performed after stratification of the obese group for the extent of obesity. The prosthesis was the same for all patients. The clinical data analyzed included Knee Society objective and functional scores, patellofemoral symptoms, activity level, and complications.

Results.—The percentages of knees with a Knee Society score of 80 or more points at an average of 80 months of follow-up were 88% and 99% in the obese and nonobese groups, respectively. Patients in the morbidly obese subgroup had a significantly higher revision rate compared to that of the nonobese group ($P = .02$).

Conclusion.—Any degree of obesity (body mass index 30 or greater) has a negative impact on the outcome of TKA.

▶ These authors are to be commended for attempting to address one of the most commonly faced issues in elective hip and knee replacement, specifically, the increased risk incurred by operating on an obese patient. The outcome of this very straightforward study does confirm the increased rate of revision and a poorer outcome in the obese patients. Others have documented similar observations. This type of information should be conveyed to patients in anticipation of joint replacement who remain obese or morbidly obese.

B. F. Morrey, MD

Total Knee Arthroplasty for Neuropathic (Charcot) Joints

Parvizi J, Marrs J, Morrey BF (Rothman Inst at Jefferson, Philadelphia; Mayo Clinic, Rochester, Minn)

Clin Orthop 416:145-150, 2003 6–8

Background.—Neuropathic arthropathy (Charcot joint) is a progressive, degenerative joint disease that can result in severe dysfunction and deformity. The outcomes of treatment with modern design, cemented, condylar TKAs performed at 1 center in patients with confirmed neuropathy of the knee were reviewed.

Methods.—Forty TKAs in 29 patients were included in the review. The mean follow-up was 7.9 years. Radiographic surveillance was done for a median 6.4 years.

Findings.—After knee arthroplasty, Knee Society pain and function scores as well as range of motion were improved significantly. Ninety-five percent of the knees had extensive bone fragmentation and bone defect. Bony defects were reinforced by metal wedge augments, autologous bone grafting, and bone allografts. Ligamentous instability necessitated long-stem components in 27 knees and rotating hinge prostheses in 5. Six reoperations were performed for periprosthetic fracture, aseptic loosening, instability, and deep infection.

Conclusions.—Selected patients with end-stage neuropathic arthropathy may benefit from TKA. Clinicians treating such patients must adhere to the basic principles of knee arthroplasty in restoring limb alignment, reinforcing bony defects by bone grafting or augmented prostheses, careful ligamentous balancing, and appropriate selection of constrained prostheses. The technical challenges of TKA in this patient population, especially in those with significant deformities, can require skills, implant systems, and methods usually reserved for complex revision arthroplasty.

▶ The reason this particular article was included is that no single surgeon or practice has much experience with this problem. It is a major question when such a patient presents to our office. This experience averages almost 8 years and provides an adequate clinical sample in our judgment to justify the conclusions. The use of the long-stemmed components even as a primary procedure should be noted. The high incidence of reoperation for periprosthetic fracture, aseptic loosening, instability, and infection should also be noted. However, 2 loosenings in the 29 patients after an average of 8 years is somewhat less than might have been predicted. We conclude that a well-done TKA selecting a design that provides some stability by virtue of its articulation employing stems for stable implant fixation is a reasonable option for this patient.

B. F. Morrey, MD

Analysis of Unicompartmental Knee Arthroplasty in a Community-Based Implant Registry

Gioe TJ, Killeen KK, Hoeffel DP, et al (St Anthony Orthopaedic Specialists, St Paul, Minn; St Joseph's Hosp, St Paul, Minn; Summit Orthopedics, St Paul, Minn)

Clin Orthop 416:111-119, 2003 6–9

Background.—There has been a resurgence of interest in unicompartmental knee arthroplasty designs. This study used a unique community implant and explant registry to assess the long-term survival of unicompartmental knee arthroplasty.

Methods.—Data were obtained on 516 unicompartmental knee arthroplasties performed since 1991 and followed up prospectively to January, 2002. The arthroplasties represented 9 different designs and were performed by 23 surgeons.

Findings.—Thirty-nine arthroplasties were revised during the follow-up period. Revisions were indicated by progression of arthritis in the uninvolved compartments in 51.3%, aseptic loosening in 25.6%, and polyethylene (PE) wear in 20.5%. Kaplan-Meier survival analysis with revision as the end point demonstrated a 92.6% survival at 5 years and an 88.6% survival at 10 years for these unicompartmental knee arthroplasties. The 10-year survival rate for primary TKAs was 94.8%.

Conclusions.—Revision of unicompartmental knee arthroplasties is usually performed for progression of arthritis in the contralateral compartment. The rate of revision was higher than with primary cemented TKA.

► Unicompartmental TKA has certainly regained favor in recent years. There are relatively few long-term studies regarding this implant and as the authors try to point out, these usually emanate from the designers of the articular device. The authors accurately highlight the value of this contribution. It represents a heterogeneous number of designs, a number of surgeons using somewhat variable selection criteria. Given all of that, it is impressive that 92.6% survived at 5 years and 88.6% survived at 10 years. This is not as good as results with conventional TKA, and it would be expected that with uniform selection factors with increased experience and with enhanced design and technique the outcome would be improved from that in this report.

B. F. Morrey, MD

Shelf Age of the Polyethylene Tibial Component and Outcome of Unicondylar Knee Arthroplasty

Collier MB, Engh AC Jr, Engh GA (Anderson Orthopaedic Research Inst, Alexandria, Va)

J Bone Joint Surg Am 86-A:763-769, 2004 6–10

Background.—In a recent report, shelf-aging of unicondylar polyethylene tibial components was associated with accelerated fatigue wear and rapid failure. The authors reviewed their experiences with another unicondylar knee system to determine the relationship between the shelf age of the polyethylene components and clinical outcome.

Methods.—Between 1990 and 1996, 100 single compartment replacement unicompartmental knee arthroplasties with cement were done. The polyethylene inserts had a median shelf age of 1.7 years. Four patients were lost to follow-up, and 16 patients died. By the time of review, 19 knees had undergone revision. At a mean 8 years postoperatively, 61 knee replacements remained in situ.

Findings.—With revision used as the end point, Kaplan-Meier survivorship analysis indicated a 6-year survival rate of 96% when the insert had a shelf age less than the median shelf age. However, when the median shelf age was exceeded, this survival rate was only 71%. Fatigue wear was seen on all retrieved components except for 2 that had shelf ages of less than 1 year and had been revised within 3 years. At 4 to 6 years of clinical follow-up, knees with inserts exceeding the median shelf age also had lower knee and function scores.

Conclusions.—Shelf aging appears to accelerate fatigue failure of polyethylene inserts sterilized with gamma irradiation in air and compromise intermediate outcomes in patients with this unicondylar knee replacement system. Clinicians must pay attention to the relationship between shelf age and clinical performance of the polyethylene component in patients treated with unicondylar knee arthroplasty implants.

▶ It is well known that polyethylene undergoes oxidation on the shelf and this adversely effects its mechanical and wear properties. This study is important in that it documents the degree of deterioration in mechanical performance of the polyethylene as it relates to survival of these implants. I found it particularly interesting that in those with a polyethylene insert that exceeded the median shelf age, a whopping 71% of patients had undergone revision at 6 years following surgery. This study provides compelling evidence to accurately assess implant inventory shelf life with cross-linked poly and newer methods of polyethylene preparation and sterilization, this issue should become less relevant.

B. F. Morrey, MD

Stiffness After Total Knee Arthroplasty: Prevalence of the Complication and Outcomes of Revision

Kim J, Nelson CL, Lotke PA (Univ of Pennsylvania, Philadelphia)

J Bone Joint Surg Am 86-A:1479-1484, 2004 6–11

Introduction.—Stiffness is an infrequent, yet disabling, problem after TKA. Its incidence is not well defined. The outcomes of revision surgery for a stiff knee after arthroplasty have not been determined in a large series of patients. The prevalence of stiffness after primary TKA was examined, along with the efficacy of revision surgery for treatment of stiffness.

Methods.—A stiff knee was considered to be a knee that had a flexion contracture of 15° or greater or 75° of flexion. Two cohorts were assessed as follows: (1) 1000 consecutive primary TKAs were reviewed to ascertain the prevalence of stiffness and (2) 56 patients who underwent revision after total TKA to treat stiffness were evaluated, along with the pain or component loosening experienced by some patients.

Results.—At an average of 32 months postoperatively, the incidence of stiffness was 1.3%. Patients with a stiff knee experienced significantly less preoperative extension and flexion compared to those without ($P < .0001$). No significant differences were observed in age, gender, implant design, diagnosis, or requirement for lateral release between patients with and without stiffness.

The second group of knees revised due to stiffness were followed up for an average of 43 months. The mean Knee Society score improved from 38.5 points preoperatively to 86.7 points at follow-up. The mean Knee Society function score rose from 40.0 to 58.4 points, and the mean Knee Society pain score increased from 15.0 to 46.9 points. The mean flexion contracture dropped from 11.3° to 3.2°, the mean flexion improved from 65.8° to 85.4°, and the mean arc of motion improved from 54.6° to 82.2°. The arc of motion improved in 93% of knees and flexion increased in 80% of knees. Extension improved in 63%; it was unchanged in 30%.

Conclusion.—The prevalence of stiffness in 1000 primary TKAs was 1.3%. Revision surgery was an acceptable option for treatment of stiffness. The Knee Society scores improved, flexion contractures decreased, and 93% of knees had an increased arc of motion. Benefits of revision surgery were considered modest.

▶ With the continued outstanding success of knee joint replacement, a knee that is stiff or with limited motion, while uncommon, does remain one of the most significant complications of this procedure. This study documents the infrequent nature of significant knee stiffness (less than 2%) and the definite, but relatively modest, improvement that might be realized by revision procedure. The editor has used arthroscopic debridement and gentle examination under anesthesia as late as 12 months in patients flexing less than 80°. Great care must be taken, however, not to exert undue force in order to avoid the potential complication of a supracondylar fracture.

B. F. Morrey, MD

Addition of Hand-Blended Generic Tobramycin in Bone Cement: Effect on Mechanical Strength

DeLuise M, Scott CP (Stryker, Mahwah, NJ)

Orthopedics 27:1289-1291, 2004 6–12

Introduction.—This study compared the mechanical strength of commercially prepared antibiotic bone cement (Simplex With Tobramycin; Stryker, Mahwah, NJ), cement with generic tobramycin (Pharma-Tek, Huntington,

TABLE.—Comparison of Tensile Test Results for Commercially Blended Antibiotic, Hand-Blended Antibiotic, and Nonantibiotic Bone Cement

Type of Bone Cement	Tensile Property Strength (MPa)	Strain (mm/mm)
Hand-blended antibiotic	29.06 ± 6.89	0.013 ± 0.003
Commercially blended antibiotic	44.10 ± 1.69	0.020 ± 0.002
Control nonantibiotic	45.49 ± 2.81	0.018 ± 0.002

(Courtesy of DeLuise M, Scott CP: Addition of hand-blended generic tobramycin in bone cement: Effect on mechanical strength. *Orthopedics* 27:1289-1291, 2004.)

NY) blended in by the orthopedic nursing staff, and standard nonantibiotic bone cement. The results showed an approximate 36% decrease in the strength of the cement with hand-mixed generic tobramycin, while the commercial antibiotic cement remained unchanged relative to the nonantibiotic control (Table). These results indicate the mechanical properties of bone cement can be severely compromised by hand-mixing antibiotics into bone cement at the time of surgery.

► This contribution is elegant in its simplicity. It addresses a common question and offers interesting insight. It is a clear demonstration of the adverse effect of the bureaucracy of the Food and Drug Administration preventing the availability of a superior product, that is, a commercially mixed antibiotic with polymethylmethacrylate. As a result, the surgeons resort to the hand-blended mixture, which at least in this demonstration shows inferior tensile properties. It is possible that this difference is not clinically significant, but it is an interesting observation nonetheless.

B. F. Morrey, MD

Minimal Incision Total Knee Arthroplasty: Early Experience

Tria AJ Jr, Coon TM (Robert Wood Johnson Med School, New Brunswick, NJ; Shasta Orthopaedics and Sports Medicine, Red Bluff, Calif)

Clin Orthop 416:185-190, 2003 6–13

Background.—TKA has been an evolving technique since 1974, when the first total knee prosthesis was introduced. Over the past 2 decades, the techniques of balancing the ligaments, equalizing the flexion and extension gaps, and adjusting the overall alignment have been perfected to the point that long-term results are quite satisfactory. In the early 1990s, the concept of minimally invasive surgery for unicondylar knee arthroplasty was introduced by Repicci. The suggestion of this approach was that less invasive surgery could provide results similar to those obtained with standard unicondylar knee arthroplasty.

Early reports in the literature have supported these conclusions. It is not surprising then that minimally invasive surgery has been applied to TKA. However, it will be important in the coming years to clearly define the meaning of minimally invasive surgery. The early outcomes in minimally invasive TKA procedures were assessed.

Methods.—Seventy minimally invasive TKA procedures were performed in a 9-month period by means of an approach detailed in this report. The average age of the patients was 67 years, with a range of 51 to 84 years. The group included 35 men and 31 women.

Results.—Early results have demonstrated that the minimally invasive approach to TKA has provided less intraoperative blood loss, shorter length of stay, increased ROM, and similar implant accuracy to standard TKA.

Conclusion.—As with any new clinical endeavor, these new minimally invasive techniques will require thorough evaluation. It must be remembered also that the primary goal of any new technology is the advancement of science without compromising the ultimate outcome for the patient. However, early findings are encouraging for the future of minimally invasive TKA.

▶ Amidst the great wave of enthusiasm for limited surgical exposures, it would seem that this particular diagnosis and procedure may be the most suited for the so-called minimally invasive surgery. In our experience, the improved instrumentation and implant design warrants further consideration of this technique. We have been impressed with the short-term outcome in our hands. The literature continues to be deficient however with regard to the true risk/benefit consideration, and this issue will not be clarified for several years, until an adequate amount of follow-up is obtained.

B. F. Morrey, MD

Uncemented Rotating-Platform Total Knee Replacement: A Five to Twelve-Year Follow-up Study

Sorrells RB, Voorhorst PE, Murphy JA, et al (Joint Replacement Clinic, Little Rock, Ark; DuPuy Orthopaedics, Warsaw, Ind; Cleveland Clinic Health System, Ohio)

J Bone Joint Surg Am 86:2156-2162, 2004 6–14

Introduction.—A dual surface articulation between a polyethylene insert and metallic femoral and tibial tray components is a defining feature of mobile-bearing total knee designs. This knee replacement is an alternative to conventional fixed-bearing TKA. Presented are the findings of a prospective, intermediate-term clinical follow-up investigation of the bicruciate ligament–sacrificing porous-coated Low Contact Stress rotating-platform total knee design.

Methods.—Between February 1984 and January 1994, 421 patients underwent 528 uncemented primary knee replacements. All patellae were resurfaced with the Low Contact Stress rotating patellar component. Average patient age at the time of the index procedure was 69 years. A total of 261 women and 160 men were evaluated at 3 months, 6 months, and yearly thereafter with the 100-point New Jersey Orthopedic Hospital knee-scoring

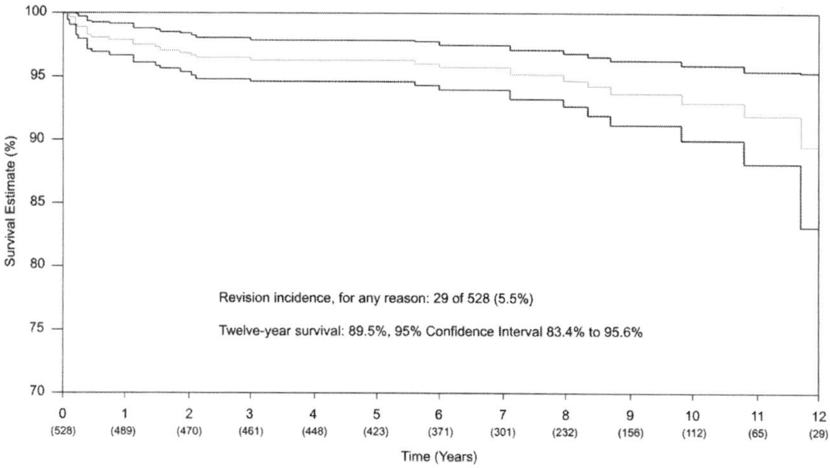

FIGURE 2.—Kaplan-Meier survivorship curve (and 95% confidence intervals) for 528 cementless Low Contact Stress rotating-platform total knee replacements that were followed up for as long as 12 years, with revision for any reason as the end point. (Republished with permission of the Journal of Bone and Joint Surgery, Inc, from Sorrells RB, Voorhorst PE, Murphy JA, et al: Uncemented rotating-platform total knee replacement: A five to twelve-year follow-up study. *J Bone Joint Surg Am* 86:2156-2162, 2004. Reproduced by permission of the publisher via Copyright Clearance Center, Inc.)

system. Patients underwent radiographic analysis of the tibial, femoral, and patellar components at each evaluation point.

Results.—Revision was performed in 29 failures. The Kaplan-Meier estimate of implant survival at 12-year follow-up was 89.5% (95% confidence interval, 83.4%-95.6%) (Fig 2). The total clinical scores improved significantly compared with preoperative scores during the initial 12 months postoperatively; thereafter, it plateaued. A total of 321 knees had adequate radiographic follow-up (average, 8.1 years; range, 5-12 years). Zonal radiographic analysis showed 93 instances of radiolucent lines (82 that measured <1 mm in width); the greatest number of radiolucent lines (39) were located around the tibial tray stem. None of the lines was considered progressive. No knee with a radiolucent line that measured more than 2 mm was revised because of failure.

Conclusion.—This first-generation, uncemented, mobile-bearing bicruciate ligament–sacrificing knee replacement was linked with a good survival rate and exhibited clinical efficacy during the 5- to 12-year follow-up interval.

► This is the largest US series with the longest documented follow-up for this particular design. The enthusiasm for this approach to knee joint replacement has waned in recent years because of the lack of evidence of the expected improvement in motion. The additional anticipation of a lower wear rate will take even longer to appreciate. I consider this particular contribution the standard by which other reports will be compared. Note that the 12-year survival rate of 90% does approximate but is not superior to the numerous previous reports of fixed bearing generic condylar implants. Thus, since the survival for this particular design is not enhanced, its value will rest on demonstration of the above 2 qualities that, as mentioned, have yet to be demonstrated.

B. F. Morrey, MD

MIS Unicondylar Knee Arthroplasty: Surgical Approach and Early Results

Gesell MW, Tria AJ Jr (Orthopaedic Ctr of New Jersey, Somerset)

Clin Orthop 428:53-60, 2004 6–15

Introduction.—Unicondylar arthroplasty of the knee has seen a resurgence of interest in the United States. The principles of unicondylar arthroplasty of the knee are different from those for total knee arthroplasty, allowing replacement of only the affected joint compartment with less bone loss. Minimally invasive surgery allows for less soft tissue dissection with the potential for less morbidity. The key question is: will the changes associated with the minimally invasive surgery procedure improve the clinical results of the standard unicondylar arthroplasty of the knee or will the changes make the procedure too difficult and lead to an increasing failure rate? This study reviews the surgical technique and presents the 2 to 4 year results of the minimally invasive unicondylar arthroplasty of the knee (47 knees) in 41 patients. The average range of motion increased from 121°-132°. The Knee Society pain score improved from 45-80 and the function score improved from 47-78. Only one knee has been revised. With proper patient selection, minimally invasive unicondylar arthroplasty of the knee allows for results that are at least equal to those of the standard open procedure at 2 to 4 years after the surgery.

▶ Commensurate with the growing clinical interest in the unicondylar knee and minimally invasive surgery is the combination of these 2 concepts. The increased interest in this topic has been reflected in several reports this year. We are including this particular one as a sample which, of necessity, has a relatively small number of knees with relatively modest follow-up. Nonetheless, the early results do at least demonstrate no catastrophic failures, thus justifying continued interest in the development of this basic surgical approach. It is felt that the technique will continue to improve, and as always, a learning curve would be expected. We have performed this procedure on a number of occasions and, to date, have been pleased with the early results. Careful patient selection is important, and an understanding of the technical features is particularly relevant.

B. F. Morrey, MD

Unicompartmental Knee Arthroplasty: 2- to 12-Year Results in a Community Hospital

Rajasekhar C, Das S, Smith A (Furness Gen Hosp, Barrow-in-Furness, England)

J Bone Joint Surg Br 86-B:983-985, 2004 6–16

Introduction.—We report the outcome of 135 knees with anteromedial osteoarthritis in which the Oxford meniscal-bearing unicompartmental arthroplasty was inserted in a district general hospital by a single surgeon. All the knees had an intact anterior cruciate ligament, a correctable varus deformity and the lateral compartment was uninvolved or had only minor osteoarthritis. The mean follow-up was 5.82 years (2 to 12). Using revision as the end-point, the outcome for every knee was established. Five knees have been revised giving a cumulative rate of survival of the prosthesis at ten years of 94.04% (95% confidence interval 84.0 to 97.8). Knee rating and patient function were assessed using the modified Knee Society scoring system. The mean knee score was 92.2 (51 to 100) and the mean functional score 76.2 (51 to 100). The survival of the implant is comparable to that reported by the designers of the prosthesis and not significantly different from that for total knee replacement. Unicompartmental knee replacement offers a viable alternative in patients with medial osteoarthritis. Appropriate selection of patients and good surgical technique are the key factors.

▶ This contribution is included as it does provide reasonably long-term follow-up in a modest sample of patients with increasingly popular unicompartmental knee replacement. The outcome of 10-year survival of 94% is impressive. This particular contribution was also included since it reflects the practice not just in this country but rather in England, thus providing insight into the emerging and accepted practice in other parts of the world.

B. F. Morrey, MD

Computer-Assisted Knee Arthroplasty Versus a Conventional Jig-Based Technique: A Randomised, Prospective Trial

Chauhan SK, Scott RG, Breidahl W, et al (Royal Perth Hosp, Western Australia)

J Bone Joint Surg Br 86-B:372-377, 2003 6–17

Introduction.—Computer navigation systems are widely used in Europe and Australia to provide more accurate implantation via digital mapping that is based on standard anatomical landmarks and kinematic analysis. Trials suggesting that this approach provides improved alignment have used standard radiography with isolated CT to measure alignment, a method that may not be sufficiently accurate. The safety and accuracy of this new computerized technology were evaluated in a prospective, randomized, controlled trial by comparing a group of patients who underwent computer-assisted TKA (CAKA) with a similar group in whom a conventional jig-based technique (JBKA) was used with a standardized CT protocol for 7 measurements of outcome.

Methods.—The study included 70 patients awaiting TKA who were selected randomly to undergo either CAKA or JBKA. Postoperative CT was conducted according to the Perth CT Knee Arthroplasty Protocol. Preoperative and postoperative Maquet views of the limb were obtained in all patients. Intraoperative and perioperative morbidity data were obtained, and blood loss was measured.

Results.—Postoperative CT revealed a significant improvement in the alignment of the components using the computer-assisted surgery in measures of femoral varus/valgus (P = .032), femoral rotation (P = .001), tibial varus/valgus (P = .047), tibial posterior slope (P = .0001), tibial rotation (P = .011), and femorotibial mismatch (P = .037). Standing alignment was also improved (P = .004), and less total blood loss was observed (P = .0001). A mean increase of 13 minutes in surgery time was noted in the computer-assisted group (P = .0001), compared with that of the conventional jib-based technique.

Conclusion.—It remains to be seen whether the individual and cumulative improvement in alignment provided by CAKA provides better long-term results. In the short term, CAKA is more accurate than JBKA and has less morbidity.

▶ There are few comments with regard to the objective value of the emerging computer-based alignment systems. This prospective study, therefore, is worthwhile in addressing an important and relevant issue for the orthopedic community. As one might expect, the study does document improved alignment in virtually all parameters studied. Of particular relevance is the enhanced varus/valgus and axial rotational position of the implant. However, it should also be noted that this study did not address whether the degree of improvement was associated with a measurable and comparable enhancement of outcome in the short-term. The real key is whether the improvements enhance function or survival and thus are worth the added costs of doing the procedure.

B. F. Morrey, MD

Navigation in Total-Knee Arthroplasty: CT-Based Implantation Compared With the Conventional Technique

Perlick L, Bäthis H, Tingart M, et al (Univ of Regensburg, Germany; Aarhus Univ Hosp, Denmark)

Acta Orthop Scand 75:464-470, 2004 6–18

Background.—Exact axial limb alignment in total-knee arthroplasty (TKA) is important for a successful outcome. We evaluated the efficiency of computer-assisted implantation in TKA and compared it with the classical surgeon-controlled technique.

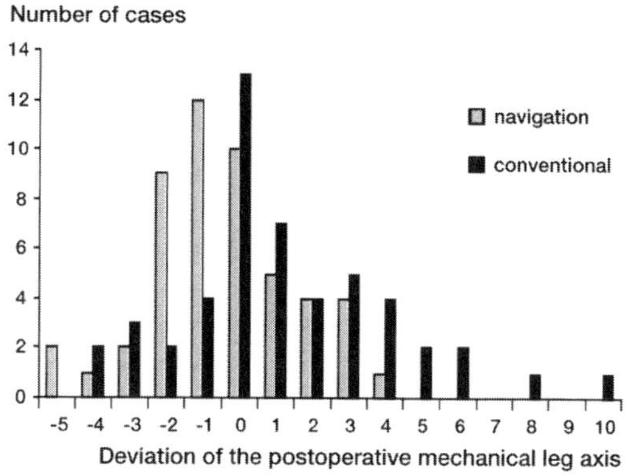

FIGURE 5.—Distribution of the postoperative mechanical leg axis. (Courtesy of Perlick L, Bäthis H, Tingart M, et al: Navigation in total-knee arthroplasty: CT-based implantation compared with the conventional technique. *Acta Orthop Scand* 75:464-470, 2004.)

Patients and Methods.—We implanted 100 TKA using either the computer-assisted technique (50) or the conventional approach (50). There were no significant differences between the groups regarding the preoperative leg deformity. Accuracy of implantation was determined in postoperative long-leg coronal and lateral radiographs.

Results.—A postoperative leg axis between 3° varus and 3° valgus was achieved in 46 patients in the group with computer-assisted implantation and 36 patients in the control group ($p = 0.01$) (Fig 5). A significant difference was also seen for the femoral component alignment in frontal plane. No complications influencing the clinical outcome were observed.

Interpretation.—A CT-based navigation system improves the accuracy of TKA, but higher costs and time-consuming planning will mean that its usage is limited to special cases. Additional tools such as ligament balancing, which are presently only available with the CT-free software module, require to be added to the CT-based system.

▶ This article is one of several that has appeared this year to document the value of application of navigation technology in joint replacement arthroplasty. For the most part, these efforts do document improved positioning of the implant, particularly the tibial component and its effect on varus valgus angulation and femoral component rotational alignment. Going forward, if navigation is to be widely applied, it must be less expensive, require less preparation, and ultimately must not significantly lengthen the time of surgery. The demonstrated value to date is not necessarily one that translates to its expected clinical utility, specifically that of providing longer-term survival due to more accurate component placement. In a word, the jury is still out. It is unlikely that the current systems will be widely adopted, but there is also little doubt that the concept will continue to be developed to a point where it will, in all likelihood, be useful in certain settings, knee arthroplasty being one of them.

B. F. Morrey, MD

Reoperations After 3200 Revision TKAs: Rates, Etiology, and Lessons Learned

Sierra RJ, Cooney WP, Pagnano MW, et al (Mayo Clinic, Rochester, Minn)

Clin Orthop 425:200-206, 2004 6–19

Introduction.—Primary TKA is an amazingly successful surgery with survivorship to aseptic loosening of as much as 93% to 97% at 20 to 23 years postoperatively. Revision TKA is a reliable and durable treatment for most failed TKAs. Reoperation rates range between 8% and 19%. The prevalence, etiology, and evolution with time of reoperations performed after index revision TKAs were examined.

Methods.—After exclusion criteria were met, 1814 index knee revisions in 1627 patients were included. Over 50% of revisions performed for loosening and extensor mechanism problems and over 80% of revisions involving the femoral, tibial, or both components were examined.

Results.—A total of 373 knees underwent reoperation 1 or more times. The average time from index revision TKA to first reoperation was 3.5 years (range, 1 day to 19 years). Of the 1814 index revision TKAs, 373 (20%) had 593 reoperations (336 patients). The cumulative risks of first reoperation at 5, 10, and 15 years were 16.1% (95% confidence interval [CI], 14.2%-17.9%), 26% (95% CI, 23.4%-28.6%), and 31.4% (95% CI, 30.2%-39%), respectively.

There was no difference in risk to first reoperation when comparing the decades in which the index revisions were performed (1970-1980, 1981-1990, and 1991-2000). There was a trend toward a higher cumulative risk of first time reoperations for deep infection, loosening, and instability in the last decade. With the numbers available, this was not statistically significant.

Conclusion.—The incidence of reoperations in this large series of index revision TKAs performed for aseptic reasons was surprisingly high. Despite marked improvements during the past 3 decades in component design, surgical technique, and prevention of infection, patients who have a revision TKA are at increased risk of having 1 or more subsequent problems that result in reoperation.

► These authors used the Mayo Clinic database to understand the potential causes of failure of a revision knee replacement procedure, asking the simple question of why the revision of a failed knee replacement also subsequently fails. The expectation of an 85% success at 5 years, a 75% success at 10 years, and a 70% outcome free of reoperation at 15 years is worthwhile information. The causes for the reoperation of a failed revision are similar to that which was defined in a smaller study by Stuart et al,[1] specifically, instability of the extensor mechanism and implant loosening.

B. F. Morrey, MD

Reference

1. Stuart MJ, Larson JE, Morrey BF: Reoperation after condylar revision total knee arthroplasty. *Clin Orthop* 286:168-173, 1993.

7 Sports Medicine

Introduction

Most literature related to sports continues to focus on the ACL. We have selected those studies that offer new rather than confirmatory contributions regarding the ACL. The major effort was to select those specific articles that cover a broad spectrum of sports medicine topics. Further, articles were chosen not so much from the viewpoint of a sports medicine subspecialist, but rather from the perspective of an orthopedic surgeon who handles a broad spectrum of injuries and athletes from the high school gymnast to the serious recreational enthusiast. We particularly enjoyed reviewing the articles on this subject this year, and hopefully the selections will be useful in your practice.

Bernard F. Morrey, MD

Nonsteroidal Anti-inflammatory Drugs and Acetaminophen in the Treatment of an Acute Muscle Injury

Rahusen FTG, Weinhold PS, Almekinders LC, et al (St Maartenskliniek, Nijmegen, The Netherlands; Univ of North Carolina, Chapel Hill; Duke Univ, Durham, NC)

Am J Sports Med 32:1856-1859, 2004 7–1

Background.—Nonsteroidal anti-inflammatory drugs are frequently used to treat muscle injuries in athletes. It is not known whether the anti-inflammatory effects of these drugs are important or whether their effectiveness is a result of their central analgesic effect.

Hypothesis.—The effects of nonsteroidal anti-inflammatory drugs are no different than the effects of an analgesic (acetaminophen) without anti-inflammatory action in an experimental, acute muscle contusion model.

Study Design.—Controlled animal study.

Methods.—A standardized, unilateral, nonpenetrating injury was created to the tibialis anterior muscle of 96 adult male mice. Four treatment groups were used: group 1, placebo treatment; group 2, treatment with rofecoxib, a nonsteroidal anti-inflammatory drug with cyclooxygenase-2 selectivity, and treatment after the injury; group 3, rofecoxib treatment starting 24 hours before the injury; and group 4, acetaminophen treatment after the injury. The muscle and the contralateral normal muscle were evaluated at 2, 5, and

7 days after injury by grading of gait, wet weight as a measure of edema, and histologic evaluation.

Results.—Group 1 had significantly more gait disturbances at day 2 than all other groups ($P < .05$). No differences were found at days 5 and 7. Wet weights showed an increase at day 2 in group 1 ($P < .01$). Again, no differences were found at days 5 and 7. Histology revealed similar inflammatory changes at day 2 in all groups, with regeneration of muscle fibers at days 5 and 7.

Conclusions.—Rofecoxib as a nonsteroidal anti-inflammatory drug and acetaminophen as a non-nonsteroidal anti-inflammatory drug analgesic have similar effects. The lack of differences in wet weights and histology suggests that the anti-inflammatory effects of rofecoxib are not an important feature of its action.

Clinical Relevance.—The routine use of nonsteroidal anti-inflammatory drugs in muscle injuries may need to be critically evaluated because low-cost and low-risk analgesics may be just as effective.

► There is great apprehension that even the brief use of nonsteroidal anti-inflammatory agents may cause serious complications. The finding that a well-known and safe analgesic has a similar effect to an anti-inflammatory agent is worthy of note. The value of the conclusions are enhanced when considering the cost-effectiveness of the analgesic.

B. F. Morrey, MD

Influence of Obesity on Outcome After Knee Arthroplasty

Harrison MM, Morrell J, Hopman WM (Queen's Univ, Kingston, Ont, Canada)

Arthroscopy 20:691-695, 2004 7–2

Background.—Women are more likely than men to sustain osteoarthritis of the knee. The prevalence of knee arthritis is 4.9% for women compared with 2.6% for men. Bilateral knee arthritis is also more common in women than in men. Several studies have identified obesity as a risk factor contributing to the development of knee osteoarthritis. The association between obesity and knee arthritis is so strong that some authors have stated that obesity is a causal factor in osteoarthritis. Obesity is also a risk factor for disability in patients with arthritis.

The short-term results of arthroscopic surgery for mild to moderate arthritis are good, and about 75% of patients have experienced initial improvement in their symptoms. The clinical outcomes for overweight women were compared with those of a group of normal-weight women 4 to 11 years after arthroscopic debridement of the knee.

Methods.—The study group was composed of 121 women between the ages of 30 and 55 years at the time of arthroscopic debridement of the knee. All patients had been initially treated conservatively with activity modification, anti-inflammatory drugs, and physiotherapy. A questionnaire consisting of the Western Ontario and McMaster Universities Osteoarthritis Index, the short form health survey SF-36, and a survey regarding satisfaction with surgery was mailed to these patients. Data obtained from the questionnaire were supplemented by chart review.

Results.—Completed questionnaires were returned by 94 of 121 (74%) patients. All of these patients scored significantly lower compared with age-matched normative data on all domains of the SF-36. Scores of the normal-weight group were better than those for the obese group, particularly in the area of physical functioning, role physical, mental health, and role emotional domains. Patients in the normal-weight group were also more satisfied with their surgery, more likely to indicate that they would have the surgery again, and had fewer recurrences of knee pain.

Conclusion.—Overweight women who undergo knee arthroscopy have poorer outcomes in terms of quality of life and satisfaction with surgery than do women of normal weight.

► It has long been recognized that obesity is felt to be associated with increased complications and possibly lessens the functional life of joint replacements of both the hip and the knee. This interesting study demonstrates the poorer outcome, even with the less invasive procedure of arthroscopy. These findings are particularly relevant since obesity is becoming a nationwide epidemic and one of the major health concerns of our population. The full impact of this health problem is yet to be demonstrated.

B. F. Morrey, MD

Ulnar Collateral Ligament Reconstruction in High School Baseball Players: Clinical Results and Injury Risk Factors

Petty DH, Andrews JR, Fleisig GS, et al (American Sports Medicine Inst, Birmingham, Ala)

Am J Sports Med 32:1158-1164, 2004 7–3

Introduction.—Injury to the ulnar collateral ligament (UCL) of the elbow produces significant disability for the throwing athlete. The incidence of this injury is rising in baseball, particularly at the high school level. Many of the injured high school baseball players describe regimens that incorporate year-round throwing; others describe excessive throwing during the regular season, a playoff, or a showcase. The clinical results of UCL reconstruction for high school athletes were examined retrospectively.

Methods.—Between 1995 and 2000, 31 UCL reconstructions on the elbows of high school baseball players were performed in a single institution. Twenty-seven athletes were available for follow-up at a point at which it could be determined whether or not they would return to baseball at the same or a higher level. All participants were males. The age range was 15.9 to 19.0 years at the time of surgery.

Follow-up examinations and questionnaires were initiated at an average of 35 months after UCL reconstruction. Six potential risk factors were assessed as follows: year-round throwing, seasonal overuse, event overuse, throwing velocity more than 80 mph, throwing breaking pitches before age 14 years, and inadequate warm-ups.

Results.—Overall, 74% of players returned to baseball at the same or a higher level at an average of 11 months. Patients averaged 3 potential risk factors for throwing injury. Eighty-five percent demonstrated at least 1 overuse category. The average self-reported fastball velocity among pitchers was 83 mph. Sixty-seven percent threw breaking pitches before the age of 14 years.

Conclusion.—The success rate of UCL reconstruction among high school baseball players is about equal to that of more mature throwers. Overuse of the throwing arm and throwing breaking pitches at an early age may increase the incidence of injuries. More attention needs to be paid to preventing serious elbow injury, particularly in elite-level teenage pitchers who throw with high velocity.

▶ Successful repair of the medial collateral ligament was pioneered by Jobe and is now recognized as an effective means of treating the mature baseball pitcher with medial collateral ligament deficiency. Very little is known with regard to the surgical procedure in the immature or high school athlete. This article is therefore of significant value, first because of the large number of patients treated and second, because of the care with which the patients were followed up.

The overall 75% return to high level of play is roughly comparable to that which was demonstrated in the older populations. These investigators did make an effort to understand the development of this injury in the high school pitcher, with the finding that frequent use of breaking pitches in an early age may have a potential causal effect.

B. F. Morrey, MD

The Effect of a Proprioceptive Balanced Board Training Program for the Prevention of Ankle Sprains: A Prospective Controlled Trial

Verhagen E, van der Beek A, Twisk J, et al (EMGO-Inst, Amsterdam; Oslo Sports Trauma Research Ctr, Norway)

Am J Sports Med 32:1385-1393, 2004 7–4

Introduction.—The high rate of ankle sprains and their negative consequences for future sports participation in volleyball necessitates the need for effective preventive measures. Some evidence supports the theory that a proprioceptive balance board program is effective in the prevention of ankle sprains in volleyball players. The effect of a proprioceptive balance board training program on the incidence of ankle sprains in volleyball players was evaluated in a prospective controlled trial.

Methods.—A total of 116 male and female volleyball teams from the second and third Dutch volleyball divisions were followed up prospectively during the 2001-2002 season. Teams were randomly assigned by 4 geographical regions to an intervention group (66 teams, 641 players) or a control group (50 teams, 486 players). Teams in the intervention group followed a prescribed balance board training program; control teams followed their normal training routine. The coaches documented exposure on a weekly basis for each player. Injuries were recorded by the players within 1 week after onset.

Results.—Significantly fewer ankle sprains were reported in the intervention than in the control group (risk difference, 0.4/1000 playing hours; 95% CI, 0.1-0.7). A significant decrease in ankle sprain risk was observed only in players with a history of ankle sprains. The incidence of overuse knee injuries in players with a history of knee injuries was higher in the intervention group.

Conclusion.—The proprioceptive balance board program is effective in the prevention of a recurrence of an ankle sprain among volleyball players. A history of knee injury may be a contraindication to participation in this intervention program.

Prophylactic Ankle Taping and Bracing: A Numbers-Needed-to-Treat and Cost-Benefit Analysis

Olmsted LC, Vela LI, Denegar CR, et al (Pennsylvania State Univ, Univ Park)

J Athl Train 39:95-100, 2004 7–5

Introduction.—Taping and bracing are believed to reduce the incidence of ankle sprains; however, few trials have addressed the effect of preventive measures on the incidence of ankle sprains. The effectiveness of ankle taping and bracing in decreasing the incidence of ankle sprains was determined by application of a numbers-needed-to-treat (NNT) analysis to previously published trials.

Methods.—Searches of PubMed, CINAHL, SPORT Discus, and PEDro were performed; reference lists of resulting articles were also reviewed. Articles that did not address the effects of ankle taping or bracing on ankle injury rates were not included.

Results.—Of 8 articles identified, 3 permitted calculation of NNT (NNT addresses the clinical usefulness of an intervention by providing estimates of the number of treatments necessary to prevent 1 injury occurrence). In a trial of collegiate intramural basketball players, the prevention of 1 ankle sprain required the taping of 26 athletes with a history of ankle sprains and 143 without a prior history. In a military academy intramural basketball program, the prevention of 1 sprain necessitated bracing of 18 athletes with a history of ankle sprains and 39 athletes with no history. A trial of ankle bracing in competitive soccer players produced an NNT of 5 athletes with a history of prior sprains and 57 without prior sprains. A cost-benefit analysis of ankle taping versus bracing showed that taping was about 3 times more expensive than bracing.

Conclusion.—A greater benefit was observed for the use of prophylactic ankle taping or bracing among athletes with a history of ankle sprains than among athletes without prior strains. The generalizability of these findings to other physically active populations is not known.

► The sprained ankle is probably the most common athletic injury. It involves both genders and is seen in a wide spectrum of sporting activity. Thus, any insight on prophylaxis for this injury is worth noting. A balance board is commonly recommended by trainers and coaches to strengthen and to condition the athlete's ankle, and the carefully done prospective study by Verhagen et al (Abstract 7–4) does provide a scientific basis for this recommendation. The use of a balance board, therefore, might be seriously considered in those sports in which the sprained ankle continues to be a major and common problem. Similarly, Olmsted et al (Abstract 7–5) provide additional insight into what is probably the most common effective prophylactic measure: ankle taping. This ritualistic technique is not effective in preventing ankle sprains but is of value in providing some measure of protection for those who have sustained a previous ankle ligament injury.

B. F. Morrey, MD

Midterm Results of a Modified Evans Repair for Chronic Lateral Ankle Instability

Baltopoulos P, Tzagarakis GP, Kaseta MA (Athens Univ, Greece)
Clin Orthop 422:180-185, 2004 7–6

Background.—More than 80 surgical procedures have been described for secondary repair of chronic lateral ankle instability. The Evans procedure has been a popular reconstructive technique that has been reported to provide good and excellent clinical results. However, biomechanical studies and functional evaluations have shown that this method leads to joint changes, including limited motion and long-term development of arthritis. The Evans technique is a nonanatomical procedure that indirectly repairs the ruptured ligaments. The midterm results of a modified Evans repair (which differs from the typical Evans method because of the anatomical view of the procedure) were investigated.

Methods.—A modification of the Evans procedure was used to treat 28 ankles of 27 patients (19 males and 8 females) with chronic instability of the ankle. The diagnosis was assessed by clinical evaluation and radiographic stress tests. All patients were active in sports such as basketball, volleyball, soccer, and running, and all had an acute ankle sprain at 7 to 32 months (average, 17 months) before surgery. The patients ranged in age from 17 to 33 years at the time of surgery.

Results.—Of the 27 patients, 25 were available for follow-up at a mean of 99.6 months (8.3 years; range, 28-117 months). Midterm results were evaluated by the ankle-hindfoot score of the American Orthopaedic Foot and Ankle Society and postoperative radiographic stress tests. The current reconstruction procedure, according to this scoring system, resulted in 92.64 points (range, 63-100 points). However, moderate restriction in hindfoot inversion was observed in 9 patients (34.61%). A positive anterior drawer sign (more than 8 mm) was present in 3 ankles (11.5%). There were mild degenerative joint changes in 5 ankles (19.2%).

Conclusion.—The modification of the Evans procedure currently in use for treatment of chronic lateral instability of the ankle provided a satisfactory clinical and functional midterm outcome as measured on a numeric scale.

▶ Several recent articles have suggested a more anatomical reconstruction of the lateral talofibular ligaments is preferable to that realized with the Evans procedure. This study suggests that the modified Evans technique can be effective in stabilizing the ankle with midterm surveillance. The restriction of hind foot inversion is noted, as well as the residual laxity. The modification does attempt to more closely assimilate the normal anatomy in its reconstruction. This may account for the favorable results reported by these investigators. The reconstruction continues to be attractive in its simplicity.

B. F. Morrey, MD

Nonoperative Treatment of Partial-Thickness Meniscal Tears Identified During Anterior Cruciate Ligament Reconstruction

Zemanovic JR, McAllister DR, Hame SL (Univ of California, Los Angeles)

Orthopedics 27:755-758, 2004 7–7

Introduction.—Partial-thickness tears of the menisci associated with ACL injury are common, yet are considerably less investigated than ACL injuries. Treatment of partial-thickness tears has not been standardized. The incidence of partial-thickness meniscal tears detected at ACL reconstruction and the success of nonoperative treatment were examined.

Methods.—During a 2-year period, 101 consecutive patients undergoing arthroscopically assisted ACL reconstruction were followed up prospectively. Patients who also had a concomitant posterior cruciate ligament injury, tibial plateau fracture, prior ACL reconstruction, or prior meniscectomy were excluded. Ninety patients (35 females, 55 males) with an average age of 28 years (range, 14-54 years) were included.

Patients underwent ACL reconstruction at an average of 18 months post injury (range, 21 days to 15 years) and were followed up for an average of 24.6 months postoperatively (range, 12-38 months). During ACL reconstruction, both menisci were examined and probed arthroscopically. All patients underwent standardized post-ACL reconstruction rehabilitation immediately postoperatively.

Participants were followed up clinically for the development of meniscal symptoms. At an average of 2 years after the procedure, patients were contacted by telephone. Modified Lysholm scores and Tegner activity scores were calculated.

Results.—A complete ACL tear was identified in all patients at the time of surgery. Meniscal pathology was detected in 55 patients (61%); 43 tears

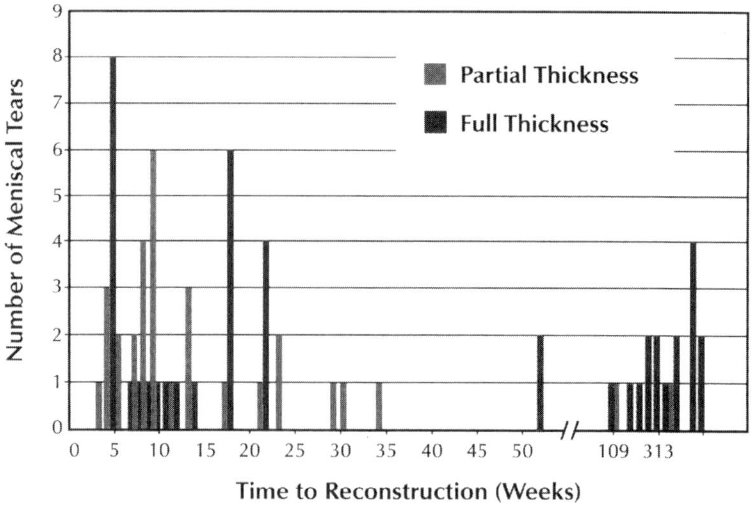

FIGURE 2.—Incidence of full-thickness and partial-thickness meniscus tears relative to time between injury and ACL reconstruction. (Courtesy of Zemanovic JR, McAllister DR, Hame SL: Nonoperative treatment of partial-thickness meniscal tears identified during anterior cruciate ligament reconstruction. *Orthopedics* 27:755-758, 2004.)

(59%) were lateral meniscal tears and 30 (41%) tears were medial meniscal tears. Thirteen and 27 patients, respectively, had isolated medial and lateral meniscal tears. Of the 73 meniscal tears identified, 31 (42%) were stable partial-thickness tears; 23 were in the lateral meniscus and 8 were in the medial thickness. One patient had 2 partial-thickness tears (both lateral meniscus) and 1 had 3 partial-thickness tears (2 lateral meniscus, 1 medial meniscus).

Partial-thickness and full-thickness tears had an average injury-to-surgery interval of 28 weeks and 120 weeks, respectively ($P = .02$) (Fig 2). The use of data from 24 of 28 patients (86%) with partial-thickness meniscus tears gave an average modified Lysholm score of 92.1. The average Tegner activity score was 5.

Conclusion.—Partial-thickness tears of the menisci are frequently observed at ACL reconstruction. The lateral meniscus was involved 3 times as often as the medial meniscus. Partial-thickness tears were observed more acutely after ACL injury; full-thickness tears were more common in delayed ACL reconstruction. Excellent knee function scores may be anticipated when partial-thickness tears detected at ACL reconstruction are treated nonoperatively.

► Most surgeons do not feel comfortable leaving partial tear of the menisci in the face of ACL reconstruction for reasons demonstrated in the study reviewed above. This interesting contribution does, however, reveal that the partial tear behaves differently than full-thickness injuries. This observation, along with the documentation that most partial tears are of the lateral compartment, is consistent with the report of Shelbourne and Heinrich (see Abstract 7–11) also reviewed here.

B. F. Morrey, MD

Eight- to 14-Year Followup of Arthroscopic Meniscal Repair

Kimura M, Shirakura K, Higuchi H, et al (Zenshukai Hosp, Ninomiya, Maebashi, Japan; Gunma Univ, Showa, Maebashi, Japan)

Clin Orthop 421:175-180, 2004 7–8

Introduction.—Repaired tissue is different from and weaker than normal meniscus. Re-tears of repaired menisci can occur after healing. It is not known whether repaired menisci are able to have normal meniscus function in the long term. The mid-term to long-term progression of arthroscopic meniscal repair was examined by second-look arthroscopy.

Methods.—Between 1984 and 1989, 97 arthroscopic meniscal repairs were performed in 96 patients. The second-look arthroscopy was performed at a mean of 10 months after repair. Fifty-three of 96 patients (54 menisci) underwent second-look arthroscopy at an average of 10 months (range, 2-30 months) after repair. A total of 28 patients (28 menisci) were examined at 8 to 14 months (mean, 10.2 years); 8 after isolated meniscal repair (Isolated group) and 20 after concomitant ACL reconstruction (ACL group).

Results.—No participants in the Isolated or ACL group had meniscal signs at long-term follow-up. The mean overall Lysholm's functional scores were 95.4 points (85-100 points); mean scores for the Isolated and ACL groups were 98.1 points (range, 90-100 points) and 94.3 points (range, 85-100 points), respectively.

Four patients in the ACL group rated their outcome as good; 24 rated their outcome as excellent. No participants in the Isolated group and 12 in the ACL group had osteoarthritic changes observed in radiographs. Four and 19 patients, respectively, had increased signal intensity on MRI scans. Ten patients in the ACL group had changes of grade 3 severity.

No meniscal signs or symptoms were detected. No significant relationship between findings of radiographs and MRI scans was seen. ACL-reconstructed knees that were changed to grade 3 severity, as observed on MRI scans, had higher sagittal instability observed on stress radiographs compared with grade 2 or less severe changes. The anterior laxity of the knees impacted the severity of meniscal signal changes on the MRI scans.

Conclusion.—Excellent mid-term to long-term progression of arthroscopic meniscal repair was observed in functional score, radiographs, and MRI scans.

► This important article continues to emphasize the relationship of the integrity of the menisci in association with ACL deficiency. The authors clearly demonstrate that the increased severity of arthritic changes correlates with sagittal instability. The emphasis, therefore, is long-term protection of the knee, which would seem to be afforded by a repaired menisci and ACL reconstruction.

B. F. Morrey, MD

Long-term Results After Combined Medial Meniscal Allograft Transplantation and Anterior Cruciate Ligament Reconstruction: Minimum 8.5-Year Follow-up Study

Graf KW Jr, Sekiya JK, Wojtys EM (Univ of Michigan, Ann Arbor; Naval Med Ctr Portsmouth, Va)

Arthroscopy 20:129-140, 2004 7–9

Introduction.—Given the important role of the meniscus in knee function, orthopedic surgeons seek to preserve the meniscus whenever possible. Partial or total meniscectomy may be necessary in cases in which retaining or repairing an injured meniscus is not always possible. Meniscal allograft transplantation is an attractive option, particularly in relatively young patients with intact chrondral surfaces. The long-term results after medial meniscal allograft transplantation combined with ACL reconstruction were examined in a retrospective clinical outcome trial.

Methods.—Between 1990 and 1992, 9 medial meniscal allograft transplantations were performed in patients with symptomatic knees with a previous total or near-total medial meniscectomy. One of the 9 patients needed transplant removal postoperatively due to a presumed low-grade infection versus immune reaction. Eight patients were evaluated. An ACL reconstruction was performed in all 8 patients. One patient also underwent a staged high tibial osteotomy. The average follow-up was 9.7 years.

Results.—All 8 patients were assessed by the standard Internal Knee Documentation Committee (IKDC) form with no normal scores. One patient had a nearly normal score, 4 had abnormal scores, and 3 had severely abnormal scores. The IKDC symptoms assessment yielded 2 normal scores, 5 nearly normal scores, and 1 abnormal score. The IKDC function test produced 5 normal scores, 1 nearly normal score, and 2 abnormal scores. Six patients reported being extremely satisfied with the function of the affected knee and were active in recreational sports. All 8 patients indicated they would recommend the procedure to a friend and would undergo the procedure again under similar circumstances.

Conclusion.—Consistent with earlier short-term follow-up reports, reliable improvement was observed in pain, swelling, stability, and knee function at an average of 9.7 years after the index procedure. The addition of a ligament-stabilizing procedure probably improved the outcome in this patient population.

► The presentation of the long-term results after combined meniscal allograft and ACL reconstruction emphasizes the validity of the findings of the first study. This strategy does demonstrate the value of allograft transplantation compared to those knees that are medial meniscus-deficient. It provides further insight with regard not only to the essential elements of long-term progressive pathology in the cruciate/meniscus–deficient knee, but also the expected outcomes of viable options for intervention.

B. F. Morrey, MD

Healing Potential of Meniscal Tears Without Repair in Knees With Anterior Cruciate Ligament Reconstruction

Yagishita K, Muneta T, Ogiuchi T, et al (Tokyo Med and Dental Univ)

Am J Sports Med 32:1953-1961, 2004 7–10

Background.—Few previous studies have documented the healing potential of meniscal tears that are left to heal without repair.

Purpose.—To determine the healing rates of meniscal tears left without repair in knees with anterior cruciate ligament reconstruction.

Study Design.—Prospective cohort study.

Methods.—One hundred and ninety-two knees were evaluated at the time of anterior cruciate ligament reconstruction and repeat arthroscopy. The healing rates of 41 medial and 42 lateral torn menisci without repair were evaluated by the same 2 surgeons in an identical fashion.

Results.—Of 41 medial torn menisci left without repair, 22 (56%) were considered completely healed, 3 (7%) were incompletely healed, 11 (24%) were unhealed, and 5 (10%) had expanded unhealed lesions. Of 42 lateral torn menisci, 31 (74%) were considered completely healed, 2 (5%) were incompletely healed, 6 (14%) were unhealed, and 3 (7%) had expanded unhealed lesions. The healing rate of a medial meniscal tear was length dependent and not related to reconstructed ligament stability.

Conclusions.—Stable meniscal tears at the time of anterior cruciate ligament reconstruction possibly could be left in situ. However, longer medial meniscal tears are thought to require additional stabilizing procedures.

▶ This article is of interest in that it shows the high percentage of healing potential of a torn meniscus at the time of ACL reconstruction. The natural history of the alternate option, specifically leaving the anterior cruciate–deficient knee untreated, is well known to place the menisci at risk. This study, therefore, further confirms the protective value of anterior cruciate function that is typically restored with a reconstructive procedure.

B. F. Morrey, MD

The Long-term Evaluation of Lateral Meniscus Tears Left In Situ at the Time of Anterior Cruciate Ligament Reconstruction

Shelbourne KD, Heinrich J (Methodist Hosp, Indianapolis, Ind)

Arthroscopy 20:346-351, 2004 7–11

Introduction.—Meniscus damage occurs in about 70% of patients at the time of ACL damage, with lateral meniscus tears being observed more com-

TABLE 2.—Subjective Scores

Type of Lateral Meniscus Tear	No.	Time After Surgery (yr)	Pain*	Activity Level†	Modified Total Score‡
Posterior horn tears	55	7.5 ± 3.8	17.0 ± 2.9	18.8 ± 2.7	92.2 ± 11.9
Radial flap tears	36	5.8 ± 2.7	17.0 ± 3.4	19.1 ± 2.2	93.4 ± 8.1
Peripheral or posterior tears left in situ	117	6.2 ± 3.5	17.3 ± 3.1	19.3 ± 1.8	94.8 ± 6.0
Peripheral or posterior tears abraded and trephined	31	7.3 ± 2.7	17.0 ± 2.9	19.1 ± 1.8	93.6 ± 7.0

Note: Scores are mean ± standard deviation.
*Subjective pain scores with maximum of 20 points = no pain.
†Activity level scores with a maximum of 20 points = normal level of activity.
‡Subjective Noyes score with a maximum of 100 points.
(Reprinted from Shelbourne KD, Heinrich J: The long-term evaluation of lateral meniscus tears left in situ at the time of anterior cruciate ligament reconstruction. *Arthroscopy* 20:346-351, 2004. Copyright 2004, with permission from The Arthroscopy Association of North America.)

monly than medial meniscal tears at the time of acute ACL reconstructions. Reviewed were the long-term subjective and objective outcomes of patients with lateral meniscus tears identified at the time of ACL reconstruction that were left in situ or abraded and trephined, not repaired or removed.

Methods.—With the use of a database of patients who underwent ACL reconstruction between 1987 and 1998, 332 patients were identified who had lateral meniscus tears that were left in situ or underwent abrasion and trephination. Excluded were patients who had undergone lateral or medial partial meniscectomy or prior knee surgery or had greater than grade II chondromalacia in any knee compartment.

Tears were classified as posterior horn tears in 70 patients, stable radial flap tears in 50, and peripheral or posterior tears in 212. Subjective assessment was performed by a modified Noyes knee questionnaire. The International Knee Documentation Committee criteria were used for objective evaluation.

Results.—At a mean of 6.6 years (range, 2-16.5 years) postoperatively, the mean modified Noyes score for 239 patients was 93.8 points (Table 2). At a mean of 5.1 years postoperatively, the objective International Knee Documentation Committee score for 163 of 170 patients (96%) was normal or nearly normal. Radiographic examination revealed that 162 patients (95%) had a normal rating, 6 had a nearly normal rating, and 2 had an abnormal rating. Of 332 patients evaluated, only 8 (2.4%) needed subsequent surgery for the lateral meniscus.

Conclusion.—Lateral meniscus tears that are posterior horn tears, stable flap tears, or peripheral or posterior third tears which do not continue further than 1 cm in front of the popliteus tendon can be treated successfully by means of abrasion and trephination or by being left in situ.

► This impressive contribution is the largest of its kind with the longest follow-up of patients with a lateral meniscus tear in conjunction with ACL reconstruction. The documentation of the type of tear and the expected long-term status of the meniscus is extremely valuable in determining the management of these patients in the acute setting. The observation that the lateral meniscus may and should be left in situ is extremely important and is now well recognized and accepted

B. F. Morrey, MD

Meniscal Transplantation in Symptomatic Patients Less Than Fifty Years Old

Noyes FR, Barber-Westin SDB, Rankin M (Cincinnati Sportsmedicine and Orthopaedic Ctr, Ohio)

J Bone Joint Surg Am 86-A:1392-1404, 2004 7–12

Background.—There has been an increase in interest in recent years in the repair of meniscal tears, including complex tears that extend into the central avascular zone. However, some meniscal tears are not repairable, particularly if there is considerable tissue damage. Transplantation of human menisci should restore some load-bearing meniscal function. However, inconsistent results have been obtained in experimental studies. Clinical investigators have disagreed on the outcome and success rates of human menisci transplantation.

The primary candidate for this procedure is a young patient who has had a total meniscectomy and has pain in the tibiofemoral compartment because of early joint arthrosis. There are few treatment options for these patients, and the goal of meniscal transplantation is to provide pain relief and to delay the progression of tibiofemoral arthrosis. The outcomes of meniscal transplantation in a consecutive series of younger patients treated for pain in the tibiofemoral compartment after a previous meniscectomy were prospectively evaluated.

Methods.—Forty cryopreserved menisci were implanted in 38 patients. Sixteen knees also had an osteochondral autograft transfer, and 9 had a knee ligament reconstruction. Clinical outcomes and the failure rate of all transplants were evaluated at a mean of 40 months postoperatively. Meniscal allograft characteristics were determined with the use of a rating system that combined subjective, clinical, and MRI factors.

Results.—The knee condition was rated as improved in 34 of 38 (89%) patients. Prior to surgery, 30 patients (79%) had pain with daily activities, but only 4 (11%) had pain with daily activities at the time of the latest follow-up.

Conclusion.—The short-term results of meniscal transplantation are encouraging in terms of pain reduction and increased function in the knee. However, the long-term effects of transplant function and any chondroprotective effects are unknown and in need of additional study.

▶ The value of the meniscus in normal knee function is well recognized. In those patients in whom the meniscus has been removed or is irreparable, the viability of meniscal transplantation has been recently considered. This study represents one of the largest experiences with intermediate term surveillance, suggesting that the outcome of meniscal transplantation can be encouraging. The authors correctly emphasize that the protective value of meniscus transplantation is only surmised and, hence, the long-term benefits, if any, have not been documented in this experience.

B. F. Morrey, MD

Arthroscopic Evaluation of the Articular Cartilage After Anterior Cruciate Ligament Reconstruction: A Short-term Prospective Study of 105 Patients

Asano H, Muneta T, Ikeda H, et al (Tokyo Med and Dental Univ)
Arthroscopy 20:474-481, 2004 7–13

Introduction.—The value of surgical repair and stabilization in decreasing the incidence of posttraumatic osteoarthritis is controversial. Several trials have reported that in many knees with reconstructed ACL, osteoarthritis develops postoperatively. No trials have reported early cartilage changes after ACL reconstruction. The articular cartilage lesion at reconstruction and second-look arthroscopy were examined in 105 patients.

Methods.—Cartilage lesions were examined arthroscopically in the 6 articular surfaces independently. Characteristics were categorized by modified Outerbridge's classification. The articular cartilage at reconstruction and at second-look arthroscopy were compared.

Results.—A significant worsening of the status of the articular cartilage was observed after ACL reconstruction. This worsening was identified at all articular surfaces except the lateral femoral condyle. Most changes involved softening or fibrillation. Anterior laxity and meniscal lesion had no association with a progression of degenerative change of articular cartilage. The patient's age was a significant factor in progression of articular cartilage damage after reconstruction.

Conclusion.—The status of articular cartilage was significantly worsened post-ACL reconstruction. Potential risk factors producing articular cartilage damage include female gender and age 30 years or older.

► With an ever increasing incidence of ligament injury and ACL reconstruction, the question of articular injury and subsequent degeneration in the ACL-deficient knee remains one that is constantly being considered and addressed. This important study does demonstrate that the articular cartilage at the time of the ACL reconstruction does tend to deteriorate, even in the short term. This observation should be shared with patients undergoing ACL reconstruction. Fortunately, most patients do well clinically long term. Nonetheless, these findings should be considered in this patient population.

B. F. Morrey, MD

The Effect of Anterior Cruciate Ligament Reconstruction on the Risk of Knee Reinjury

Dunn WR, Lyman S, Lincoln AE, et al (Hosp for Special Surgery, New York; Veterans Affairs Med Ctr, Washington, DC; Johns Hopkins Bloomberg School of Public Health, Baltimore, Md; et al)

Am J Sports Med 32:1906-1913, 2004 7–14

Background.—Although there is evidence that very active, young patients are better served with anterior cruciate ligament reconstruction, there is a lack of objective data demonstrating that future knee injury is prevented by these procedures.

Hypothesis.—Anterior cruciate ligament reconstruction protects against reinjury of the knee that would require reoperation.

Study Design.—Retrospective cohort study.

Methods.—A cohort of 6576 active-duty army personnel who had been hospitalized for anterior cruciate ligament injury from 1990 to 1996 were identified. Using the Total Army Injury and Health Outcomes Database, the authors followed these individuals for up to 9 years and collected clinical, demographic, and occupational data. These data were evaluated with bivariate and multivariable analyses to determine the effect of anterior cruciate ligament reconstruction on the rate of knee reinjury that required operation.

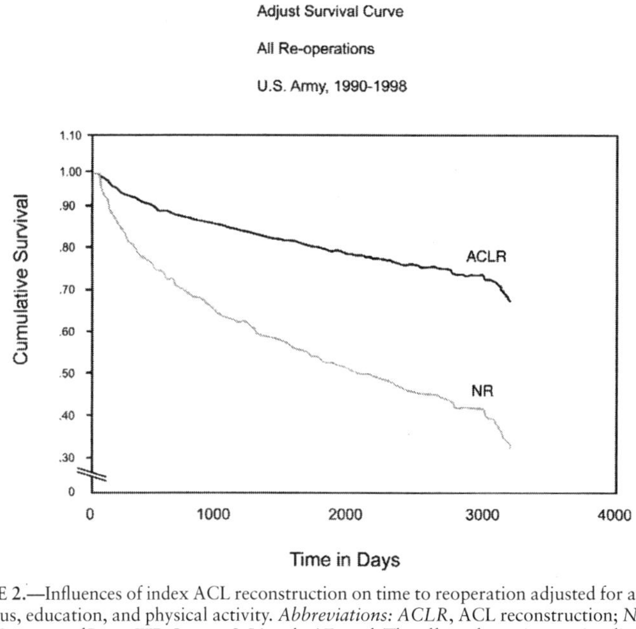

FIGURE 2.—Influences of index ACL reconstruction on time to reoperation adjusted for age, race, sex, marital status, education, and physical activity. *Abbreviations: ACLR*, ACL reconstruction; *NR*, no reconstruction. (Courtesy of Dunn WR, Lyman S, Lincoln AE, et al: The effect of anterior cruciate ligament reconstruction on the risk of knee reinjury. *Am J Sports Med* 32:1906-1913, 2004.)

Results.—Of the 6576 study subjects, 3795 subjects (58%) underwent anterior cruciate ligament reconstruction and 2781 (42%) did not. The rate of reoperation was significantly lower among the anterior cruciate ligament reconstruction group (4.90/100 person-years) compared with those treated conservatively (13.86/100 person-years; $P < .0001$) (Fig 2). Proportional hazard regression analyses adjusted for age, race, sex, marital status, education, and physical activity level confirmed that anterior cruciate ligament reconstruction was protective against meniscal and cartilage reinjury ($P < .0001$). Secondary medial meniscal injury was more common than secondary lateral meniscal injury ($P < .003$). Younger age was the strongest predictor of failure of conservative management leading to late anterior cruciate ligament reconstruction ($P < .0001$).

Conclusions.—Anterior cruciate ligament reconstruction protected against reoperation in this young, active population; younger subjects were more likely to require late anterior cruciate ligament reconstruction.

Clinical Relevance.—Strong consideration should be given to anterior cruciate ligament reconstruction after anterior cruciate ligament injury in young, active individuals.

▶ The editor has long been waiting for a definitive answer for this question that requires a large cohort with reasonable follow-up. Such an opportunity exists in the military, which is the source of this article. Consistent with the theme of other reviewed articles in this volume, this study clearly demonstrates a protective effect of the ACL, not for a subsequent injury of the meniscus, but on the risk of knee reinjury in general. Once again, strong evidence to support the value of ligament reconstruction, particularly in the presence of a positive pivot shift test.

B. F. Morrey, MD

Functional Bracing After Anterior Cruciate Ligament Reconstruction: A Prospective, Randomized, Multicenter Study

McDevitt ER, Taylor DC, Miller MD, et al (United States Naval Academy, Annapolis, Md; United States Military Academy, West Point, NY; Univ of Virginia, Charlottesville; et al)

Am J Sports Med 32:1887-1892, 2004 7–15

Background.—Bracing after anterior cruciate ligament reconstruction is expensive and is not proven to prevent injuries or influence outcomes.

Purpose.—To determine whether postoperative functional knee bracing influences outcomes.

Study Design.—Prospective, randomized, multicenter clinical trial.

Methods.—One hundred volunteers from the 3 US service academies with acute anterior cruciate ligament tears were randomized into braced or nonbraced groups. Only those subjects with anterior cruciate ligament tears treated surgically within the first 8 weeks of injury were included. Patients with chondral injuries, significant meniscal tears, or multiple knee ligament injuries were excluded. Surgical procedures and the postoperative physical therapy protocols were identical for both groups. The braced group was instructed to wear an off-the-shelf functional knee brace for all cutting, pivoting, or jumping activities for the first year after surgery.

Results.—Ninety-five subjects were available with a minimum 2-year follow-up. There were no statistically significant differences between groups in knee stability, functional testing with the single-legged hop test, International Knee Documentation Committee scores, Lysholm scores, knee range of motion, or isokinetic strength testing. Two braced subjects had reinjuries, and 3 nonbraced subjects had reinjuries.

Conclusions.—In this young, active population, postoperative bracing does not appear to change the clinical outcomes after anterior cruciate ligament reconstruction.

▶ This interesting study from 3 service academies would appear to offer valid insights referable to the postoperative management of an ACL. Although I personally feel as though the findings are valid and the methodology appears to be reasonable, it is unlikely that the orthopedic sports medicine community is ready for the findings. On the other hand, as greater attention is paid towards functional and repetitive rehabilitation programs, there is little doubt that this study will be repeated and, in all likelihood, the findings will be confirmed. Ultimately, this study may well alter the manner in which patients are treated postoperatively after ACL reconstruction.

B. F. Morrey, MD

Relationships Between Objective Assessment of Ligament Stability and Subjective Assessment of Symptoms and Function After Anterior Cruciate Ligament Reconstruction

Kocher MS, Steadman JR, Briggs KK, et al (Steadman Hawkins Sports Medicine Found, Vail, Colo; Harvard Med School, Boston; Harvard School of Public Health, Boston)

Am J Sports Med 32:629-634, 2004 7–16

Introduction.—The objective evaluation of ACL injury by instrumented knee laxity, Lachman examination, and pivot-shift examination is helpful in the diagnosis of ACL injury. These tests are commonly emphasized and reported after ACL reconstruction. The association between objective evaluation of ligament laxity and subjective evaluation of symptoms and function after ACL reconstruction has not been established. The relationship between objective evaluation of ligament stability and subjective evaluation of symptoms and function after ACL reconstruction was examined.

Methods.—A total of 202 patients undergoing ACL reconstruction with 2-year minimum follow-up were evaluated. At follow-up, patients underwent objective determinations of instrumented laxity, Lachman examination, and pivot-shift examination. Subjective variables of symptoms evaluated at follow-up were pain, swelling, giving way, locking, crepitus, stiffness, and limping. Subjective function measures evaluated at follow-up included walking, squatting, stair climbing, running, cutting, jumping, twisting, activity limitation, sports level, activities of daily living, work level, knee function, sports participation, Lysholm score, and satisfaction with outcome.

Results.—Instrumented knee laxity and Lachman examination had no significant ($P < .05$) association with any subjective variables of symptoms and function. Pivot-shift examination had significant correlations with satisfaction ($P = .03$), partial giving way ($P = .01$), full giving way ($P = .01$), difficulty cutting ($P = .01$), difficulty twisting ($P = .01$), activity limitation ($P = .01$), overall knee function ($P = .03$), sports participation ($P = .02$), and Lysholm score ($P = .01$).

Conclusion.—The pivot-shift examination may be a superior measure of "functional instability" compared to instrumented knee laxity or Lachman examination after ACL reconstruction.

► This article was included possibly because it simply confirms my clinical impression. In the final analysis, the presence or absence of a Lachman is the single most significant finding that relates to a patient's knee function in the presence of ACL deficiency. This article simply provides a scientific basis for this previously held clinical impression.

B. F. Morrey, MD

Positive Pivot Shift After ACL Reconstruction Predicts Later Osteoarthrosis: 63 Patients Followed 5-9 Years After Surgery

Jonsson H, Riklund-Åhlström K, Lind J (Univ Hosp of Northern Sweden, Umeå)

Acta Orthop Scand 75:594-599, 2004 7–17

Background.—Rupture of the anterior cruciate ligament (ACL) may cause osteoarthrosis (OA) and functional impairment. We wanted to find out whether the degree of knee stability obtained after ACL reconstruction correlates with radiographic and clinical outcome.

Patients and Methods.—We examined 63 patients 2 and 5-9 years after anterior cruciate ligament (ACL) reconstruction. Knee stability was assessed 2 years after surgery by recording AP laxity using radiostereometric technique (RSA) and by performing the pivot shift test. Degeneration of the knee joint was evaluated with bone scintigraphy, and radiographically. Functional outcome was assessed with Lysholm score, Tegner activity scale and with the one-leg hop test.

Results.—Radiographic signs of osteoarthrosis at the most recent follow-up (5-9 years) did not correlate with knee stability. Patients with positive pivot shift test 2 years after surgery showed increased scintigraphic activity of the subchondral bone at the most recent follow-up (Fig 4), and inferior subjective functional outcome 2 years after surgery. Knees having had meniscus resections had more often OA. Radiographical signs of OA were associated with higher scintigraphic uptake in the operated knee relative to the contralateral knee.

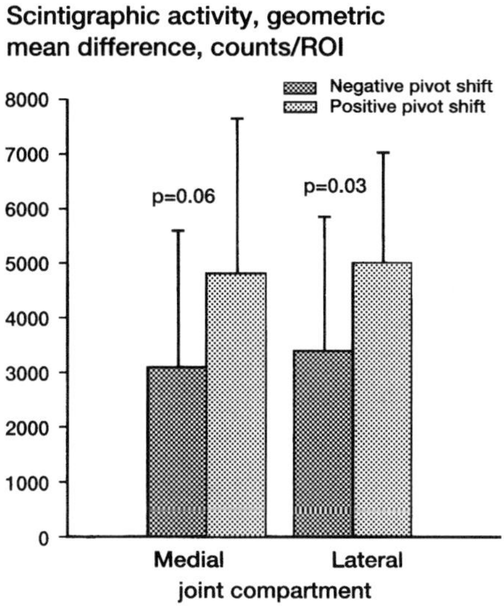

FIGURE 4.—Results of pivot shift test 2 years after surgery in 50 patients and difference in scintigraphic uptake (geometric mean) 5 to 9 years after surgery. ACL reconstructed–contralateral knees (mean values and SD). *Abbreviation: ROI*, Region of interest. (Courtesy of Jonsson H, Riklund-Åhlström K, Lind J: Positive pivot shift after ACL reconstruction predicts later osteoarthrosis: 63 patients followed 5-9 years after surgery. *Acta Orthop Scand* 75:594-599, 2004.)

Interpretation.—The ability to obliterate the pivoting by ACL reconstruction appears to be more important than normalizing the AP laxity in order to prevent later OA.

► It is the editor's opinion and confirmed by numerous subsequent studies that the most sensitive clinical finding referable to a systematic anterior cruciate–deficient knee is that of a positive pivot shift maneuver. This contribution is, therefore, felt to be important in that the same finding after reconstruction also correlates to subsequent radiographic OA. It should be noted that this is a relatively small sample and that the inclusion criteria as well as the extent of injury of the cohort are not well described. Nonetheless, the conclusions would appear to be valid given the long-term follow-up that was achieved.

B. F. Morrey, MD

Primary Repair of Posterior Cruciate Ligament Avulsion Fracture: The Effect of Occult Injury in the Midsubstance on Postoperative Instability
Inoue M, Yasuda K, Kondon E, et al (NTT East Japan Sapporo Hosp, Japan; Hokkaido Univ, Sapporo, Japan)
Am J Sports Med 32:1230-1237, 2004 7–18

Background.—Restoring posterior cruciate ligament (PCL) function in knees with an avulsion fracture requires surgical intervention, specifically, open reduction and internal fixation of the bony fragment. This is recommended during the acute phase of the injury to obtain satisfactory results. Even with this approach, about 60% of the injured knees exhibit a mild but significant posterior instability. This residual instability has been attributed to hidden or occult injuries inside the PCL midsubstance that produce dysfunction. This hypothesis was tested with the use of MRI to find occult midsubstance injury and determine its contribution to residual posterior instability.

Methods.—A prospective comparative clinical study design was used to evaluate 31 patients during 2 to 8 years. MRI scans obtained immediately after injury were used to divide the group into those having an occult injury (15 knees) and those having no injury (16 knees).

Results.—The group with occult injury had an average side-to-side difference in total AP laxity of 3.2 mm, and the noninjured group had a measurement of 3.0 mm of the same variable. No significant difference was noted in total AP laxity between the groups. Nine (60%) patients in the occult group and 10 (62.5%) in the noninjured group had a side-to-side difference exceeding 3 mm. Sixty-six percent of the occult group and 69% of the noninjured group had mild residual posterior instability, but these values did not differ significantly. Range of knee motion averaged 135° and 133° in the occult and noninjured groups, respectively. Neither the knee score nor that range of knee motion differed significantly between the 2 groups. The average Lysholm score was 89.4 points for the occult group and 91.9 points for the noninjured group. No significant correlation was found between the MRI results and the Lysholm score.

Conclusions.—Orthopedic surgeons need not worry about an occult midsubstance injury in the treatment of avulsion fracture of the PCL. The results obtained with these patients show that occult injury of the PCL midsubstance has no significant effect on postoperative posterior knee instability.

► The need for immediate repair of PCL tears remains somewhat controversial. This interesting study takes the question 1 step further and investigates the relevance of a substance tear occurring with the avulsed fragment. The observation that there is no additional residual instability even in the presence of the midsubstance tear is comforting. It allows the surgeon to treat the injury by direct repair without a concern for residual stretching or instability. The prospective and randomized nature of this study strengthens the validity of these observations.

B. F. Morrey, MD

8 Foot and Ankle

Introduction

A tremendous volume of literature has appeared this year referable to foot and ankle pathology and surgery. An effort was made to cover a spectrum of topics that are of particular relevance to the busy orthopedic practice. The selections, therefore, include what we feel are reliable long-term studies of various reconstructive options of the foot and ankle. The emerging value of joint replacement arthroplasty is also recognized with the inclusion of articles with a reasonably large sample of patients followed for a sufficient period to begin to understand the expectation and potential problems of the newer ankle replacement designs. Nonoperative techniques are also included to round out this section.

Bernard F. Morrey, MD

Recall of the Risks of Forefoot Surgery After Informed Consent

Shurnas PS, Coughlin ML (Regional Orthopaedic Health Care, Mountain Home, Ark; Oregon Health Sciences Univ, Portland)

Foot Ankle Int 24:904-908, 2003 8–1

Background.—One of the major reasons cited for litigation against physicians and surgeons is a lack of informed consent. Another major cause of claims for compensation is the issue of complications related to surgery. It is assumed in the concept of informed consent that the patient is competent to understand the explanation of the nature, risks, and benefits of proposed surgery and alternatives to this surgery. It is also assumed that these points are explained in terms that the patient can understand. Previous studies have reported that providing more detailed and complete information has no advantage over a simple explanation in terms of patient anxiety and comprehension of a proposed surgical procedure.

One aspect of the informed consent process is a patient's understanding of the risks of his or her proposed surgery. When patients acknowledge that they understand the risks of the proposed procedure, can they recall those risks? This study set out to determine the number of risks a patient can recall from the informed consent process before surgery, to determine whether recall can be improved with a visual aid, and to assess patient satisfaction with the informed consent process utilized.

RISKS OF SURGERY OF THE FOREFOOT

1. *DEFORMITY* **DOES NOT GO AWAY COMPLETELY**
2. *DEFORMITY* **COMES BACK AGAIN**
3. *INCISION* **HEALING PROBLEM**
4. *INFECTION* **OF THE SKIN, DEEP TISSUE, JOINTS OR BONE**
5. *PAIN* **DOES NOT GO AWAY OR IS WORSE**
6. *LOSS* **OF TOES OR FOOT,** *AMPUTATION*
7. *SCAR* **FORMATION**
8. *STIFFNESS* **DOES NOT GO AWAY OR GETS WORSE**
9. **LOSS OF** *FUNCTION*
10. **NEED FOR** *MORE SURGERY*
11. *DEATH*

I HAVE READ, FULLY DISCUSSED AND UNDERSTAND THESE RISKS ________________________

FIGURE 1.—Visual aid demonstrating the standard 11 risks of forefoot surgery. (Courtesy of Shurnas PS, Coughlin MJ: Recall of the risks of forefoot surgery after informed consent. *Foot Ankle Int* 24:904-908, 2003. Copyright 2003 by the American Orthopaedic Foot and Ankle Society. Reproduced with permission.)

Methods.—From among all patients requiring forefoot surgery, randomly selected patients from August 2001 through October 2001 were assigned to 1 of 2 groups All patients were read the same standard risks of surgery, but only 1 group (group B) was given a visual aid which they read and signed (Fig 1). All patients were asked to recall the risks of surgery and to rate their satisfaction with the informed consent process at their final routine postoperative visit.

Results.—Nineteen patients were assigned to each group. All patients expressed satisfaction with the preoperative informed consent discussion at their final visit. The mean number of the 11 risks recalled per patient was 1 for group A and 0.94 for group B.

Conclusion.—The use of a visual aid had no apparent effect on improving recall of risks of specific surgery in this patient population. At the final routine postoperative visit, patients in both groups had poor or no recall of the 11 risks described for their specific surgery.

► This is an interesting study and demonstrates that the recollection of the risks and benefits discussion prior to this type of surgery reveals surprisingly poor recall. As the authors note, these observations have been made before other types of surgery. The interesting feature of this article is that even in life threatening elective circumstances, patient recall with regard to understanding the risks of surgery is surprisingly limited.

B. F. Morrey, MD

Volume of Ambulatory Care Visits and Patterns of Care for Patients Diagnosed With Plantar Fasciitis: A National Study of Medical Doctors

Riddle DL, Schappert SM (Virginia Commonwealth Univ, Richmond; Ctrs for Disease Control and Prevention, Hyattsville, Md)

Foot Ankle Int 25:303-310, 2004 8–2

Background.—Plantar fasciitis is a relatively common disorder, but little is known about its prevalence; the types of physicians that see patients with the disorder; or how, in national terms, patients are typically managed. National estimates were generated of the volume of patient visits and characteristics of care given to patients given a diagnosis of plantar fasciitis.

Methods.—Data were obtained from the National Ambulatory Medical Care Survey (NAMCS) and the National Hospital Ambulatory Medical Care Survey (NHAMCS) for the years 1995 to 2000. These tools are multistage probability sample surveys of visits to office-based physicians (NAMCS) and visits to nonfederal, short-stay, and general hospitals (NHAMCS) to consult doctors of medicine and osteopathy.

Sample data have been weighted to produce national estimates. Univariate analyses were used to summarize data describing the number of patient visits for plantar fasciitis and the characteristics of the care provided during those visits. Data were combined for the 6 years of the study to increase the reliability of the estimates and were presented as annual averages.

Results.—There were approximately 1 million patient visits per year to office-based physicians and hospital outpatient departments for the diagnosis and treatment of plantar fasciitis during the study period, with about 62% of these visits to primary care practitioners and 31% to orthopedic surgeons. Patient visits for plantar fasciitis accounted for approximately 1% of all patient visits to orthopedic surgeons. The most frequently used intervention (47% of visits) was pain medication, including nonsteroidal anti-inflammatory drugs. Exercise counseling was provided in about 26% of visits, and physical therapy was ordered or provided at 19% of visits.

Conclusion.—Plantar fasciitis is a relatively common condition that is seen by physicians in several specialties. There is no consistent approach to management of plantar fasciitis. Instead, a large amount of variation exists in the way these patients are managed. Additional research is needed to identify effective interventions for plantar fasciitis and to determine whether specialty influences the outcome of treatment.

Extracorporeal Shock Wave Therapy for the Treatment of Plantar Fasciitis

Theodore GH, Buch M, Amendola A, et al (Harvard Med School, Boston; Othopäedische Klinik Kassel, Germany; Univ of Iowa, Iowa City; et al)

Foot Ankle Int 25:290-297, 2004 8–3

Background.—Plantar fasciitis is a common disorder that likely involves a traction degeneration of the plantar fascia band at its origin in the medial calcaneal tuberosity. Many treatments have been developed, and variable success has been reported. Extracorporeal shock wave therapy (ESWT) is evolving as a treatment option for this disorder. Preliminary studies have reported success rates between 4% and 81% in eliminating heel pain. The clinical effectiveness of high-energy ESWT for the treatment of plantar fasciitis in a single therapeutic session was evaluated.

Methods.—A total of 150 patients were enrolled in this multicenter, randomized, placebo-controlled trial. The study group (76 patients) was treated with electromagnetically generated shocks using US guidance during a single treatment session. The control group (74 patients) received a sham treatment under similar clinical conditions. The groups were demographically similar in regard to age, height, and weight. The average duration of symptoms was nearly 2 years in both groups. All of the patients were evaluated by the visual analogue scale for pain, American Orthopaedic Foot and Ankle Society scores, Roles and Maudsley Score, SF-12 health status questionnaire, and physical examination.

Results.—The study group had 56% success at 3 months and 94% success at 12 months after treatment. The control group had 47% success at 3 months after treatment. Data were not collected at 12 months for the control group because they were unblinded at 3 months and offered treatment.

Conclusion.—ESWT is a safe modality for the treatment of chronic proximal plantar asciitis.

► We have included Abstract 8–2 in this year's YEAR BOOK because it highlights a very common condition in most orthopedic surgeon's practice. Furthermore, the fact that there is no universally accepted treatment modality is clearly demonstrated by this large sample survey. The conclusion of this article is that more research is needed in order to determine what treatment influences outcome. The second article in this pair (Abstract 8–3) provides a prospective randomized study regarding ESWT for such patients. The enhanced clinical value of this methodology is noted and thus the conclusions would seem to be reliable and valid.

It is disappointing, however, to note that the study did not allow the 12-month or intermediate-to–long-term follow-up of the control group to be documented since these patients were offered ESWT after the 3-month interval. The editor would emphasize the fact that the 9 percentage points difference at 3 months is often neutralized or diminishes at a 12-month assessment when this modality is used for tennis elbow. Hence, our interpretation of this study is that the ESWT is of value long term, but the other modalities may be equally successful. For the acute "hot" plantar fasciitis, this more expensive modality might be considered, but the data do not allow an accurate statement or documentation of the true long-term benefit.

B. F. Morrey, MD

Infectious and Healing Complications After Elective Orthopaedic Foot and Ankle Surgery During Tumor Necrosis Factor-Alpha Inhibition Therapy

Bibbo C, Goldberg JW (Marshfield Clinic, Wis; Univ of Wisconsin, Madison)

Foot Ankle Int 25:331-335, 2004 8–4

Background.—In patients with rheumatoid arthritis, significant deformities of the ankle and foot can develop, and in these patients multiple surgical procedures are required to achieve long-lasting, balanced corrections. Often these patients are taking multiple medications which possess systemic side effects. Biological response modifiers are assuming a larger role in the management of these patients.

The tumor necrosis factor–α (TNF-α) inhibitors etanercept and infliximab improve patient symptoms and function, but these drugs have been associated with a risk for healing and infectious complications due to systemic blockade of TNF-α, a ubiquitous mediator required in the normal inflammatory response in tissue healing and infection surveillance. The risk of healing and infectious complications was assessed in patients undergoing elective foot and ankle surgery while being treated with etanercept and infliximab.

Methods.—Patients with rheumatoid arthritis who underwent elective foot and ankle surgery over 12 months were prospectively followed up for the development of complications in the postoperative period. All of the patients continued with their antirheumatic medication schedule with no changes in the perioperative period. The data collected included age, all medications used to treat rheumatoid arthritis, smoking history, and number of orthopedic foot and ankle procedures performed.

The 31 patients were then stratified into 2 groups on the basis of the use of immunomodulation via TNF-α inhibition (group 1; 16 patients) versus patients who did not receive TNF-α inhibition therapy (group 2; 15 patients). The groups were followed up and compared for the development of infectious/healing complications.

Results.—The 2 groups were comparable for sex distribution; number of orthopedic procedures performed; and use of steroids, methotrexate, leflunamide, and nonsteroidal anti-inflammatory drugs. Group 1 had 6 times as many smokers as group 2. At a mean follow-up of 10.6 months (group 1) and 9.7 months (group 2), healing or infectious complications were similar in the 2 groups. However, when total complications were analyzed, the patients in group 1 had a lower complication rate.

Conclusion.—The data suggest that in patients with rheumatoid arthritis undergoing elective foot and ankle surgery, TNF-α inhibition agents may be used safely without increasing the risk of healing or infectious complications.

▶ We continue to be impressed with the effectiveness of the disease-remitting agents. The impact to most orthopedic practices is that we see fewer patients with rheumatoid arthritis needing intervention. If these patients are seen, however, frequently they will have been treated with a TNF-α agent. The fact that patients with such treatment and having foot surgery can be safely managed is extremely important. What remains unclear is the value and duration of maintaining patients free of these agents before surgical intervention.

B. F. Morrey, MD

Comprehensive Reconstruction of the Lateral Ankle for Chronic Instabilty Using a Free Gracilis Graft

Coughlin MJ, Schenck RC Jr, Grebing BR, et al (Private Practice Foot and Ankle Orthopedic Surgery, Boise, Idaho; Univ of New Mexico, Albuquerque; Private Practice of Orthopedic Surgery, Belleville, Ill)
Foot Ankle Int 25:231-241, 2004 8–5

Introduction.—The incidence of persistent instability following an acute lateral ankle sprain varies between 15% and 48%. Over 50 surgical procedures have been reported that address restoration of lateral ankle stability. Described were the results of a novel surgical technique for treating chronic lateral ankle instability that uses both a direct repair of the anterior talofibular ligament and a free gracilis tendon transfer (Fig 3) to reconstruct anatomically the anterior talofibular and calcaneofibular ligaments.

Methods.—Medical records were retrospectively reviewed between December 1998 and February 2002. A total of 28 patients (29 ankles) underwent an anatomical reconstruction of the lateral ankle ligaments for chronic ankle instability. Patients underwent clinical and radiologic follow-up evaluations at an average of 23 months postoperatively (range, 12-52 months).

Outcomes were examined by comparing preoperative and postoperative American Orthopedic Foot and Ankle Society (AOFAS) scores and visual analogue pain scores and postoperative Karlsson scores. A subjective self-assessment rating was also performed. All participants underwent preoperative and postoperative radiographic evaluation, including talar tilt and anterior drawer stress radiographs.

Results.—All 28 patients returned for final evaluation. Good or excellent outcomes were achieved on patient subjective self-assessment, pain scores, AOFAS, and Karlsson scores at final follow-up in all participants. The ankle ROM was not affected by the lateral ankle reconstruction. Talar tilt was decreased from a mean of 13° to 3° ($P < .0001$), and the anterior drawer was decreased from a mean of 10 mm to 5 mm ($P < .0001$) by the lateral ankle ligamentous reconstruction.

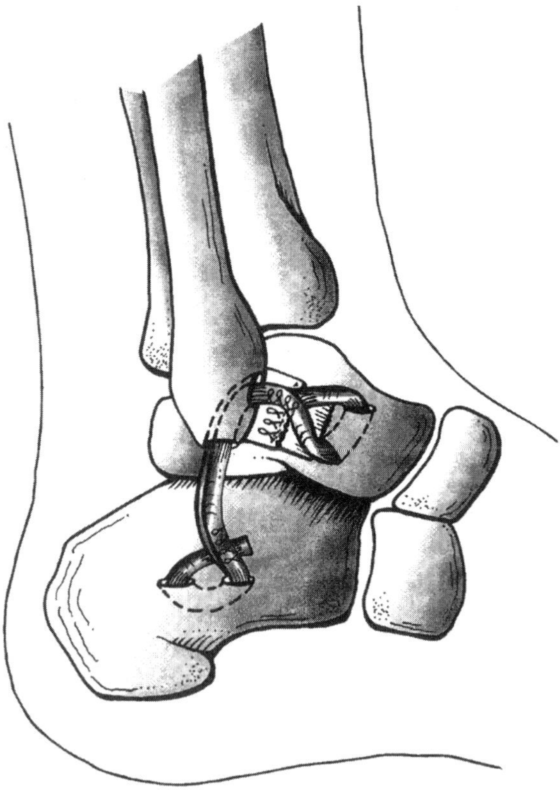

FIGURE 3.—The finished reconstruction. The anterior talofibular ligament has been imbricated and the double loop of gracilis tendon has been used to create an anatomical reconstruction of the anterior talofibular and DF ligaments. (Courtesy of Coughlin MJ, Schenck RC Jr, Grebing BR, et al: Comprehensive reconstruction of the lateral ankle for chronic instability using a free gracilis graft. *Foot Ankle Int* 25:231-241, 2004. Copyright 2004 by the American Orthopaedic Foot and Ankle Society. Reproduced with permission.)

Conclusion.—Lateral ankle reconstruction with a direct anterior talofibular repair and free gracilis tendon graft augmentation resulted in a high percentage of successful results, excellent ankle stability with a minimal loss of ankle or hindfoot motion, and substantial reduction of pain at an average follow-up of about 2 years.

► Most orthopedic surgeons remain fascinated with the topic of lateral ankle ligament reconstruction. This study provides what appears to be a relatively straightforward simple solution to this vexing problem. As noted in Fig 3, using a gracilis free graft, there is sufficient tissue to allow reconstruction of both the talocalcaneal and the talofibular ligament. This provides a very anatomical reconstruction. The only concern is the relatively short-term follow-up does not allow consideration of the observation of other investigators of late degenerative changes, usually in the subtalar joint. Nonetheless, the technique and the gratifying relatively early result prompted the selection of this article for this year's YEAR BOOK.

B. F. Morrey, MD

Arthroscopic Drilling With Debridement of Remaining Cartilage for Osteochondral Lesions of the Talar Dome in Unstable Ankles

Takao M, Uchio Y, Kakimaru H, et al (Shimane Univ, Japan; Hiroshima Univ, Japan)

Am J Sports Med 32:332-336, 2004 8–6

Introduction.—Arthroscopic drilling for treatment of osteochondral lesions of the talar dome (OLT) improves clinical symptoms, including ankle pain and disability. The regenerative cartilage that appears after drilling does not always cover the cartilage defect adequately. The results for patients who underwent arthroscopic drilling for OLT and in whom the remaining cartilage was removed were compared with those for patients in whom the remaining cartilage was kept.

Methods.—Thirty-nine patients participating in a prospective randomized trial underwent arthroscopic drilling that kept the remaining cartilage at the lesion (group A), together with 30 patients who underwent arthroscopic drilling that removed the remaining cartilage at the lesion (group B). At 1 year postoperatively, ankle arthroplasty was performed to assess the cartilage condition.

Results.—Follow-up arthroscopy showed that in group A, 11 cases (28.2%) were improved, 12 (30.8%) were unchanged, and 16 (41.0%) had deteriorated. In group B, 27 cases (93.1%) were improved and 2 were unchanged. Groups A and B were significantly different in the rate of cases in which the cartilage condition was improved on arthroscopic examination ($P < .0001$).

Conclusion.—Removing the remaining degenerative cartilage may be of some benefit in the treatment of patients with OLT.

Osteochondral Defects of the Talus Treated With Autologous Bone Grafting

Kolker D, Murray M, Wilson M (Harvard Med School, Boston)

J Bone Joint Surg Br 86-B:521-526, 2004 8–7

Introduction.—Several reports have described the use of autologous bone for treatment of osteochondral defects in the knee. Few have investigated the efficacy of using autologous bone grafting in the treatment of osteochondral defects of the talus. A standardized outcome analysis was performed that assessed the management and prognosis of osteochondral defects of the talus treated with autologous bone grafts.

Findings.—Thirteen patients who had undergone open antegrade autologous bone grafting of the talus for symptomatic osteochondral defects of the dome of the talus were evaluated retrospectively. The defect of the talar dome was located medially in 10 patients and laterally in 3. The mean age of the 7 men and 6 women was 38.4 years. The defects included the full thickness of articular cartilage, extended through the subchondral plate, and were linked with subchondral cysts. Six patients (46%) were clinical failures and needed further surgery. Among the remaining 7 patients, functional outcome results were obtained at a mean of 51.9 months postoperatively.

For all patients, CT and plain radiographs showed incorporation of the bone graft into the host bed with subchondral union. The mean outcome score for the Musculoskeletal Outcomes Data Evaluation and Management System foot and ankle questionnaire was 87; for the American Orthopaedic Foot and Ankle Society ankle-hindfoot scale, it was 84.3. The overall patient satisfaction rate was 46.2%.

Conclusion.—It is recommended that the described technique of autologous bone grafting be used with extreme caution when considered as the primary treatment of adult patients with a symptomatic advanced osteochondral defect of the talus.

► The findings of the experience documented by Takao et al (Abstract 8–6) are interesting and are consistent with what has been recommended without as much clinical data. The very strong statistically significant difference between those undergoing a drilling procedure leaving the osteochondral defect of the talus intact, compared with the dramatic improvement of those in whom the lesion was removed before drilling, is convincing. It would seem as though this article does provide the scientific basis for the optimum management of these patients, that is, the osteochondral lesion should be removed and the base drilled.

In contrast, the removal of the defect and management with autologous bone grafting (Abstract 8–7) was surprisingly unsuccessful in more than 50% of the patients. The experience reported in these studies provides clear data on the optimum management of this lesion, specifically that recommended and demonstrated by Takao et al.

B. F. Morrey, MD

Triple Arthrodesis in Adults With Non-paralytic Disease: A Minimum Ten-Year Follow-up Study

Smith RW, Shen W, DeWitt S, et al (Long Beach Mem Med Ctr, Calif; Balance Orthopaedic Foot and Ankle Ctr, Long Beach, Calif)

J Bone Joint Surg Am 86:2707-2713, 2004 8–8

Introduction.—Triple arthrodesis was initially developed to correct a variety of hindfoot problems, particularly deformities resulting from paralytic diseases. As the prevalence of paralytic diseases has diminished, it has been used more frequently for treatment of posttraumatic arthritis, rheumatoid arthritis, and dysfunction of the posterior tibial tendon and their related de-

TABLE 1.—Radiographic Evidence of Arthrosis at the Time of Final Follow-up in 26 Feet at a Mean of 14 Years

Joint	None (Grade 0)	Mild/Moderate (Grade 1)	Severe (Grade 2)*
Ankle	14	5	7 (includes 3 fused)
Naviculocuneiform	14	5	7 (includes 1 fused)
Tarsometatarsal	14	6	6 (includes 1 fused)

*Some patients had severe arthrosis at more than 1 level.

(Republished with permission of the Journal of Bone and Joint Surgery, Inc, from Smith RW, Shen W, DeWitt S, et al: Triple arthrodesis in adults with non-paralytic disease: A minimum ten-year follow-up study *J Bone Joint Surg Am* 86:2707-2713, 2004. Reproduced by permission of the publisher via Copyright Clearance Center, Inc.)

formities. The long-term outcome of triple arthrodesis was examined in patients with degenerative disease.

Methods.—A total of 27 adult patients (31 feet) who underwent triple arthrodesis for treatment of chronic hindfoot pain and were followed up for a minimum of 10 years completed an outcomes questionnaire. Of these, 22 patients (26 feet) underwent physical examination, radiographs, and functional testing. The mean patient age at the time of surgery was 45 years; the mean duration of follow-up was 14 years (range, 11-18 years).

Results.—Twenty-five (93%) patients reported satisfaction with outcome. Only 11 patients (41%) reported they could perform moderate activity with mild or no pain in the foot and ankle. Twenty patients (74%) indicated having moderate to severe difficulty with or inability to negotiate uneven surfaces. The mean SF-36 physical component outcomes score was 35.2 points, well below the mean of 50 points for the US population. The SF-36 score was significantly lower among patients with systemic inflammatory disease (primarily rheumatoid arthritis). There was an average 12× (27%) loss of plantar flexion. No significant loss of dorsiflexion was present in the treated versus nontreated foot. Severe arthrosis developed in 7 ankles, in 7 naviculocuneiform joints, and in 6 tarsometatarsal joints. Some patients had severe arthrosis at more than 1 level (Table 1); 3 later underwent ankle arthrodesis. No nonunions or revisions of the triple arthrodeses occurred. Average patient performances on both the 6-minute walk and the 3-meter up-and-go functional tests were well below age-controlled means.

Conclusion.—Triple arthrodesis may provide patients with marked long-term relief of preoperative symptoms. Adverse effects, especially degenerative changes in adjacent joints, may also occur; these consequences may be reason for orthopedic surgeons to consider alternatives to triple arthrodesis when feasible.

► Triple arthrodesis remains one of the stalwarts of the salvage armamentarium for difficult foot and ankle problems. This contribution is of value, therefore, in providing long-term follow-up of the outcome of this salvage procedure. The article does demonstrate the increasing number of adverse consequences, particularly the degenerative changes that occur in the proximal and distal joints. Thus, while this intervention may be effective, it should be considered a last resort with other alternatives, including limited arthrodesis being first considered when appreciable.

B. F. Morrey, MD

Percutaneous Versus Open Tendo Achillis Repair

Haji A, Sahai A, Symes A, et al (Basildon Univ Hosp, England)

Foot Ankle Int 25:215-218, 2004 8–9

Introduction.—There is no consensus in the literature concerning optimal management of acute Achilles tendon rupture. Open repair and percutaneous repair of ruptured Achilles tendon were retrospectively compared over a 14-year period.

Findings.—Of 108 patients identified, 70 underwent traditional open repair and 38 underwent a modified Ma & Griffith repair. The mean operating time with a percutaneous repair was 28.5 minutes, compared with 45.9 minutes for the open repair group ($P < .0001$). Comparable results were seen in a subjective analysis of ROM, stiffness, and power in both groups at the time of clinic discharge. There were 4 cases of rupture (5.7%), 4 deep infections (4.7%), 2 palpable suture knots (2.9%), and 1 sural nerve lesion (1.4%). There were 10 complications with percutaneous repair: 1 rerupture (2.6%), 5 palpable suture knots (13.2%), and 4 transient nerve lesions (10.5%). There were no significant between-group differences in any measures.

Conclusion.—Percutaneous repair is advocated in experienced hands as a suitable alternative to traditional open techniques.

Percutaneous Repair of Acute Achilles Tendon Rupture

Gorschewsky O, Pitzl M, Pütz A, et al (Klinik Sonnenhof, Bern, Switzerland; Orthopädische Universitätsklinik Magdeburg, Germany)

Foot Ankle Int 25:219-224, 2004 8–10

Introduction.—The treatment of Achilles tendon rupture remains debatable, but opinion is leaning toward an operative approach. Described was a percutaneous repair technique that combines the advantages of surgical and nonsurgical management, has a low re-rupture rate, and has improved conditions for early mobilization.

Methods.—Sixty-four patients (average age, 42 years; range, 28-58 years) with a diagnosis of new Achilles tendon rupture underwent percutaneous repair.

> *Surgical Technique.*—The procedure is performed with the patient in the prone position and a roll support below the ankle to ensure free mobility. No tourniquet is used. After a longitudinal incision is made directly over the rupture, the proximal and distal tendon stumps are identified. Two incisions of 1 cm are made at 12 to 15 cm above the

rupture site and 4 cm medially and laterally on the dorsal midline. Dissection of the soleus fascia is performed to avoid the sural nerve.

A curved guide wire with a Lengemann extension is placed through the lateral 1-cm incision into the soleus muscle and directed to the proximal stump of the Achilles tendon, at which time spikes of the Lengemann wire are hooked at the fascia of the soleus muscle. With the use of a big, curved needle, the wire is positioned in the distal stump of the tendon and advanced out laterally above the calcaneus. This is repeated medially. The stumps of the ruptured tendon are approximated by pulling the 2 wires distally. Two balls of lead are used to block the wires distally so that a fibrin sealant can be applied at the rupture site.

The proximal end of the Lengemann wire is advanced out through the skin with the use of a small curved needle (Fig 4). The paratenon is closed with a resorbable 2.0 thread and the skin is closed with 2.0 PDS intracutaneously. The 1-cm incisions are closed and the wires

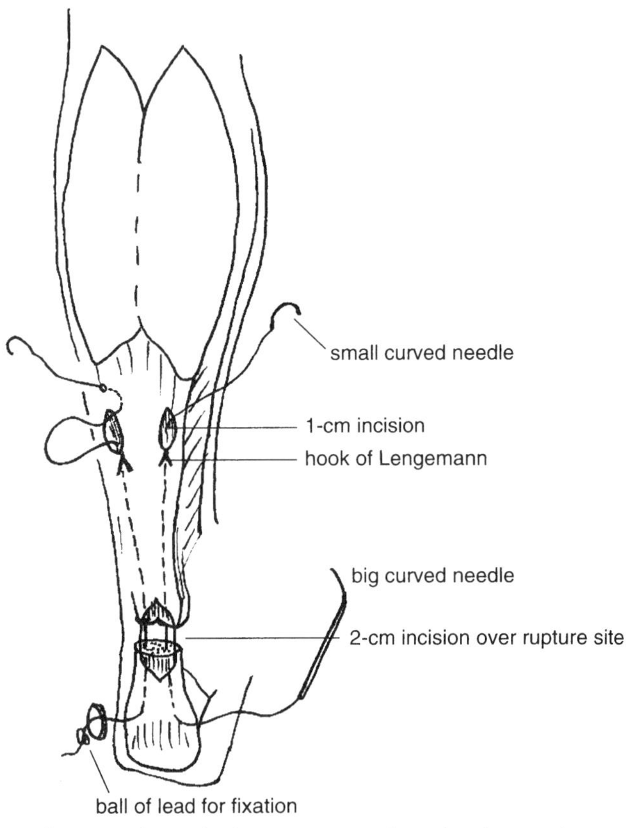

FIGURE 4.—Illustration of surgical technique. (Courtesy of Gorschewsky O, Pitzl M, Pütz A, et al: Percutaneous repair of acute Achilles tendon rupture. *Foot Ankle Int* 25(4):219-224, 2004. Copyright 2004 by the American Orthopaedic Foot and Ankle Society. Reproduced with permission.)

are proximally fixed via steristrips. After closure, below-knee plaster is applied in the neutral position of the ankle. The wires are removed during the sixth postoperative month.

Results.—There was 1 complication at 3 weeks postoperatively. A patient experienced re-rupture after a further injury. Outcome was regarded as very good in 98% of patients.

Conclusion.—Percutaneous tenodesis with Lengemann wires is an acceptable and alternative method that can be recommended in the treatment of new Achilles tendon rupture.

Immediate, Full Weightbearing Cast Treatment of Acute Achilles Tendon Ruptures: A Long-term Follow-up Study

Josey RA, Marymont JV, Varner KE, et al (Baylor College of Medicine, Houston; Foundation for Orthopedic, Athletic, and Reconstructive Research, Houston; Joe W King Orthopedic Inst, Houston; et al)

Foot Ankle Int 24:775-779, 2003 8–11

Introduction.—There are no known trials that have comprehensively examined the nonoperative treatment of Achilles tendon ruptures. The long-term follow-up of a consecutive series of patients treated by a single surgeon using an identical, nonoperative protocol was examined retrospectively.

Methods.—Thirty-two patients (33 ruptures) were available for comprehensive examination, including a questionnaire, physical examination, and manual and objective (Kin-Com) strength testing. Data excluding Kin-Com strength testing were used in an additional 7 patients (7 ruptures). A total of 39 patients (40 ruptures) were evaluated. All patients had undergone treatment initiated within 11 days of injury. Included in the treatment protocol was a maximum, unforced equinus cast with a heel lift used for 1 month. Patients were permitted to bear full body weight as tolerated by pain; two crutches were used when needed.

The cast was changed at 1 month to a resting position, gravity equinus (about 20° plantarflexion), weight-bearing cast with an appropriate heel lift used for 1 month. The patient progressed to a built-up shoe with a 1½-inch heel rise. No physical therapy or stretching was allowed. At 4 months after injury, a gentle, self-directed rehabilitation program was initiated to include a stationary bicycle. The patient was permitted to return to full activity at 6 months.

Results.—The average follow-up was 55 months (range, 24-133 months). Ninety-five percent (38/39) of patients reported that they were completely satisfied with their treatment. The American Orthopedic Foot and Ankle Society ankle hindfoot scores were over 80 in 97.4% of the cohort. The incidence of re-rupture was 6.25% (3/48). Calf circumference and ankle ROM were similar for both legs. The injured leg tended to be somewhat weaker than the uninjured leg. The difference was not significant for many of the quantitative measurements of strength.

Conclusion.—When considering the risk and expense of surgery, the risk of re-rupture, return to prerupture function, and patient satisfaction, the nonoperative treatment of acute Achilles tendon rupture using an immediate, full weight-bearing cast is a satisfactory treatment modality.

► Since the optimum management of Achilles tendon ruptures has not been clearly documented in the literature, the surgeon is left with the lack of scientific basis regarding the optimum management of these patients. The first article of this trilogy by Haji et al (Abstract 8–9) demonstrates that percutaneous repair of the Achilles tendon rupture is as effective as is the open procedure. This is particularly relevant since the operative time is almost half and is statistically significantly different.

The impressive results and recommendations offered by Haji et al are confirmed by the experience of Gorschewsky et al (Abstract 8–10). These authors demonstrate a 95% satisfactory outcome with the percutaneous repair technique. The third article of this trilogy by Josey et al (Abstract 8–11) emphasizes cast treatment for such injuries. The conclusions are valid that many patients treated by cast will do well and do not require an open operation. The bulk of the literature therefore, in our judgment, suggests that the formal open repair is probably no longer appropriate.

The remaining question is whether or not the percutaneous repair provides sufficient benefit to be considered the treatment of choice in the majority of patients. If so, the specific selection critieria need yet to be defined.

B. F. Morrey, MD

Open Reduction for Intra-articular Calcaneal Fractures: Evaluation Using Computed Tomography

Kurozumi T, Jinno Y, Sato T, et al (Jinno Hosp, Himeji, Japan; Okayama Univ, Japan)

Foot Ankle Int 24:942-948, 2003 8–12

Background.—Displaced intra-articular calcaneal fractures represent a diagnostic and therapeutic dilemma, and the results achieved with both operative and nonoperative treatments remain unpredictable. One study has found no significant differences in treatment outcomes between operative and nonoperative treatment, but another study found that in surgically treated calcaneal fractures, the overall clinical results were better in patients with anatomical reduction of the subtalar joint. These conflicting findings prompt consideration of whether the key to the difference in findings is in the quality of the anatomical reduction.

Numerous studies over 20 years have found good to excellent results in most cases of open reduction for displaced intra-articular calcaneal fractures with the use of a lateral approach to performing open reduction and internal fixation. Few studies have published prognostic factors of such fractures with the use of CT. The prognostic factors that influence the late functional

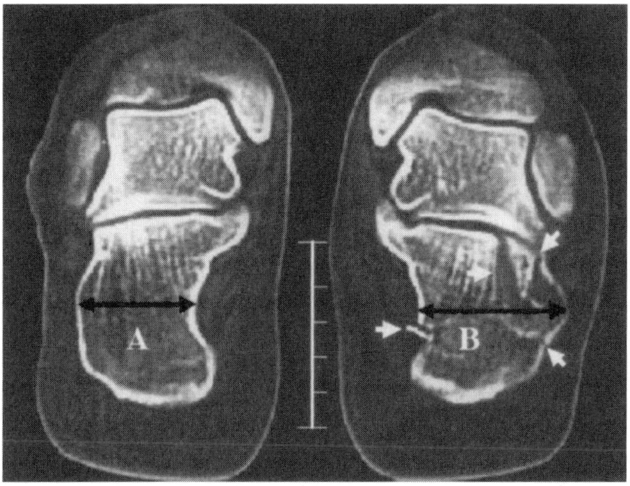

FIGURE 2.—Fracture width in posterior facet excluding lower tuberous region on coronal image. Width = B/A. (Courtesy of Kurozumi T, Jinno Y, Sato T, et al: Open reduction for intra-articular calcaneal fractures: Evaluation using computed tomography. *Foot Ankle Int* 24:942-948, 2003. Copyright 2003 by the American Orthopaedic Foot and Ankle Society. Reproduced with permission.)

results of open reduction for intra-articular calcaneal fractures using plain radiographs and CT images were evaluated.

Methods.—Radiographic and CT features of unilateral intra-articular calcaneal fractures after open reduction and internal fixation were compared with late functional outcomes in 67 patients treated between 1997 and 2002.

Results.—Of the 67 patients evaluated, 61 could walk painlessly postoperatively at an average of 19.7 months after surgery. Functional results, as determined by Laasonen's criteria, were excellent or good in 92.5% of patients. Factors associated with better functional results were lower age, greater Böhler angle at the time of injury, lower Sanders' grade, increased height of fractured regions, better reduction of the posterior facet, and better

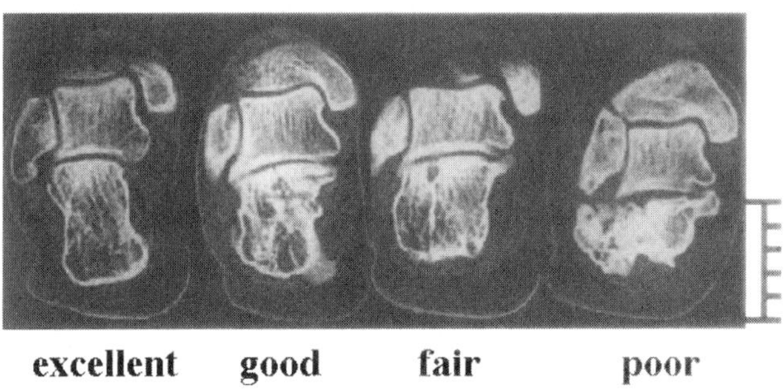

FIGURE 5.—Reduction of the posterior facet on coronal image. (Courtesy of Kurozumi T, Jinno Y, Sato T, et al: Open reduction for intra-articular calcaneal fractures: Evaluation using computed tomography. *Foot Ankle Int* 24:942-948, 2003. Copyright 2003 by the American Orthopaedic Foot and Ankle Society. Reproduced with permission.)

reduction of the calcaneocuboid joint. However, only better reduction of the posterior facet and the calcaneocuboid joint were found to be surgical diagnostic factors (Figs 2 and 5).

Conclusion.—The optimal treatment of intra-articular fractures of the calcaneus has not been clearly determined. However, this study has demonstrated a strong correlation of functional results with radiographic characteristics.

▶ Fracture of the calcaneus remains one of the most difficult of all fractures to effectively manage. With this prospective study, the authors have shown strong correlation with functional results and radiographic characteristics. Although previously described, it is worthwhile to emphasize the improved functional outcome with restoration of Böhler's angle, increased height of the fractured region, and the adequacy of the reduction of the posterior facet and of the calcaneocuboid joint. The challenge remains the technical execution of a procedure that attains these radiographic features, that is, restores the anatomy.

B. F. Morrey, MD

The Role of Limited Joint Mobility in Diabetic Patients With an At-Risk Foot

Zimny S, Schatz H, Pfohl M (Evangelisches Krankenhaus Bethesda, Duisburg, Germany; Ruhr-Universität Bochum Medizinische Klinik und Poliklinik, Bochum, Germany)

Diabetes Care 27:942-946, 2004 8–13

Background.—Foot ulceration is a significant problem for patients with diabetes, often resulting in amputation of a lower limb and an increased death rate. Diabetic neuropathy is the most important etiologic factor, but there is a complex relationship among a number of other factors, including limited joint mobility (LJM), altered foot pressures, glycemic control, and ethnic background. The role of LJM in abnormal high plantar pressures in the forefoot of diabetic patients with an at-risk foot was assessed.

Methods.—The study group for this cross-sectional investigation was composed of 70 patients with type 1 or 2 diabetes and 30 control subjects. Subgroups were composed of 35 diabetic patients with an at-risk-foot (defined as a foot with neuropathy but without ulceration or previous ulceration) and 35 diabetic control subjects without neuropathy. Joint mobility was assessed in the foot at the ankle and metatarsophalangeal 1 (first MTP) joints. The FastScan plantar pressure analyzer was used to measure the pressure-time integrals (PTIs) as dynamic variables. The clinical assessment included standard measures of peripheral neuropathy.

Results.—Mobility at the ankle and first MTP joint were significantly reduced in the foot-at-risk group compared with the diabetic control group and the control subjects. The PTIs were significantly higher in the foot-at-risk group compared with the other 2 groups. There was a strong inverse correlation between the mobility of the ankle of the first MTP joint and the PTI of the diabetic patients. The vibration perception threshold was positively correlated with the PTI of the patients with diabetes.

Conclusion.—Diabetic patients with an at-risk foot have LJM and elevated PTIs on the plantar forefoot, which place them at risk for subsequent ulceration. Limited joint mobility may be a factor in the development of high plantar pressures and may contribute to foot ulceration in the susceptible neuropathic at-risk foot.

4.5-Gram Monofilament Sensation Beneath Both First Metatarsal Heads Indicates Protective Foot Sensation in Diabetic Patients

Saltzman CL, Rashid R, Hayes A, et al (Univ of Iowa, Iowa City)
J Bone Joint Surg Am 86-A:717-723, 2004 8–14

Background.—From 12 to 16 million persons in the United States have diabetes mellitus, and more than 500,00 new cases are diagnosed annually. However, many new cases remain undiagnosed. Serious infections of the foot occur in approximately 20% of patients with diabetes. In addition, patients with diabetes have a 15-fold higher rate of lower extremity amputation than do persons without diabetes. The cost associated with the treatment of diabetic patients with ulcers has been reported to be 5.4 times greater than that associated with the treatment of diabetic patients without ulcers.

The loss of protective plantar foot sensation is the major cause of diabetic foot ulcerations and ultimate limb loss. Thus, the identification of patients without protective sensation could reduce the risk of unrecognized foot injury. The current recommended screening protocol specifies 10-g monofilament testing of 10 sites in the foot with use of a forced-choice paradigm. Whether testing of fewer than 10 sites could provide accuracy comparable with that obtained by testing all 10 sites was investigated.

Methods.—This cross-sectional comparative study of plantar sensory levels in diabetic patients with and without plantar ulceration was conducted in a tertiary care teaching hospital. The study group was composed of 47 diabetic patients with a history of foot ulceration and 45 diabetic patients with no history of ulceration. Plantar sensory threshold values at 5 sites on the sole of each foot were measured with a quasi-continuous range of applied forces, and receiver operating characteristic analysis techniques were used.

Results.—Screening based solely on the maximum force threshold for the left and right first metatarsal head sites provided comparable or better performance at high levels of sensitivity compared with either the mean or the maximum force threshold across all 10 sites. A sensory threshold of 4.5 g for both the left and right first metatarsal head sites were predictive of the risk of ulceration, with a sensitivity of 100% and a specificity of 67%.

Conclusion.—The testing of diabetic patients for protective sensation may be simplified by testing under both first metatarsal heads with a 4.5-g monofilament. A patient who cannot sense the application of a 4.5-g monofilament under either first metatarsal head has probably lost protective sensation and should be considered to be at risk for undetected injury.

► These 2 articles (Abstracts 8–13 and 8–14) are offered to emphasize a growing need to understand the opportunities to prophylactically avoid the devastating problem of ulceration of the diabetic foot. Both studies have demonstrated a positive correlation with the specific feature studied. Limited motion of the first MTP joint does have a correlation to plantar ulceration and to the neurologic findings. In addition, a practical estimation of the "foot at risk" is the simple use of a 4.5-gram monofilament under the metatarsal head. These are readily available office assessments. It would seem that the combination of these 2 articles would provide valuable information to the orthopedic surgeon dealing with such problems.

B. F. Morrey, MD

Role of First Ray Hypermobility in the Outcome of the Hohmann and the Lapidus Procedure: A Prospective, Randomized Trial Involving One Hundred and One Feet

Faber FWM, Mulder PGH, Verhaar JAN (Leyenburg Hosp, The Hague, The Netherlands)

J Bone Joint Surg Am 86-A:486-495, 2004 8–15

Background.—The role of hypermobility of the first tarsometatarsal joint in the etiology of hallux valgus deformity is a controversial issue. As a result, the necessity of an arthrodesis of this joint in the surgical treatment of hallux valgus has been questioned. The role of arthrodesis of the first tarsometatarsal joint in the outcome of surgical treatment of hallux valgus was evaluated.

Methods.—The study included 101 feet of 87 patients. A Hohmann procedure was performed on 50 feet, and a Lapidus procedure was performed on 51 patients. The mobility of the first tarsometatarsal joint was assessed in the preoperative clinical examination. Two subgroups were identified on the basis of this examination: 68 feet with a hypermobile first tarsometatarsal joint and 33 feet with a nonhypermobile first tarsometatarsal joint. The patients underwent clinical and radiographic assessment at 2 years after the operation.

Results.—A significant improvement was observed in the score on the great toe metatarsophalangeal-interphalangeal scale of the American Orthopaedic Foot and Ankle Society and in the pain score after both procedures. No significant difference was observed between the 2 procedures or between the subgroups of feet with a hypermobile first tarsometatarsal joint and those with a nonhypermobile joint. The radiographic results of the 2 methods were also similar, with the exception of shortening of the first metatarsal which was significantly greater in the Hohmann group, and plantar flexion of the first metatarsal, which was greater in the Lapidus group.

Conclusion.—The short-term outcomes in this finding were satisfactory and were comparable with results in previous isolated reports on these 2 procedures. These findings did not support the theory that patients with a hallux valgus and a hypermobile first tarsometatarsal joint should be managed with a Lapidus procedure.

▶ The editor found this level 1 prospective randomized study of interest in that it provides insight into the rationale of selecting surgical procedures based on real or perceived pathologic and physiologic characteristics. The fact that first ray hypermobility had no impact on either the Hohmann or the Lapidus procedure is a very interesting observation. It appears that both operations, with different philosophies, are equally effective regardless of the heretofore considered-important characteristic of first ray hypermobility. This study simply underscores the fact that, in many instances, the reasons for selecting a certain procedure are based on logic. This is not necessarily demonstrable by rigorous clinical study.

B. F. Morrey, MD

The Agility Total Ankle Arthroplasty: Seven to Sixteen-Year Follow-up

Knecht SI, Estin M, Callaghan JJ, et al (Univ of Iowa, Iowa City)

J Bone Joint Surg Am 86-A:1161-1171, 2004 8–16

Background.—A previous study reported the intermediate-term results with the early version of the Agility total ankle arthroplasty (DePuy, Warsaw, Ind). The main feature of the Agility design is that it makes use of arthrodesis of the tibiofibular syndesmosis for tibial component support. Longer-term results with the Agility total ankle replacement in the treatment of patients with disabling ankle arthritis were reported.

Methods.—An independent review was conducted of all Agility total ankle replacements performed by a single surgeon from 1994 to 2004. Follow-up included completion of a validated ankle osteoarthritis scale and a brief questionnaire as well as a review of the radiographs. All radiographs were evaluated for evidence of the development of progressive hindfoot arthritis, nonunion of the tibiofibular syndesmosis, progressive radiolucent lines, osteolysis, and component subsidence.

Results.—A total of 132 arthroplasties were performed for 126 patients (Fig 3). After a mean follow-up of 9 years, 33 patients (36 implants) had died, 14 patients (11%) had a revision of the implant or an ankle arthrodesis, and 1 patient underwent amputation of the limb for unrelated causes. Of the remaining 78 patients (81 ankles), 67 (69 ankles) were followed up clinically.

Over 90% of these patients reported decreased pain and satisfaction with the outcome of surgery. Of the 117 ankles that had been followed up radiographically for at least 2 years, 22 (19%) had progressive subtalar arthritis, 17 (15%) had progressive talonavicular arthritis, and 9 (8%) had a syndesmosis nonunion (Fig 8). There was some evidence of peri-implant radiolucency in 89 of 117 ankles (76%).

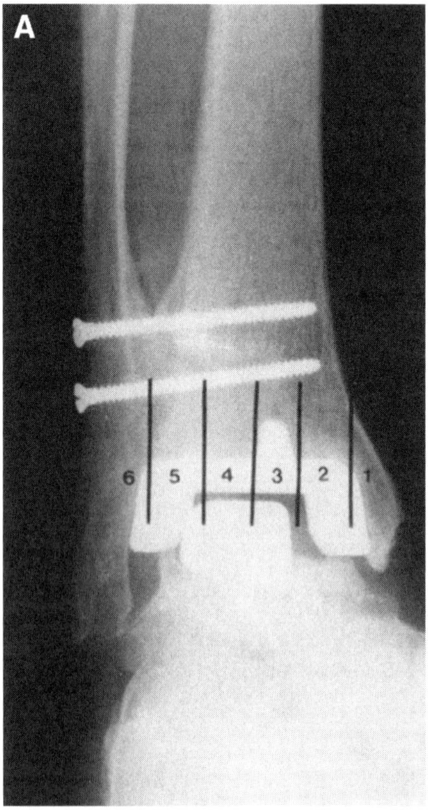

FIGURE 3.—A, The tibial component was divided into 6 zones on the AP and mortise radiographs for the purpose of describing the presence of periprosthetic lucencies and lysis. Lucency was defined as a radiolucent line of 2 mm or less in width, and lysis was defined as a radiolucent area of more than 2 mm. (Republished with permission of the Journal of Bone and Joint Surgery, Inc, from Knecht SI, Estin M, Callaghan JJ, et al: The agility total ankle arthroplasty: Seven to sixteen-year follow-up. *J Bone Joint Surg Am* 86-A:1161-1171, 2004. Reproduced by permission of the publisher via Copyright Clearance Center, Inc.)

Conclusion.—The radiographic and clinical outcomes of the Agility total ankle replacement are affected by arthrodesis of the tibiofibular syndesmosis. The relatively low rates of radiographic hindfoot arthritis and revision procedures at an average of 9 years after arthroplasty are encouraging. The Agility total ankle arthroplasty is a viable and long-lasting option for the treatment of ankle arthritis in selected patients.

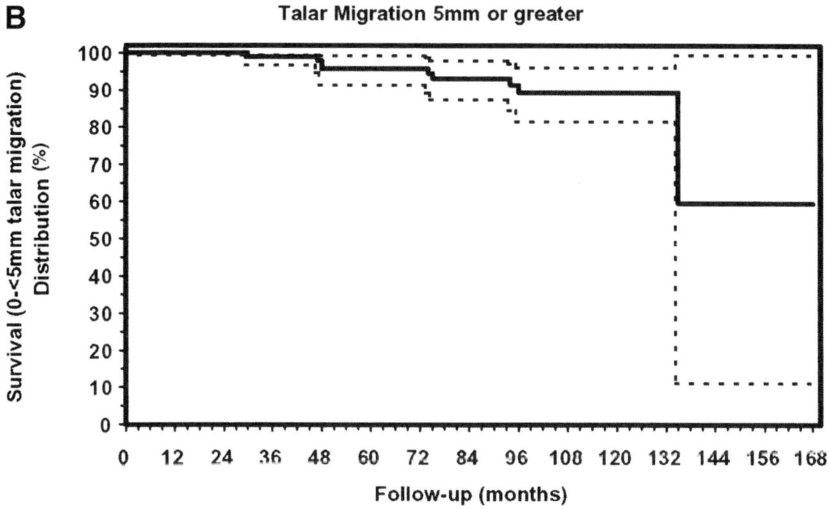

FIGURE 8.—B, Survivorship curve with talar migration of 5 mm or more as the end point. The *hatched lines* show the 95% confidence intervals. (Republished with permission of the Journal of Bone and Joint Surgery, Inc, from Knecht SI, Estin M, Callaghan JJ, et al: The agility total ankle arthroplasty: Seven to sixteen-year follow-up. *J Bone Joint Surg Am* 86-A:1161-1171, 2004. Reproduced by permission of the publisher via Copyright Clearance Center, Inc.)

Scandinavian Total Ankle Replacement: A 3.7-Year Average Followup of 65 Patients

Valderrabano V, Hintermann B, Dick W (Univ of Basel, Switzerland)
Clin Orthop 424:47-56, 2004 8–17

Background.—Short-term results in studies of total ankle arthroplasty have been encouraging, but medium- and long-term results have revealed many complications, including ankle pain, painful malleolar impingement, tibial component loosening, and talar component subsidence. The major factors implicated in loosening have been highly constrained designs and cement fixation.

More recent approaches to total ankle replacement have allowed semiconstrained to nonconstrained motion and rely on bone ingrowth for stability of the implant. One of the more popular of these prostheses is the Scandinavian Total Ankle Replacement (S.T.A.R.) (Waldemar Link, Hamburg, Germany). The midterm results of a series of total ankle replacements done with the S.T.A.R. prosthesis were evaluated.

Methods.—A total of 68 total ankle replacements were done for 65 patients with the S.T.A.R. prosthesis. This prosthesis comprises 3 components with 2 anchorage bars, a high-density PE inlay, and a convex cylindrical talar component resurfacing the entire talus. The patients ranged in age from 22 to 85 years, with a mean age of 56.1 years at surgery. The patients were evaluated at a mean of 3.7 years (range, 2.4-6.2 years).

Results.—Of the 65 patients evaluated, 35 (54%) were completely pain free. The overall clinical score was graded as excellent or good for 67 ankles. The American Orthopaedic Foot and Ankle Society hindfoot score improved from a mean of 24.7 points (range, 2 to 44 points) preoperatively to 84.3 points (range, 44 to 100 points) at follow-up. A ballooning bone lysis was present on the tibial side in 3 patients (3 ankles, 4.4%). Periarticular hypertrophic bone formation was present in 43 ankles (63%) despite prophylaxis and was associated with a decrease in dorsiflexion and plantar flexion.

Revision surgery was performed in 9 ankles (13%, 9 patients) because of problems with the components; secondary or additional operations were performed in 14 patients (21%). All of the revision and secondary operations were successful, and no ankle had to be converted to an ankle arthrodesis.

Conclusion.—Early outcomes for patients treated with the Scandinavian Total Ankle Replacement are encouraging. However, this study found more complications and potential problems than have previously been reported.

► These 2 articles (Abstracts 8–16 and 8–17) serve to update the status of joint replacement arthroplasty from 2 rather different perspectives. The Agility total ankle arthroplasty (Abstract 8–16) provides significant 7- to 16-year surveillance in a large sample of over 125 patients. Although, as typically noted, over 90% of the patients in whom the implant had not been revised report satisfactory subjective outcome, the 25% with evidence of periprosthetic radiolucency is of concern for the long-term viability of this design.

The assessment by Valderrabano (Abstract 8–17) reports on the outcome of what is probably the most popular ankle implant, the so-called S.T.A.R. prosthesis (Scandinavian Total Ankle Replacement). This report is of a much smaller sample with significantly less surveillance (averaging only 3½ years), thus must be considered a preliminary assessment. The high incidence of revision (13%) and reoperation (21%) with an average follow-up of less than 4 years is more in keeping with what has been anticipated in the past with the ankle replacement.

Overall, these 2 articles serve to summarize the current status of total ankle replacement, that is, improved and more reliable outcomes compared to previous experiences with earlier designs. However, replacement of this joint cannot be done with the same confidence as that of a hip and knee replacement, nor of the shoulder and elbow patient, in the majority of patients.

B. F. Morrey, MD

9 Forearm, Wrist, and Hand

Introduction

Much of the past year's contributions to the literature on disorders of the forearm, wrist, and hand continue to be weighted toward the process verification and scientific scrutiny of procedures and methods long held up as sound by anecdotal or poorly investigated retrospective data. I have included several selections that deserve our review to take a closer look at a varied array of commonly performed procedures about the wrist and hand.

True innovation was seen this past year in the design and methods of volar fixed-angle plate fixation of complex distal radius fractures. I have also included several studies that bring forth new information from diagnostic and operative wrist arthroscopy, both in the acute and chronic setting, that further our understanding of sources of wrist pain.

As the numbers of elderly patients continue to rise in our practices (reflecting the aging of the population), clinically specific and relevant information on this subgroup is increasingly important. Several informative selections have been chosen on surgical outcomes, and hopefully these will be useful to you in providing care to our older patients.

Stephen D. Trigg, MD

Evaluation and Diagnosis

Radiation Exposure With Use of the Mini-C-Arm for Routine Orthopaedic Imaging Procedures

Badman BL, Rill L, Butkovich B, et al (Univ of Florida, Gainesville)
J Bone Joint Surg Am 87-A:13-17, 2005 9–1

Background.—Substantial concerns have been raised about health care providers' radiation exposure from mobile fluoroscopic devices used during orthopedic procedures. Previous studies have documented the increased risk associated with large c-arm device use. The amount of radiation exposure that surgeons receive while using a mini-c-arm device was investigated.

Methods and Findings.—Tissue-equivalent anthropomorphic phantoms were used. Measures were made with a radiation dosimeter to determine quantitatively exposure rates at various locations and distances from the mini-c-arm during 2 common upper and lower extremity procedures. Results indicated that exposure rates associated with the mini-c-arm were lower than those reported for the large c-arm device by 1 to 2 orders of magnitude. Exposures were lower regardless of position, distance, or relative duration of exposure.

Conclusions.—Whenever feasible, the mini-c-arm device should be used for orthopedic imaging procedures instead of the large c-arm device. The use of the mini-c-arm addresses health care providers' concerns about cumulative radiation hazards, positioning, relative distance from beam, and the need for protective shielding.

▶ Mini-c-arm fluoroscopic devices have become increasingly more common over the past decade. Many of us consider them to be a routine and integral piece of surgical equipment for procedures of the elbow, wrist, and hand. The manufacturers of these devices reported early on that the radiation exposure for unshielded surgeons is minimal, no doubt a major contributing factor to their burgeoning popularity. The authors of this study report that, apart from the manufacturers' data, the radiation risks to the surgeon and patient have not been documented. Their findings are both informative and comforting to those who use these devices routinely.

S. D. Trigg, MD

The 45° Pronated Oblique View for Volar Fixed-Angle Plating of Distal Radius Fractures

Smith DW, Henry MH (Univ of Texas, Houston)

J Hand Surg [Am] 29A:703-706, 2004 9–2

Background.—Subchondral support just below the articular surface optimizes distal fracture fragment stabilization. Placing these plate supports too proximal may result in metaphyseal bone loss, osteopenia, or comminution, leading to a lack of implant purchase and subsequent fracture collapse. However, the margin between too proximal and too distal is narrow. Standard posteroanterior and lateral radiographic views cannot reliably confirm proper positioning. A 45° pronated oblique view can display the relation between dense subchondral bone and support hardware to verify absence of joint penetration.

> *Technique.*—To obtain a pronated oblique view, the clinician centers the wrist in the path of the horizontally oriented x-ray beam, similar to that for a posteroanterior view. The wrist is then pronated 45°. The clinician can also obtain this view with a vertically oriented x-ray beam and the wrist supinated 45° from full pronation.

Patients and Outcomes.—Forty-eight patients with unstable distal radius fractures treated with volar fixed-angle plate stabilization between July

2002 and March 2003 participated in the development of this technique. In all patients, 5 image intensifier views were obtained during surgery to evaluate reduction and plate placement. The views were standard posteroanterior, standard lateral, 10° tilted posteroanterior, 20° inclined lateral, and 45° pronated oblique. The addition of the 45° pronated oblique view enabled definitive interpretation in all patients.

Conclusions.—The 45° pronated oblique view enables clinicians to verify that volar hardware placed at the immediate subchondral bone level avoids the radiocarpal joint. This is important when volar fixed-angle plating of distal radius fractures is planned.

► The use of volar fixed-angle plates for the treatment of unstable fractures of the distal radius continues to grow at a rapid pace. Several of the most frequently used designs now have several rows of locking peg or screw holes that allow for a multiple-angle splay to increase support of the distal subchondral bone or to fixate fracture fragments. This study shows the optimum radiographic view to best image the position of the pegs.

S. D. Trigg, MD

Ultrasound for the Early Diagnosis of Clinically Suspected Scaphoid Fracture

Senall JA, Failla JM, Bouffard JA, et al (Henry Ford Hosp, Detroit)
J Hand Surg [Am] 29A:400-405, 2004 9–3

Background.—Most scaphoid fractures are apparent on initial radiography. In patients with symptoms but no radiographic evidence of such fracture, the diagnosis must be suspected clinically. The ability of US to diagnose clinically suspected occult scaphoid fractures was evaluated.

Methods.—This prospective controlled study included 18 patients with 18 injured wrists assessed in an emergency department. The patients, aged 10 to 77 years, had a single traumatic wrist injury, snuffbox tenderness, swelling, and negative findings on wrist radiography. All underwent physical examination and high-resolution US in addition to the initial radiograph. Treatment consisted of immobilization in a thumb spica. Patients were then followed up 1 to 14 days later.

Findings.—Nine wrists were eventually positive for scaphoid fracture on plain radiography. US correctly identified 7 of these cases. US was interpreted as negative correctly in 8 of 9 radiograph-negative cases, which was statistically significant. The patient with the false-positive result had radioscaphoid arthrosis and radial wrist swelling. The sensitivity and specificity of US examination were 78% and 89%, respectively. Positive and negative predictive values were 88% and 80%, respectively.

Conclusions.—High-frequency US should be used to assess occult suspected scaphoid fractures. This technique enables early diagnosis and eliminates the need for more invasive or costly diagnostic tests in most patients.

▶ MRI has arguably proven to be the most sensitive imaging technique for the detection of acute scaphoid fractures not visible on plain radiographs. However, both MRI and, alternatively, CT scans are expensive and therefore may not be allowable or covered procedures by many insurance plans, resulting in delays in diagnosis. The authors present their early experience to support that high-frequency US may prove to be a diagnostically sensitive yet less-expensive alternative imaging technique for the early diagnosis of acute occult scaphoid fractures.

S. D. Trigg, MD

Nerve

Functional Outcomes in Young, Active Duty, Military Personnel After Submuscular Ulnar Nerve Transposition

Fitzgerald BT, Dao KD, Shin AY (Naval Med Ctr San Diego; Westminster, Calif; Mayo Clinic, Rochester, Minn)

J Hand Surg [Am] 29A:619-624, 2004 9–4

Background.—No adequate documentation yet exists of the functional outcomes after submuscular ulnar nerve transposition (SMUNT) for young, physically active patients who suffer cubital tunnel syndrome (CuTS). One prospective study reported the lack of a statistically significant difference between the outcomes with simple decompression and those with subcutaneous or submuscular transposition. None of the reports has involved patients younger than 45 years. SMUNT is more technically demanding and requires more extensive soft tissue dissection than other surgical options for CuTS. Active duty military personnel who are young and have physically demanding occupations and athletic interests would be expected to have mild to moderate stage disease and could benefit from transposing the ulnar nerve under the protection of the flexor/pronator origin to reliably achieve a return to their previous pursuits. The effectiveness of this surgical procedure was retrospectively investigated.

Methods.—The study included an evaluation of 20 patients (20 extremities) 20 months after SMUNT surgery. All of the patients were military active-duty personnel. Documentation included the Disability of the Arm, Shoulder, and Hand (DASH) questionnaire, Bishop-Kleinman scores, physical examination, analysis of rates for the return to work, complications, and overall patient satisfaction ratings.

Results.—The average DASH score showed a statistically significant improvement to 6.2 points postoperatively from 32.5 points preoperatively. The Bishop-Kleinman rating of results were excellent in 19 patients and good in 1 patient who was unable to return to his work as a fireman/heavy laborer. Four patients who had an abnormal 2-point discrimination preoperatively also had it after surgery. Grip strength increased 26% to 48 kilogram-force (kgf) from 41 kgf preoperatively. Key pinch strength increased 30% to 9.4 kgf from 7.3 kgf preoperatively. These increases were both statistically significant. None of the patients had a decline in strength after surgery. Ten elbows had full ROM, and 10 had a decrement in average flexion contracture of 8° and a decrement in average flexion of 7°. Between 30 and 45 days (average, 33 days) after surgery, patients were able to return to work with activity restrictions, then could assume full duty 3 to 7 months (average, 4.8 months) postoperatively. Nineteen returned to their military occupation, and 1 was discharged because of an inability to comply with physical requirements. Nineteen patients were satisfied with the procedure and would choose to have it again, but 1 was not satisfied with the choice. He had an ultimate elbow flexion contracture of 20° and persistently poor 2-point discrimination but maintained full active-duty military status. Three patients had reduced sensation in the medial antebrachial cutaneous nerve distribution postoperatively; 2 had improvement within 6 months. None of the patients required revision decompression or suffered elbow instability.

Conclusions.—These patients were the youngest and most active groups reported to have undergone SMUNT. Their baseline good health and mandatory physical fitness requirements were an excellent background for evaluating functional status. All but 1 patient had excellent functional outcomes and resumed their full active-duty military careers. Complications were few, and the patients were highly satisfied with the results.

► The surgical treatment of CuTS has been extensively studied, but no consensus has been reached on the most appropriate technique. Surgeon bias for neurolysis in situ, medial epicondylectomy, subdermal transposition, intramuscular transposition or submuscular transposition prevails. Many consider submuscular transposition to be a preferred technique for laborers, athletes, and younger individuals, because it affords for more soft tissue protection of the nerve. The authors of this study correctly point out that the functional outcomes of younger patients after SMUNT have not been well documented, and therefore, their experience and findings warrant our review.

S. D. Trigg, MD

Long-term Clinical and Neurologic Recovery in the Hand After Surgery for Severe Cubital Tunnel Syndrome

Matsuzaki H, Yoshizu T, Maki Y, et al (Niigata Chuo Hosp, Japan; Niigata Hand Surg Found, Japan)

J Hand Surg [Am] 29A:373-378, 2004 9–5

Background.—For patients having cubital tunnel surgery, with more severe preoperative ulnar neuropathy, the functional recovery may be less adequate and require tendon transfers. The extent of functional recovery, duration of the process of recovery, and need to restore intrinsic muscle function in patients who have severe cubital tunnel syndrome postoperatively were investigated.

Methods.—The records of 15 patients who had cubital tunnel release were studied retrospectively. Characteristics of the patients included marked intrinsic muscle atrophy, claw-hand deformity, electrically silent sensory and motor nerve conduction velocities (MCVs), and results of the Semmes-Weinstein test (SWT) between purple (3.84-4.31) and red (4.56-6.65). The long-term postoperative recovery of these severely impaired nerves was documented, noting how long the recovery process took. Tests of hand function (manual muscle testing [MMT] of index-finger abduction, SWT, and MCV tests) were used to determine whether restoring intrinsic muscle function was needed to improve the performance on activities of daily living (ADLs).

Results.—At a median of 4.5 years postoperatively, 5 patients had no numbness in the ring and small fingers, 9 had a substantial reduction in this measure, and 1 had no difference from the preoperative value. The preoperative difficulty with chopstick use, buttoning, and writing declined; 1 patient had impaired chopstick use, 6 had difficulty with buttoning, and 9 had no restrictions in ADLs postoperatively. SWT results improved to nearly normal levels, considering the patients' ages (50% older than 70 years). MCV was measurable in all patients. Three patients had excellent results; 6, good; and 6, fair.

Conclusions.—The 3 questions to be answered in this study included the extent of recovery of ulnar nerve function to be expected, the duration of the postoperative recovery process, and whether restoring intrinsic muscle function is needed to improve performance on ADLs. Even in severely impaired patients, a long-term satisfactory result should be anticipated. Improvement continued for more than 2 years after surgery, but an exact endpoint was not determined. Weakness of the index finger abduction was the most important problem to be overcome in intrinsic muscle impairment. It was not determined whether reconstruction index finger abduction should accompany cubital tunnel release. Fourteen of the 15 patients recovered to grade 3 or better in MMT of index finger abduction, and ADLs were improved. With older patients, intrinsic muscles required more time to recover; patients who were younger than 70 years recovered faster than those 70 years or older. Patients who had excellent or good results had a mean age of 64 years, whereas those who had a fair result had a mean age of 67 years. Age and duration of symptoms may not be independently linked to outcomes, but must be considered as functioning in a total or synergistic effect.

▶ The long-term postsurgical recovery of hand function and the duration for recovery for severe cubital tunnel syndrome have not been extensively investigated. Consequently, the indications and timing for later surgical restoration of intrinsic muscle function is underreported. Patients presenting with severe cubital tunnel syndrome remain a surprisingly all-too-frequent problem, particularly unrecognized until late in older patients. This study furthers our knowledge for the treatment of such patients.

S. D. Trigg, MD

Patient-Reported Outcome After Carpal Tunnel Release for Advanced Disease: A Prospective and Longitudinal Assessment in Patients Older Than Age 70

Leit ME, Weiser RW, Tomaino MM (Univ of Rochester, NY; Univ of Pittsburgh, Pa)

J Hand Surg [Am] 29A:379-383, 2004 9–6

Background.—Carpal tunnel syndrome is the most common compression neuropathy of the upper extremity and its incidence increases with age. Despite being common among older patients, the efficacy of carpal tunnel release procedures among elderly patients with advanced stage disease has not been well studied. The surgical outcome for older patients with advanced disease was assessed from the patient's perspective.

Study Design.—This prospective longitudinal study included 13 patients (14 hands) who were older than 70 years and had advanced carpal tunnel syndrome. Entry criteria included absence of sensory response after stimulation, increase in median distal motor latency of greater than 6.0 ms and abductor pollicis brevis fibrillation potentials. All patients had undergone open carpal tunnel release between October 2000 and January 2002. Each participant completed the Brigham Hospital carpal tunnel syndrome questionnaire before surgery and then again 6 and 12 months after surgery. Each patient also characterized their satisfaction level and stated whether they thought the surgery was worthwhile. Grip strength was assessed with a dynamometer before and 1 year after surgery.

Findings.—Six months after surgery, the average symptom severity score decreased from 29 to 15, and the average functional status decreased from 18 to 11. One year after surgery, average symptom severity decreased further to 14, and the average functional status score decreased further to 9. These changes were significant. The average grip strength did not change, but patients were satisfied with results in 13 of 14 hands.

Conclusions.—The findings of this prospective longitudinal study suggest that within 1 year of open release carpal tunnel surgery, older patients with advanced disease had symptomatic improvement and functional restoration, and they were satisfied with results, despite lack of improvement in grip strength. Therefore, carpal tunnel release surgery can be recommended for this population, even though a complete recovery does not appear to occur.

▶ Meaningful outcome data after carpal tunnel release in elderly patients are notably scant, particularly so owing to the commonality of this condition in patients older than 50 years. This prospective study provides us with valuable information to share with our older patients with advanced carpal tunnel syndrome.

S. D. Trigg, MD

Forearm and Wrist

Volar Fixed-Angle Plate Fixation for Unstable Distal Radius Fractures in the Elderly Patient

Orbay JL, Fernandez DL (Miami Hand Ctr, Fla; Lindenhof Hosp, Berne, Switzerland)

J Hand Surg [Am] 29A:96-102, 2004 9–7

Background.—Distal radius fractures are a major source of morbidity among the elderly. Experience with a volar fixed-angle internal fixation plate in the treatment of distal radius fractures in elderly persons was reported.

Methods.—For this retrospective analysis, the authors identified 26 patients older than 75 years treated for unstable distal radius fractures with a volar fixed-angle plate. Postoperatively, management consisted of immediate finger motion, early functional use of the hand, and a wrist splint for a mean of 3 weeks. Follow-up data were available on 23 patients with 24 unstable radius fractures. The mean follow-up was 63 weeks.

Findings.—Final volar tilt was a mean of 6°. Radial tilt was 20°, and radial shortening averaged less than 1 mm. The mean final dorsiflexion was 58°; volar flexion, 55°; pronation, 80°; and supination, 76°. Average grip strength was 77% of the contralateral side. No plate failures of significant loss of reduction were documented. However, 3 patients had a 1- to 3-mm settling of the distal fragment.

Conclusions.—In elderly patients, volar fixed-angle plate treatment for unstable distal radius fractures provides stable internal fixation and early function. This approach enables early return to function and carries a low rate of complications.

► The quest for optimal methods of surgical treatment for displaced, impacted, and malaligned fractures of the distal radius continues at a rapid pace. The development of volar fixed-angle plates, which use noninterfragmentary smooth subchondral bone support pegs, is a novel approach that can yield stable enough internal fixation. The use of this plate for fractures in the elderly with comminuted osteoporotic bone is particularly appealing.

S. D. Trigg, MD

Arthroscopic Findings in Wrists With Severe Post-traumatic Pain Despite Normal Standard Radiographs

Adolfsson L, Povlsen B (Univ Hosp, Linköping, Sweden; Guy's Hosp, London)

J Hand Surg [Br] 29B:208-213, 2004 9–8

Background.—Early diagnosis of carpal ligament injuries is important to permit direct repair. However, pain can limit clinical investigations, and the results of radiographic evaluations can be normal even with serious ligament damage. Radiographic findings later show the injury to be better, possibly, because the injured ligaments progressively fail until carpal instability occurs. Secondary changes at this later stage, including malalignment of the carpal ligament, can hinder direct repair. Most patients who have normal standard radiographs after wrist injury have only soft tissue injuries, and these heal spontaneously, so arthroscopy cannot be recommended for every case. The incidence of lesions that will produce symptomatic carpal instability is unknown. Guidelines to identify patients whose injuries involve the carpal ligament and who need further evaluation are required. The arthroscopic findings in wrists that had normal standard radiographs but severe symptoms both acutely and subacutely were evaluated.

Methods.—The study included 43 patients for whom conservative management had proved ineffective. All had wrist pain that eventually was assessed, using a stability test and arthroscopy within 12 weeks of their injury.

Results.—On clinical evaluation, the patients had severe tenderness over the dorsum of the wrist and pain with movement. Only 2 of the 43 patients had no intra-articular injury, the other 41 exhibiting injuries of varying severity. Seventeen injuries could have benefited from acute repair. Seven had total scapholunate rupture with marked instability. Of the partial lesions noted, partial scapholunate ligament injury was the most common. Six patients had partial lesions of the radioscaphocapitate ligament, and 3 of these also had scapholunate instability and capsular rupture and bleeding in the scapho–trapezium-trapezoid joint.

Conclusions.—No study has yet identified the benefits of intervening early for patients who have torn wrist ligaments. However, whether surgical repair or conservative treatment is appropriate depends on obtaining an accurate diagnosis in the acute stage of the injury. Identifying the injuries in the acute and subacute phases of the injury can also help clinicians understand the natural history and pathomechanical progression involved in carpal instability. The criteria used to choose patients for arthroscopy in this study were both valid and feasible. The consequences attending the lesions that were found were not defined, but surgical repair would have been appropriate for about one third of the patients for up to 4 weeks after injury. Treatment strategies are more accurately assessed when the injuries are clearly identified.

▶ Patients who present with persistent wrist pain and swelling several weeks after an injury but who have normal radiographs present us with a considerable treatment challenge. Frequently, a meaningful clinical examination is limited by global wrist pain making specific testing for carpal instability unreliable. MRI testing is expensive, and accurate diagnostic information is dependent on equipment, technique, and radiologist experience. Wrist arthroscopy remains the most sensitive and accurate method for diagnosis of carpal soft tissue injury. This study furthers our knowledge about the range of carpal injuries that might be detected with arthroscopy in the acute and subacute setting. More importantly, this information begins to set guidelines for selection criteria for those patients that should undergo early diagnostic wrist arthroscopy so that soft tissue repair can be performed early before static carpal instability and arthrosis ensue.

S. D. Trigg, MD

Arthroscopic Resection of Arthrosis of the Proximal Hamate: A Clinical and Biomechanical Study

Harley BJ, Werner FW, Boles SD, et al (Univ of New York, Syracuse)

J Hand Surg [Am] 29A:661-667, 2004 9–9

Background.—On the basis of anatomical studies, type I lunates have no medial facet for articulation with the proximal pole of the hamate and this lunate occurs in 35% to 53% of specimens. In a type II lunate, the medial facet is obvious, and this lunate is found in 47% to 65% of cases. Some patients who undergo treatment for isolated tears of the triangular fibrocartilage complex (TFCC) or lunotriquetral (LT) ligament have inexplicable residual ulnar-sided pain and/or instability. A relationship has been found between proximal hamate arthrosis and a tear of the LT interosseous ligament (LTIL). Arthritic change of the proximal pole of the hamate is present in some patients with persistent wrist pain. The specific surgical treatment options for this have been unclear. A series of patients with arthrosis of the proximal hamate had arthroscopic resection. The effect of proximal hamate resection on carpal loading was investigated in a biomechanical study.

Methods.—Of the 23 patients having arthroscopic proximate hamate resection to manage proximal hamate arthrosis, 21 were available for an average follow-up of 4.7 years postoperatively. The procedure provided full exposure of the proximal hamate and involved an average excision of 2.2 mm of the proximal hamate. Evaluation included a modified wrist score, including measures of pain relief, patient satisfaction, ROM, and grip strength. In the biomechanical study, proximal hamate resection was done in 6 cadaver wrists with type II lunates, measuring loads across the carpal and midcarpal joints via pressure-sensitive film applied before and after the intervention.

Results.—All patients had erosive changes of the proximal pole of the hamate with exposed subchondral bone and midcarpal synovitis, and 21 had an associated tear of the LT ligament. Ninety-five percent had a type II lunate, and 7 (33.3%) had perforation or tear of the TFCC. For 14 (66.7%) patients, excellent clinical outcomes were obtained; for 4 (19.0%), good; for 1 (4.8%), fair, and for 2 ((9.5%), poor. All patients with an associated TLIL tear and midcarpal synovitis achieved excellent results, as did 66% of the patients with TFCC perforations, TLIL tears, and midcarpal synovitis. Patients with preexisting radiocarpal arthritis or hamate arthrosis after previous arthroscopic surgery also had excellent results. One patient with proximal hamate erosion needed TFCC repair, LT ligament repair with suture anchors, and LT joint pinning to achieve a good result. At final follow-up, 18 patients had minimal to no change in work or recreational status; 3 required a job change or ceased work because of wrist problems. Further salvage surgery was done for 4 patients. In the biomechanical study, resection of 2.4 mm of the proximal hamate relieved the pressure on the hamatolunate articulation but did not change the load at the triquetrohamate joint.

Conclusions.—The acronym HALT, for hamate arthrosis lunotriquetral ligament tear, has been used to describe patients with LT instability and proximal hamate arthrosis. Whether LT instability contributes to the development of degenerative changes at the proximal hamate in wrists with type II lunates has not been established. Fairly conservative treatment is appropriate for these wrists, including arthroscopic removal of the proximal pole of the hamate and debridement or no treatment of the LT joint. The patient then has early postoperative wrist motion, leading to good or excellent results and a return to employment in most cases. The results of the biomechanical study supported those of the clinical evaluation, indicating that it is necessary to completely unload the medial facet of the lunate to properly treat arthrosis of the proximal pole of the hamate.

► This study furthers our knowledge of the association of proximal hamate arthrosis and tears of the LTIL as a source for ulnar-sided wrist pain. The potential for proximal hamate degeneration is particularly important to recognize in patients with type II lunates. Their proposed treatment of arthroscopic resection of the proximal hamate warrants further study.

S. D. Trigg, MD

Complications of Wrist Arthroscopy

Beredjiklian PK, Bozentka DJ, Leung YL, et al (Univ of Pennsylvania, Philadelphia)

J Hand Surg [Am] 29A:406-411, 2004 9–10

Background.—Wrist arthroscopy is used to assess and treat patients who have conditions such as tears of the triangular fibrocartilage complex (TFCC), dorsal ganglion cysts, articular fractures of the distal radius, carpal fractures and instability, and inflammatory arthritis of the radiocarpal joint. The incidence and type of complications that occur with wrist arthroscopy were retrospectively investigated.

Methods.—Data from the outpatient records and surgical reports of 211 patients who had wrist joint arthroscopy were evaluated, noting type of procedure done, type of anesthetic used, portals used, incidence of complications, and nature of adverse events.

Results.—The complication rate was 5.2% (11/211) in the 211 surgeries. Two patients had major complications (0.9%): 1 had permanent wrist stiffness and significant functional disability, and the other had a ganglion cyst over the 3-4 portal 3 months after arthroscopic TFCC tear debridement. The remaining 9 minor complications included 3 cases of transient superficial dorsal ulnar sensory neurapraxia, 2 with transient wrist- and finger-joint stiffness, 1 with an ulnar neurapraxia, 1 with a superficial portal site infection, 1 with a first-degree burn to the forearm caused by contact with a hot arthroscopic distraction tower, and 1 with extensor carpi ulnaris (ECU) tendinitis. These minor complications resolved with conservative care. None of the adjunctive arthroscopic procedures was associated with a complication. Forty-five percent of the complications were identified in the immediate postoperative period, and 55% were delayed.

Conclusions.—Only 2 major and 9 minor complications developed in the 211 patients, for an overall complication rate of 5.2%. Forty-five percent were identified immediately after surgery, and for 55%, the identification was delayed. Conservative care was sufficient to manage the minor complications. Wrist arthroscopy is safe, and the incidence of major and minor complications is low.

► Over the past decade, we have witnessed expanding indications for diagnostic and operative wrist arthroscopy procedures for disorders of the wrist. Complications from knee and shoulder arthroscopy have been well documented, but there is little reported data on complications after wrist arthroscopy. This information is important for the surgeon to be aware of and to discuss with patients preoperatively when wrist arthroscopy has been recommended.

S. D. Trigg, MD

Treatment of Isolated Perilunate and Lunate Dislocations With Combined Dorsal and Volar Approach and Intraosseous Cerclage Wire

Trumble T, Verheyden J (Univ of Washington, Seattle; Harborview Med Ctr, Seattle, Wash)

J Hand Surg [Am] 29A:412-417, 2004 9–11

Background.—Isolated perilunate dislocations are relatively rare and difficult to treat. Strong repair of the scapholunate interosseous ligament has been proposed to be the key to successful long-term outcomes. In addition, an intraosseous cerclage wire can restore normal scapholunate alignment and reduce tension on the scapholunate interosseous ligament repair during ligamentous healing. The clinical outcomes of patients with perilunate and lunate dislocations treated with a combination dorsal and volar approach as well as intraosseous cerclage wire were reported.

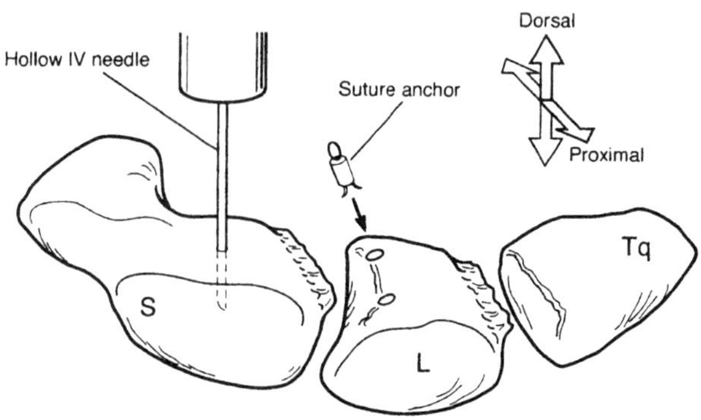

FIGURE 1.—Placement of 18-gauge IV catheter in proximal pole of scaphoid and placement of suture anchors for later repair of scapholunate ligament disruption. *Abbreviations: L*, Lunate; *S*, scaphoid; *T*, triquetrum. (Reprinted from Trumble T, Verheyden J: Treatment of isolated perilunate and lunate dislocations with combined dorsal and volar approach and intraosseous cerclage wire. *J Hand Surg [Am]* 29A:412-417, 2004. Copyright 2004, with permission from The American Society for Surgery of the Hand.)

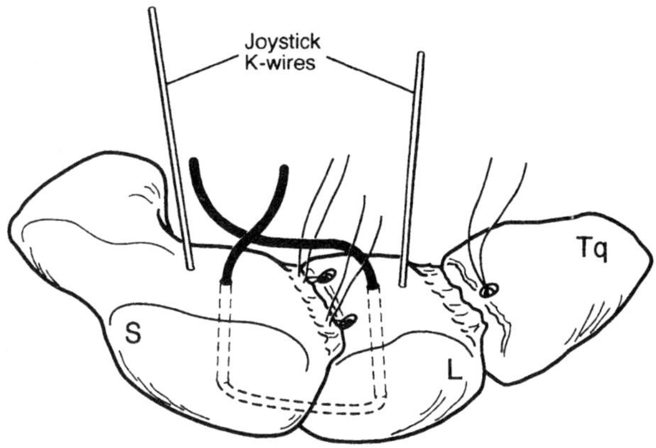

FIGURE 3.—K-wires are used as joysticks to reduce the scaphoid and lunate anatomically. Sutures from bone anchors are passed through scapholunate ligament but are not tied. (Reprinted from Trumble T, Verheyden J: Treatment of isolated perilunate and lunate dislocations with combined dorsal and volar approach and intraosseous cerclage wire. *J Hand Surg [Am]* 29A:412-417, 2004. Copyright 2004, with permission from The American Society for Surgery of the Hand.)

Methods.—Twenty-two patients with a total of 22 isolated perilunate and lunate dislocations were treated a mean 3 days after injury (Figs 1, 3, and 4). The mean follow-up was 49 months. Subjective assessment included the Disabilities of the Arm, Shoulder, and Hand questionnaire and patient ratings. Objective evaluation included range-of-motion measures, grip-strength measures, and scapholunate angle and gap comparisons on initial postoperative and final radiographs.

Findings.—Fifteen patients reported a high level of satisfaction with their results. Seven reported problems with activities of daily living after injury. Only 10 patients were able to return to the jobs they had before injury. All 22

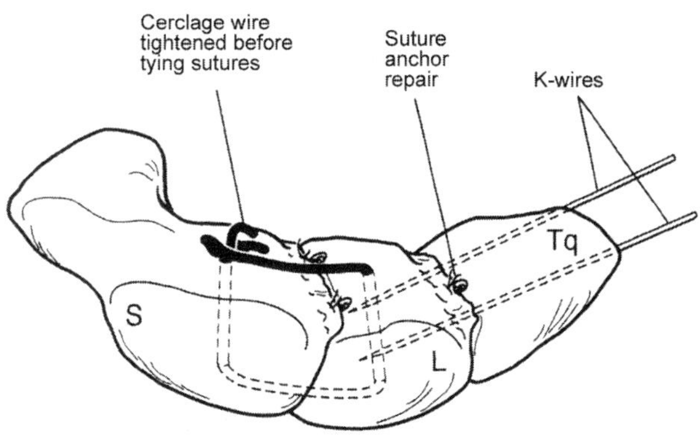

FIGURE 4.—With scaphoid and lunate reduced anatomically, cerclage wire is tightened. Next, sutures from bone anchors are tightened. In a similar fashion the triquetrum is reduced to lunate and held in place with K-wires before bone anchor sutures are tied. (Reprinted from Trumble T, Verheyden J: Treatment of isolated perilunate and lunate dislocations with combined dorsal and volar approach and intraosseous cerclage wire. *J Hand Surg [Am]* 29A:412-417, 2004. Copyright 2004, with permission from The American Society for Surgery of the Hand.)

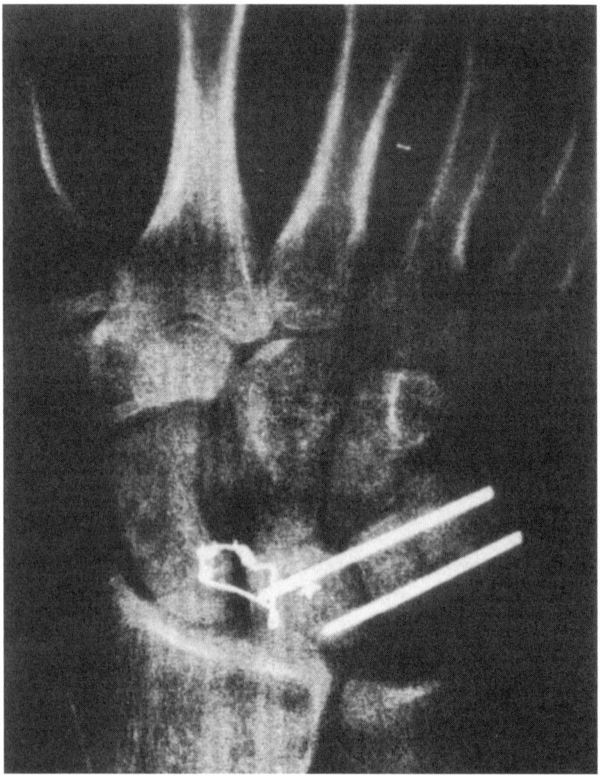

FIGURE 6.—Postsurgical posteroanterior and lateral radiographs of volar lunate dislocation treated with combined dorsal and volar approach with a 20-gauge intraosseous cerclage wire. (Reprinted from Trumble T, Verheyden J: Treatment of isolated perilunate and lunate dislocations with combined dorsal and volar approach and intraosseous cerclage wire. *J Hand Surg [Am]* 29A:412-417, 2004. Copyright 2004, with permission from The American Society for Surgery of the Hand.)

were able to return to some type of work. Sixteen patients said they could resume their previous activity levels. The average wrist flexion-extension arc strength was 80% and grip strength was 77% compared with the opposite side. No significant change in scapholunate angle or gap was seen over time on follow-up radiographs (Fig 6). The scapholunate cerclage wire often broke, as expected. Cerclage wire needed to be removed because of breakage in 12 patients and because of pain in 4.

Conclusions.—The combined dorsal and volar approach with an intraosseous wiring technique can restore normal intercarpal relations in patients with isolated perilunate and lunate dislocations. This treatment provides acceptable pain relief, functional motion, and grip strength.

▶ This study is likely the largest reported series on open reduction and internal fixation of isolated perilunate and lunate dislocations, an injury with distinctly different treatment challenges from the more common perilunate fracture-dislocations. The reported experience with combined dorsal and volar surgical approach and the use of a compressive cerclage wire to protect the scapholunate interosseous ligament repair resulted in restoration of carpal anatomy as well as acceptable functional outcomes for these challenging injuries. Their method is not without complications; a majority required removal of the broken cerclage wire, which was acknowledged to be a predictable event. The authors, however, correctly state that an acceptable resorbable and nonirritating alternative material to cerclage wire is currently not available. Their reported experience with this technique is nonetheless useful information.

S. D. Trigg, MD

The Sauve-Kapandji Procedure and the Darrach Procedure for Distal Radio-Ulnar Joint Dysfunction After Colles' Fracture

George MS, Kiefhaber TR, Stern PJ (Univ of Cincinnati, Ohio; Hand Surgery Specialists, Cincinnati, Ohio)

J Hand Surg [Br] 29B:608-613, 2004 9–12

Background.—Authorities disagree on the best way to treat posttraumatic distal radio-ulnar joint (DRUJ) derangement in younger, active patents. The Darrach procedure and the Sauve-Kapandji procedure were compared in such patients.

Methods.—This retrospective analysis included patients younger than 50 years who underwent the Darrach or Sauve-Kapandji procedure for the treatment of DRUJ derangement after malunion of dorsally displaced, unstable, intra-articular fractures of the distal radius. Twelve of 18 patients in the Sauve-Kapandji group and 21 of 30 in the Darrach group completed the Disabilities of the Arm, Shoulder and Hand (DASH) survey a mean 4 and 6 years after treatment, respectively. Data from a follow-up examination at a mean of 2 years were available for 9 of the Sauve-Kapandji recipients and at a mean of 4 years for 13 of the Darrach recipients.

Findings.—The 2 treatment groups did not differ in forearm or wrist range of motion or in mean DASH scores. On radiographic examination, all wrists in the Sauve-Kapandji group demonstrated definite DRUJ fusion. In the Darrach group, 6 patients had evidence of significant regrowth of the ulnar stump. Complication rates did not differ significantly between groups.

Conclusions.—The Darrach procedure and Sauve-Kapandji procedure produce comparable results in patients younger than 50 years with Colles' fracture on both subjective and objective measures. Neither procedure yielded predictable outcomes.

▶ Malunion of displaced distal radius fractures frequently results in painful degenerative arthritis of the DRUJ and associated ulnar abutment pain. Both the Sauve-Kapandji and Darrach procedures have been advocated for treatment of posttraumatic DRUJ degenerative arthritis, but both of the procedures suffer from well-recognized complications noted over the long term. This retrospective study (with recognition of limitations of number of patients and differing follow-up) is the first to compare these procedures in patients younger than 50 years. Their findings provide us with worthwhile information to review when considering these procedures.

S. D. Trigg, MD

Proximal Row Carpectomy: Study With a Minimum of Ten Years of Follow-up

DiDonna ML, Kiefhaber TR, Stern PJ (Univ of Cincinnati, Ohio)

J Bone Joint Surg Am 86A:2359-2365, 2004 9–13

Background.—Proximal row carpectomy (PRC) is an accepted treatment for degenerative wrist conditions, but few data on the long-term clinical and radiographic outcomes are available. The functional outcomes and patient satisfaction at least 10 years after PRC were investigated.

Methods.—The study included 21 patients with degenerative arthritis who underwent PRC in a total of 22 wrists between 1980 and 1992. The mean follow-up was 14 years.

Findings.—Four failures (18%) necessitating fusion occurred at a mean 7 years after the procedure. All were in patients aged 35 years or younger at the time of surgery. Among wrists that did not have failed procedures, the mean flexion-extension arc was 72°, correlating with a mean grip strength of 91% of that on the contralateral side. The patients with no wrist failures said they were very satisfied with the results of their treatment, and those with wrist failures reported being satisfied. According to patient ratings, 9 wrists were not painful, 4 were mildly painful, and 5 were moderately painful. None of

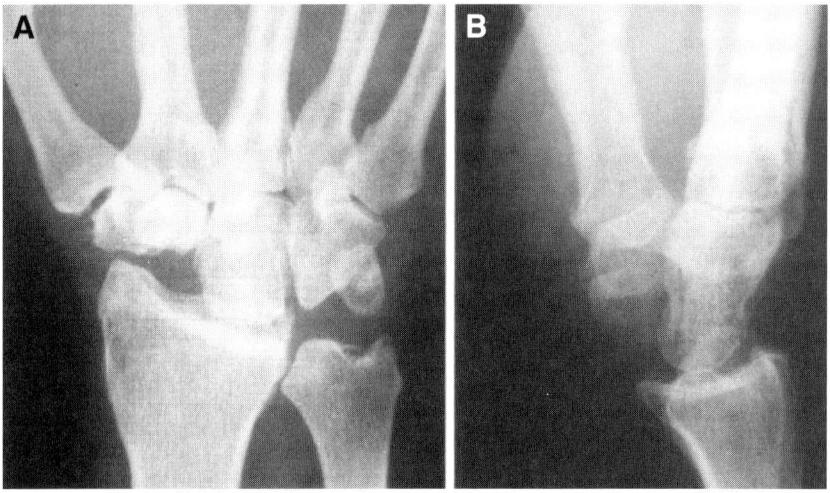

FIGURE 1.—Posteroanterior and lateral radiographs showing no narrowing of radiocapitate space in wrist 12 years after proximal row carpectomy. (Republished with permission of the Journal of Bone and Joint Surgery, Inc, from DiDonna ML, Kiefhaber TR, Stern PJ: Proximal row carpectomy: Study with a minimum of ten years of follow-up. *J Bone Joint Surg Am* 86A:2359-2365, 2004. Reproduced by permission of the publisher via Copyright Clearance Center, Inc.)

the wrists was rated as severely painful. The average score on the Disabilities of the Arm, Shoulder, and Hand scale was 9 points. Of the 17 wrists with radiographs, no loss of the radiocapitate space was apparent in 3, reduced space was seen in 7, and complete loss of space was noted in 7 (Fig 1). Loss of joint space on radiographs did not correlate with subjective or objective function.

Conclusions.—In this series, all patients older than 35 years at the time of a PRC maintained satisfactory range of motion, grip strength, and pain relief in the long term. Patients also continued to be satisfied with the result. Degeneration of the radiocapitate joint on the radiographs on 14 wrists did not preclude a successful clinical outcome.

► PRC remains an enigma in the minds of many wrist surgeons. The procedure is seemingly inelegant and yields an incongruent, shortened, simplified hinge joint that would likely be discounted by all if it were proposed as a new procedure today. However, PRC continues to stand up against the test of time compared with other procedures for similar indications. The data presented in this study further the collective experience of PRC, both validating the long-term effectiveness of the procedure and additionally providing new information about indications and long-term outcome.

S. D. Trigg, MD

Hand

Dynamic Intradigital External Fixation for Proximal Interphalangeal Joint Fracture Dislocations

Badia A, Riano F, Ravikoff J, et al (Miami Hand Ctr, Fla; Cornell Univ, Ithaca, NY)
J Hand Surg [Am] 30A:154-160, 2005 9–14

Background.—Fracture dislocations of the proximal interphalangeal (PIP) joint can be mistaken for a jammed finger and treatment may be delayed, an occurrence that can produce stiffness, pain, and posttraumatic arthritis. Generally, the injury occurs as a result of a direct force applied to the fingertip, causing hyperextension and axial loading of the PIP joint that produces impaction of the volar articular lip of the middle phalanx against the condyles of the proximal phalanx. Both nonsurgical and surgical treatments have been used. For a surgical treatment, Gaul and Rosenberg developed a simple frame to provide traction without needing rubber bands or complicated connecting pieces. A modification of this approach with a simple intradigital dynamic fixator that could be applied under a digital block in an office setting was used, and the outcomes were reported.

Methods.—The study included 6 patients (ages 21-42 years; average, 27 years) who had fracture dislocations of the PIP joint. All were treated with the simple dynamic fixator with no rubber bands. The middle finger was affected in 3 patients, the ring finger in 1, and the small finger in 2. From 35% to 60% involvement of the base of the middle phalanx was reported (average, 48%). Surgery was performed 1 to 14 days after injury (average, 6 days), and follow-up lasted 7 to 43 months (average, 24 months). This approach permitted immediate active flexion extension. The fixator was removed in 3 to 4 weeks.

Results.—The PIP joint had an average ROM of 5° to 89°, varying from 0° to 100°. The distal interphalangeal ROM at final assessment averaged 2° to 80° (range, 0°-90°). Pin tract infections developed in 2 patients but responded to oral antibiotics. Final AP and lateral radiographs confirmed appropriate reduction and congruency of the joint. One patient had mild pain with extreme flexion. None of the PIP joints evidenced instability at the final assessment.

Conclusions.—The simple dynamic fixator produced good results with only minor complications. Reduction was maintained and digital ROM was restored in the 6 cases reported.

► The optimum treatment for displaced intra-articular fracture dislocations of the PIP joint continues to be a work in progress. To date, the most favorable outcomes have resulted from early operative intervention with application of dynamic traction devices, which restores length and reduces the dislocation. Many of the reported traction devices are both ingenious and effective but can be bulky, complicated, and expensive. The search for a simple cost-effective alternative continues. The technique and data presented in this limited study appear to satisfy some of the criteria for a simpler cost-effective treatment.

S. D. Trigg, MD

Basal Joint Osteoarthritis of the Thumb: A Prospective Trial of Steroid Injection and Splinting

Day CS, Gelberman R, Patel AA, et al (Washington Univ, St Louis; Univ of Pittsburgh, Pa)

J Hand Surg [Am] 29A:247-251, 2004 9–15

Background.—The components of nonsurgical management for trapeziometacarpal (TM) osteoarthritis include splinting, the administration of oral nonsteroidal anti-inflammatory drugs (NSAIDs), and intra-articular injections of corticosteroids. The effectiveness of a single corticosteroid injection plus 3 weeks of splinting for TM arthritis was investigated and documented using an established radiographic staging system for TM osteoarthritis. It was believed that the injection and splinting would temporarily relieve symptoms regardless of the radiographic stage of the patient's TM arthritis.

Methods.—The study included 30 patients (30 thumbs) who were assessed prospectively. Each was given a single injection of corticosteroid into the TM joint, then the thumb was immobilized in a thumb spica splint for 3 weeks. The Disabilities of the Arm, Shoulder, and Hand questionnaire was distributed to the patients to determine outcomes. Evaluations were completed before the injection, 6 weeks later, and at a minimum of 18 months of follow-up. Three independent observers recorded the Eaton radiographic stage of disease.

Results.—The radiographic grades of disease were stage 1 for 6 thumbs, stage 2 for 7, stage 3 for 10, and stage 4 for 7. The pain at the thumb base had been present for 6 to 96 months (average, 18 months) before the patient came to the clinic. Four weeks after injection, 13 (43.3%) patients had a mean improvement in pain intensity of 5.5 points (range, 4-7 points) and 17 (56.7%) had no relief. The relief was maintained for 12 of the 13 who had initial relief until the final follow-up evaluation (average, 21 months). The patients who had relief of pain experienced a corresponding improvement in the ability to perform daily activities, improving from severely difficult to minimally difficult. Grip strength averaged 95% and key-pinch strength, 90% of the contralateral hand among the 12 patients who had sustained relief. The 1 patient who had no long-term relief required a tendon interposition arthroplasty procedure 12 months after receiving the injection. No further improvement occurred in the 17 patients who had no pain relief after the corticosteroid injection, with 11 patients eventually requiring either a tendon arthroplasty or arthrodesis of the TM joint. A significant difference in the grip- and pinch-strength values between these patients and those who had long-term relief was noted. Among the 6 patients with stage I disease, 5 had long-term relief. Of those with stage 2 and stage 3 disease, 7 had relief after 4 weeks and 6 at final follow-up. Basal joint surgery was done in 9 patients. No pain relief was reported by 6 of the 7 patients with stage 4 disease, and 3 required surgery.

Conclusions.—For Eaton stage I disease, nonsurgical treatment can reliably provide sustained relief in most cases. When osteophytes or joint narrowing is present radiographically, such conservative management is less reliable in achieving relief. Patients who have no scaphotrapezial arthritis can achieve long-term relief with a single corticosteroid injection and splinting if they have obtained short-term relief; however, such long-term relief occurs in only about 35% of the cases.

▶ Corticosteroid injection and splinting alone or in combination for TM osteoarthritis is frequently recommended as initial nonsurgical treatment. Most of the information of the efficacy of corticosteroid injections for TM osteoarthritis is largely retrospective or anecdotal. This prospective study provides us with clinically useful and predictive information that we can implement into our practices.

S. D. Trigg, MD

Ligament Reconstruction With Trapezium Retention Arthroplasty for Carpometacarpal Arthritis

Mo JH, Gelberman RH (Washington Univ, St Louis)

J Hand Surg [Am] 29A:240-246, 2004 9–16

Background.—The joint pain associated with carpometacarpal arthritis is nearly always relieved by excisional arthroplasty of the trapezium, but thumb strength and stability may not be restored. A modification of the procedure has been made to prevent proximal migration of the thumb metacarpal. However, ligament reconstruction and tendon interposition (LRTI) arthroplasty can still fall short of success in restoring thumb strength. A qualitative and quantitative analysis of the results of a trapezium-retaining interposition arthroplasty used in patients with carpometacarpal arthritis was undertaken.

Methods.—The study included 16 patients with basal joint arthritis who underwent the trapezium-retaining interposition arthroplasty. Follow-up at least 12 months later (mean, 20 months) included 14 patients. Measures included clinical outcome, presurgical and postsurgical radiograph comparisons, and determinations of ROM, grip strength, and pinch strength. Patients completed the Disabilities of the Arm, Shoulder, and Hand (DASH) questionnaire to assess upper-extremity function and disability.

Results.—Before surgery, the average grip strength was 22.63 kg, pinch strength was 5.34 kg, and the ROM was 0.6 cm. After surgery, these values improved to 28.48 kg, 5.90 kg, and 0.2 cm, respectively. Significant improvement was obtained only in grip strength. No significant correlation was noted between postoperative trapezial height ratio and postoperative grip strength, pinch strength, or ROM values. Ninety-three percent of the patients expressed satisfaction with the results on the DASH questionnaire. The DASH scores showed significant correlations with grip strength and pinch strength postoperatively, but not with either ROM or trapezial height ratio.

Conclusions.—Trapezial height was successfully maintained using the ligament reconstruction with trapezium retention arthroplasty of the basal joint. Patients received this approach well, with 93% expressing satisfaction with the result.

▶ Trapezium resection LRTI arthroplasty is one of the most commonly performed joint reconstructive procedures in hand surgery. Despite a high percentage of successful outcomes with respect to pain relief, restoration of pinch strength, and thumb stability, the incidence of metacarpal subsidence is less consistently reported. This study provides us with preliminary information on a technique of partial trapezium sparing designed to mitigate proximal thumb migration and improve pinch strength.

S. D. Trigg, MD

Optimizing Biomechanical Performance of the 4-Strand Cruciate Flexor Tendon Repair

Dona E, Gianoutsos MP, Walsh WR (Univ of New South Wales, Sydney, Australia; Wales Hosp, Sydney, Australia)

J Hand Surg [Am] 29A:571-580, 2004 9–17

Background.—Various multistrand core techniques for zone 2 flexor tendon repair have been developed to achieve early mobilization. The 4-strand core technique may be ideal, combining biomechanical integrity with technical simplicity. Either a grasping- or a locking-loop configuration can be used at each corner. Whether increasing the size of the locking loop increases the repair strength of the cruciate 4-strand suture technique was investigated. In addition, the biomechanical properties of the various peripheral suture techniques in the cruciate 4-strand suture method were determined.

Methods.—Deep flexor tendons were harvested from adult sheep hind limbs, then divided randomly into 7 groups of 8 tendons each. The cruciate core technique with no peripheral suture was used to repair 4 groups. Locking loops used 10%, 25%, 33%, or 50% of the tendon width and were loaded to failure using a distraction rate of 20 mm/min. The optimal locking-loop size that resulted from this assessment was used in 3 groups for repair, and they were combined with a simple running, cross-stitch, or interlocking horizontal mattress (IHM) suture, respectively. Repairs were tested until they failed. The load at the 2-mm gap, the load at failure, and the stiffness were documented.

Results.—Cruciate repair using a 10% locking loop had the poorest performance on load to failure but was best for load to 2-mm gap formation. The 50% locking loop performed poorly on load to 2-mm gap formation and had low stiffness values. The optimal size was 25% of the tendon's width. A repair site gap of 2 mm developed at 12.8 newtons and failure occurred with a load of 46.3 newtons with the 25% locking loop. The stiffness was 3.9 newtons/mm. The IHM/cruciate combination with a 25% locking loop was substantially better than the cross-stitch/cruciate and simple running/cruciate combinations.

Conclusions.—The best core technique used a 25% locking loop. The biomechanical properties of the repair require that peripheral sutures be included. The best improvement in biomechanical properties was achieved using the IHM peripheral suture technique.

► In case you have not noticed, there have been a plethora of in-vitro biomechanical studies purporting the merits of a variety of multistrand flexor tendon laceration repair techniques that have been published in recent years. While most of these studies make for dry reading, the information is nonetheless important if we are to reach the goal of safely allowing early active digit ROM to optimize function after zone 2 repairs. Multistrand 4- and 6-strand repairs are essentially 2 and 3 times stronger, respectively, than the most commonly performed 2-strand Kessler repair. The 6- strand repairs have been generally difficult to perform in vivo without adding unwanted bulk at the repair site. The cruciate 4-strand repair, presented here, has been judged by many to be perhaps an ideal method, which is nearly as easy to perform as most 2-strand repairs. This study clearly elucidates the technique for optimizing this repair for both the core and peripheral sutures.

S. D. Trigg, MD

Seventeen-Year Survivorship Analysis of Silastic Metacarpophalangeal Joint Replacement

Trail IA, Martin JA, Nuttall D, et al (Wrightington Hosp, Wigan, England)
J Bone Joint Surg Br 86-B:1002-1006, 2004 9–18

Introduction.—We reviewed the records and radiographs of 381 patients with rheumatoid arthritis who had undergone silastic metacarpophalangeal joint replacement during the past 17 years. The number of implants was 1336 in the course of 404 operations. Implant failure was defined as either revision or fracture of the implant as seen on radiography (Figs 1 and 2). At 17 years, the survivorship was 63% (Fig 6), although on radiographs two-thirds of the implants were seen to be broken (Fig 7). Factors which improved survival included soft-tissue balancing, crossed intrinsic transfer and realignment of the wrist. Surgery to the thumb and proximal interphalangeal joint had a deleterious effect and the use of grommets did not protect the implant from fracture.

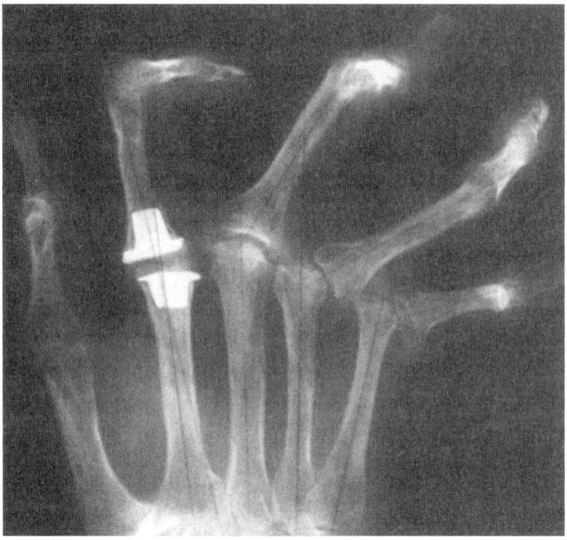

FIGURE 1.—Severe ulnar drift (>45°) of the metacarpophalangeal joints of the ring and little fingers. (Courtesy of Trail IA, Martin JA, Nuttall D, et al: Seventeen-year survivorship analysis of silastic metacarpophalangeal joint replacement. *J Bone Joint Surg Br* 86-B:1002-1006, 2004.)

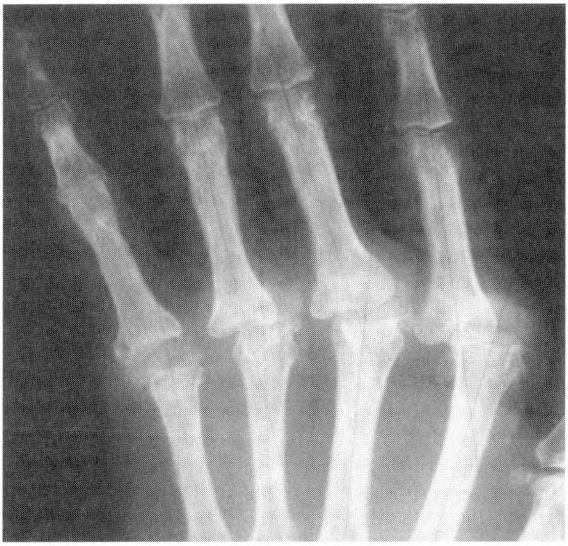

FIGURE 2.—Severe translation (>50°) of the metacarpophalangeal joint of the index finger. (Courtesy of Trail IA, Martin JA, Nuttall D, et al: Seventeen-year survivorship analysis of silastic metacarpophalangeal joint replacement. *J Bone Joint Surg Br* 86-B:1002-1006, 2004.)

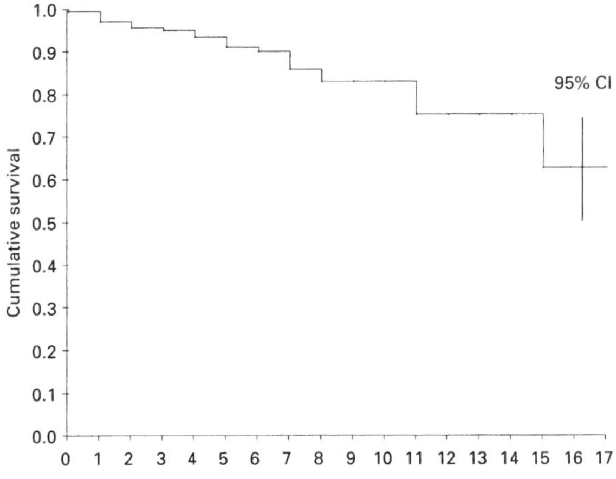

FIGURE 6.—Graph showing the cumulative survival of 1336 metacarpophalangeal joint replacements with failure defined as revision surgery to the finger. (Courtesy of Trail IA, Martin JA, Nuttall D, et al: Seventeen-year survivorship analysis of silastic metacarpophalangeal joint replacement. *J Bone Joint Surg Br* 86-B:1002-1006, 2004.)

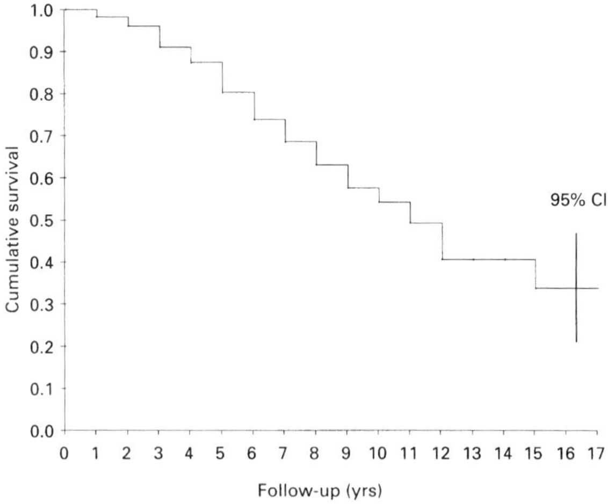

FIGURE 7.—Graph showing the cumulative survival of 1336 metacarpophalangeal joint operations with failure defined as fracture to the implant. (Courtesy of Trail IA, Martin JA, Nuttall D, et al: Seventeen-year survivorship analysis of silastic metacarpophalangeal joint replacement. *J Bone Joint Surg Br* 86-B:1002-1006, 2004.)

Long-term Assessment of Swanson Implant Arthroplasty in the Proximal Interphalangeal Joint of the Hand

Takigawa S, Meletiou S, Sauerbier M, et al (Mayo Clinic, Rochester, Minn)
J Hand Surg [Am] 29A:785-795, 2004 9–19

Purpose.—The purpose of this study was to evaluate the clinical results of Swanson silicone implant arthroplasty of the proximal interphalangeal (PIP) joint, specifically evaluating clinical results with long-term assessment.

Methods.—A retrospective review of 70 silicone implants of the PIP joint in 48 patients was performed with an average follow-up period of 6.5 years (range, 3-20 y). Clinical assessment included motion, stability, and alignment. Radiographic assessment included implant fracture, deformity, and cystic bone resorption. The pathology consisted of degenerative joint disease in 14, posttraumatic arthritis (TA) in 11, rheumatoid arthritis (RA) in 13, and idiopathic arthritis (IA) associated with collagen disease in 12 patients. Swan neck and boutonniere deformities were assessed separately. Statistical analysis of preoperative risk factors was compared with the postoperative assessment of pain, motion, and function (return to work).

Results.—There was no significant change in the active range of motion (ROM) before and after PIP arthroplasty (26° vs 30°). Correction of swan neck and boutonniere deformities was difficult, usually leading to poor results. There was improvement in maximum active extension before surgery lacking 32° to after surgery lacking 18°. From a statistical standpoint rheumatoid joint involvement with PIP arthroplasty had poorer results than degenerative or posttraumatic arthritis with respect to pain relief and ROM. Pain relief was present in 70% of replaced PIP joints with residual pain and loss of strength in 30%. Radiographic analysis showed abnormal bone formation (cystic changes) in 45%. There were 11 implant fractures and 9 joints that required revision surgery.

Conclusions.—Silicone replacement of the PIP joint is effective in providing relief of pain from arthritis but does not provide improvement in motion or correction of deformity. It provided a poorer outcome in rheumatoid disease in comparison with degenerative, posttraumatic, or idiopathic arthritis.

► Every few years in the literature, a retrospective long-term assessment study of silicone arthroplasties of the metacarpophalangeal and proximal interphalangeal joints is published. Much of the information confirms previous findings (which in and of itself is relevant), but more importantly they reveal important new information. Both of these studies (Abstracts 9–18 and 9–19) come from large, reputable clinical groups who have extensively reported on these procedures in the past. Their findings and recommendations warrant our review.

S. D. Trigg, MD

10 Elbow

Introduction

This year's articles on the elbow covered a spectrum from the most common issue of tennis elbow to more difficult problems of joint replacement arthroplasty. The few articles in this section have been specifically selected to provide practical insight and decision-making for the more common problems as well as to inform the reader of the current state of more advanced reconstructive options. The body of information regarding elbow reconstructive surgery is expanding rather rapidly, with the most significant contributions being on the management of acute trauma and arthritis. The debate of the value of extracorporeal shock wave therapy is also addressed.

Bernard F. Morrey, MD

Repetitive Low-Energy Shock Wave Treatment for Chronic Lateral Epicondylitis in Tennis Players

Rompe JD, Decking J, Schoellner C, et al (Johannes Gutenberg Univ, Mainz, Germany)

Am J Sports Med 32:734-743, 2004 10–1

Background.—Lateral epicondylalgia or epicondylitis (tennis elbow) is a repetitive overuse injury that produces microtears in the tendons that attach the extensor muscles to the epicondyle. In tennis players, this most often results from overload during a backhand stroke. Lateral epicondylalgia is more likely to occur in unskilled tennis players who use a racket that is too stiff, who hit the ball late, who frequently "frame" the ball, or whose forearm muscles are weak.

Players older than 40 years have been shown to be more susceptible to lateral elbow epicondylalgia. Extracorporeal shock wave treatment (ESWT) has been used for chronic tennis elbow, but variable results have been reported in several prospective studies. The hypothesis that treatment with repetitive low-energy ESWT is superior to repetitive placebo ESWT was investigated.

Methods.—A total of 78 patients were enrolled in this placebo-controlled trial. All patients were tennis players with recalcitrant MRI-confirmed tennis elbow of at least 12 months' duration. The patients were randomly assigned to receive either active low-energy ESWT given weekly for 3 weeks (treatment group) or an identical placebo ESWT (sham group). The main outcome measure was pain during resisted wrist extension at 3 months. The secondary outcome measures were greater than 50% reduction of pain and the score on the Upper Extremity Function Scale.

Results.—At 3 months, there was a significantly higher improvement in pain during resisted wrist extension in the treatment group compared with the sham group (mean [SD] improvement, 3.5 [2.0] vs 2.0 [1.9]) and in the Upper Extremity Function Scale (mean [SD] improvement, 23.4 [14.8] and 10.9 [14.9]). A reduction in pain of at least 50% was achieved by 65% of patients in the treatment group compared with 28% of patients in the sham group.

Conclusion.—Low-energy ESWT was more effective than sham ESWT for treatment of chronic tennis elbow.

▶ This article represents one of many that has appeared over the last couple of years assessing the efficacy of this modality for the most common elbow ailment, epicondylitis. This particular study is noteworthy because it does represent a placebo-controlled prospective assessment. The finding that low-energy ESWT was effective in the doses and intensity administered is in contrast to much of the literature, which demonstrates its value to be equivocal at 1 year. It is not uncommon, however, to have improvement at the 3-month period, as demonstrated by these authors. The overall true value of this modality, particularly from a cost-effectiveness standpoint, remains to be elucidated.

B. F. Morrey, MD

A Comparison of Open and Percutaneous Techniques in the Surgical Treatment of Tennis Elbow

Dunkow PD, Jatti M, Muddu BN (Tameside Hosp, Manchester, England)
J Bone Joint Surg Br 86-B:701-704, 2004 10–2

Background.—The syndrome of pain centered over the common origin of the extensor muscles of the fingers and wrist at the lateral epicondyle, termed *tennis elbow or lateral epicondylitis*, is found more often in nonathletes than in athletes. The peak incidence is in the fifth decade. The precise etiology and pathology are unclear, but tennis elbow is usually diagnosed by localizing pain when the patient pinches with the wrist in extension and with resisted extension of the middle finger. Rest, modification of activity, local splinting, and steroid injection are sufficient treatment in 90% of cases. Surgery is needed for up to 8% of patients. Two operative techniques, the open technique and a percutaneous division of the common extensor origin, were compared for their effectiveness in managing tennis elbow.

Methods.—The 45 patients (47 elbows) were assessed preoperatively with the use of the American Academy of Orthopaedic Surgeons Disability of Arm, Shoulder and Hand (DASH) score. Twenty-four patients underwent the open technique, and 23 had the percutaneous operation. Follow-up lasted a minimum of 12 months.

Results.—Both the open and the percutaneous groups had a median preoperative normalized DASH score of 70. Postoperatively, the median normalized DASH scores were 17 for the open group and 20 for the percutaneous group, which was a highly significant difference. On the sport function section of the DASH score, preoperative median scores were 68 and 70 for the open and percutaneous groups, respectively, and the changes in median scores were 11 and 19 for the open and percutaneous groups, respectively. This difference was also highly significant. On the high performance work section of the DASH score, the open group had a median score of 68 preoperatively and 52 postoperatively; these scores for the percutaneous group were 72 and 49, respectively. The change in the median score was 14 for the open group and 24 for the percutaneous group. Significant differences between the groups were also noted with respect to patient satisfaction levels. In the open group, 2 patients were dissatisfied, 16 were satisfied, and 6 were very pleased with the outcome of the surgery. In the percutaneous group, none of the patients were dissatisfied, 9 were satisfied, and 14 were very pleased.

Conclusions.—When surgery is being considered for the management of tennis elbow, the percutaneous procedure may give significantly better results than the open procedure. The percutaneous procedure is accomplished more quickly and can be done under local anesthesia. No significant complications developed in the patients in this study.

► Tennis elbow is the most common elbow ailment for which an orthopedic opinion is sought. The assessment of patients treated with percutaneous techniques is in contrast to a growing trend in treating these patients with a rather aggressive arthroscopic debridement. The findings of this particular group are supported by the few previous studies that, for reasons that may not be entirely clear, have demonstrated that percutaneous release is comparable in effectiveness to any one of several open techniques. I have not yet, however, had confidence in these data to attempt the approach in my clinical practice.

B. F. Morrey, MD

Ulnohumeral Arthroplasty: Results in Primary Degenerative Arthritis of the Elbow

Sarris I, Riano FA, Goebel F, et al (Univ of Pittsburgh, Pa)

Clin Orthop 420:190-193, 2004 10–3

Introduction.—Several surgical approaches have been described for treatment of primary osteoarthritis of the elbow. Presented were the results of ulnohumeral arthroplasty performed to treat early primary degenerative arthritis of the elbow.

Methods.—Seventeen patients were evaluated retrospectively at an average follow-up of 36 months (range, 24-50 months). The average age of this all-male cohort was 52 years (range, 40-74 years).

Surgical Technique.—With the patient positioned in the lateral decubitus position, all bony prominences were well padded, a sterile tourniquet was applied, and a posterior incision was made, beginning 6 to 8 cm proximal to the tip of the olecranon and extending 4 cm distal to the olecranon. The triceps tendon was split longitudinally in line with the incision until the posterior elbow was seen. A capsulotomy was performed, and the posterior osteophyte and a portion of the posterior olecranon were removed with an osteotome to minimize impingement in extension. The edges were smoothed with a rongeur.

A hole was created in the olecranon fossa to gain access to the coronoid and anterior elbow compartment. A 1.5-cm neurosurgical dowel was attached to a drill bit and a drill hole was made. The hole was used to remove debris and loose bodies from the anterior elbow. The anterior osteophyte was removed from the coronoid process during maximal elbow flexion. It was sometimes necessary to strip the anterior capsule from the anterior humerus using a blunt periosteum elevator to regain better extension.

The wound was closed, and the elbow was manipulated to maximize the total arc of motion. A splint was applied with the elbow placed in 15° extension. Continuous passive motion was not used to gain ROM; rather, active ROM was initiated 7 days postoperatively.

Results.—At final follow-up, 15 patients had complete pain relief at end ROM and 2 had moderate pain after prolonged activity. Extension and flexion were improved by a mean of 12° and 20°, respectively. The average arc of motion improved from 26° to 98° preoperatively to 14° to 118° postoperatively. Postoperative radiographs revealed a correctly placed drill hole with complete osteophyte resection. There were no neurologic or other complications. Good stability of the elbow was seen in all patients.

Conclusion.—Ulnohumeral arthroplasty requires a single approach that is safe and simple and provides adequate exposure of the coronoid process and anterior capsule. It is recommended for patients with painful limitation of motion caused by osteophyte formation in the elbow.

Arthroscopic Capsulolabroplasty for Posteroinferior Multidirectional Instability of the Shoulder

Kim S-H, Kim H-K, Sun J-I, et al (Sungkyunkwan Univ, Seoul, Korea)
Am J Sports Med 32:594-607, 2004 10–4

Introduction.—The arthroscopic treatment of posteroinferior multidirectional instability of the shoulder has not been well documented. The pathologic lesions of posteroinferior multidirectional instability and the results of arthroscopic capsulolabroplasty were prospectively examined in a nonrandomized clinical trial.

Methods.—At a mean follow-up of 51 months, 31 patients with posteroinferior multidirectional instability were prospectively assessed after arthroscopic capsulolabroplasty. The procedure was a battery of 3 major procedures: arthroscopic posteroinferior labroplasty, superior shift of the posteroinferior and anteroinferior capsule, and rotator interval closure. The labral lesion and height were measured in both the MRI arthrogram and arthroscopic examination.

Results.—All 31 participants had a labral lesion and variable capsular stretching in the posteroinferior aspect. Of 31 shoulders, there were 11 type I labral lesions (incomplete detachment), 12 type II (the Kim's lesion: incomplete and concealed avulsion), 6 type III (chondrolabral erosion), and 2 type IV (flap tear). All patients who had type II or III lesions had chondrolabral retroversion. Lost labral height was identified in the MRI arthrogram and arthroscopic examination. The Rowe score was excellent, good, and fair in 21, 9, and 1 shoulders, respectively. Every patient had improved shoulder scores and function and pain scores; 30 had stable shoulders and 1 had recurrent instability.

Conclusion.—Patients who had symptomatic posteroinferior multidirectional instability had posteroinferior labral lesions, including retroversion of the posteroinferior labrum, which were previously unnoticed. Restoration of the labral buttress and capsular tension via arthroscopic capsulolabroplasty successfully stabilized shoulders in these patients.

Débridement Arthroplasty for Primary Osteoarthritis of the Elbow

Wada T, Isogai S, Ishii S, et al (Sapporo Med Univ, Japan)

J Bone Joint Surg Am 86-A:233-241, 2004 10–5

Introduction.—Formal and aggressive debridement procedures have been described in the treatment of advanced primary osteoarthritis (OA) of the elbow. Few data are available regarding long-term follow-up. The outcomes of debridement arthroplasties performed via a posteromedial approach were examined at an average of 10 years postoperatively.

Methods.—Thirty-three elbows (32 patients) with primary OA who were treated via debridement arthroplasty underwent clinical follow-up examinations. The mean patient age at the time of surgery was 50 years. The mean duration of follow-up was 121 months; 19 elbows were followed up for more than 10 years.

> *Surgical Technique.*—The flexor-pronator muscle origin was reflected from the medial epicondyle, using a posteromedial approach. The joint was opened and the anterior oblique bundle of the medial collateral ligament was preserved. The ulnar nerve was decompressed in all procedures. Osteophytes were excised from the anterior, medial, and posterior sides of the elbow joint. In 9 elbows, osteophytes from the lateral compartment were removed via an additional lateral approach (Fig 2).

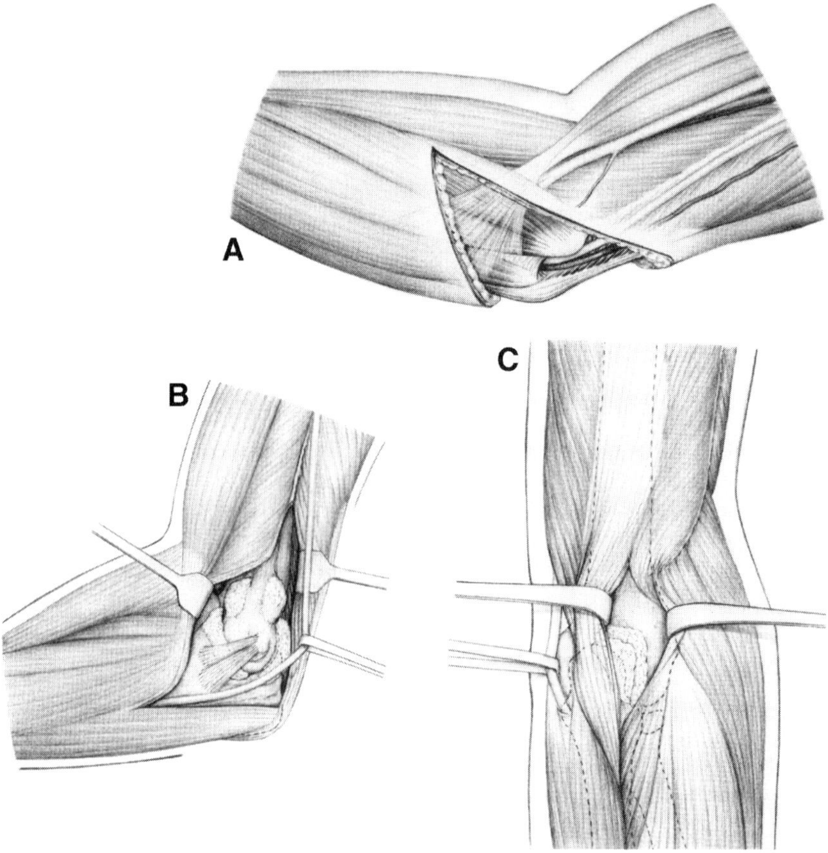

FIGURE 2.—The operative technique. A, The skin incision. B, Elevation of the pronator-flexor muscle origin. The anterior, medial, and posterior aspect of the ulnohumeral joint is exposed. The anterior oblique bundle of the medial collateral ligament is preserved. C, Osteophytes of the lateral aspect of the olecranon and the olecranon fossa are exposed and excised. (Republished with permission of the Journal of Bone and Joint Surgery, Inc, from Wada T, Isogai S, Ishii S, et al: Débridement arthroplasty for primary osteoarthritis of the elbow. *J Bone Joint Surg Am* 86-A:233-241, 2004. Reproduced by permission of the publisher via Copyright Clearance Center, Inc.)

Results.—The mean preoperative limitation of extension was reduced from 31° to 24°, and the mean preoperative flexion was improved from 101° to 118° ($P < .001$). The mean arc of movement was expanded by 24°. The mean Japanese Orthopedic Association elbow score was 83 points at latest follow-up examination, compared with that of 60 points preoperatively ($P < .001$). Of 25 patients who had performed heavy manual labor, 19 (76%) returned to their previous or equivalent job. At latest evaluation of the 19 elbows followed up for more than 10 years, the limitation of extension increased by 7°, compared with that documented at 1 year ($P < .009$); the mean arc of flexion remained the same (Fig 4). Three elbows underwent reoperation. Overall, patients indicated that 85% of elbows were satisfactory.

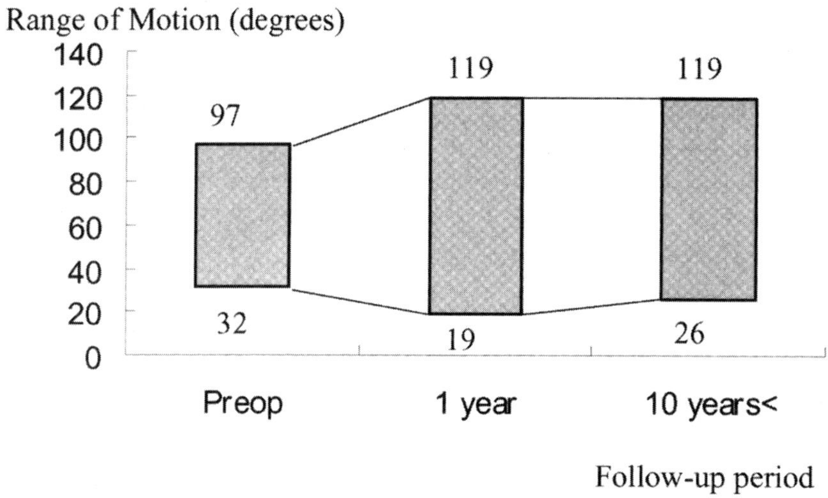

FIGURE 4.—Sequential changes in the extension-flexion arc of the elbow in the 19 patients followed for more than 10 years. (Republished with permission of the Journal of Bone and Joint Surgery, Inc, from Wada T, Isogai S, Ishii S, et al: Débridement arthroplasty for primary osteoarthritis of the elbow. *J Bone Joint Surg Am* 86-A:233-241, 2004. Reproduced by permission of the publisher via Copyright Clearance Center, Inc.)

Conclusion.—Debridement arthroplasty, with the use of a posteromedial approach, can provide both stable and reliable long-term pain relief, gains in ROM, and can hasten the patient's ability to return to previous occupation. A modest loss of extension was detected at 10 years; however, the arc of flexion remained consistent.

▶ These 2 contributions (Abstracts 10–4 and 10–5) each have one feature in common, documenting the effectiveness of debridement for the selected patient with primary osteoarthritis. The ulnohumeral arthroplasty (Abstract 10–3) has been documented to be a safe, reliable procedure in the majority of patients with a low complication rate, modest improvement in motion, and predictable relief of pain. We have found this in our experience as have others. The article from Japan (Abstract 10–5) documents the value of a more aggressive procedure, and the long-term expectation of osteophyte removal. It is encouraging to note that while progression does occur, it occurs slowly and even at 10 years, 85% were still satisfied with their procedure.

The article by Kim et al (Abstract 10–4) adds yet an additional dimension for the management of these patients. Arthroscopic debridement is more demanding but for those experienced with elbow arthroscopy, it is considered rather straightforward. It does provide the opportunity to improve the arc of motion by arthroscopically releasing the capsule. We would emphasize, however, that with all these techniques, preoperative assessment of the status of the ulnar nerve is essential to ensure that ulnar nerve pathology is considered and appropriately addressed, otherwise the outcome will be unsatisfactory.

B. F. Morrey, MD

A Biomechanical Evaluation of Methods of Distal Humerus Fracture Fixation Using Locking Compression Plates Versus Conventional Reconstruction Plates

Korner J, Diederichs G, Arzdorf M, et al (Univ of Mainz, Germany; AO Research Inst, Davos, Switzerland; Univ of Leipzig, Germany)

J Orthop Trauma 18:286-293, 2004 10–6

Background.—Fractures of the distal humerus are among the most demanding challenges in orthopedic trauma surgery. Open reduction and internal fixation has become the treatment of choice for adults and has provided biomechanically good results. Previous biomechanical studies on internal fixation of distal humerus fractures have shown that double-plate osteosynthesis with 3.5-mm reconstruction plates provides adequate stability under in vitro conditions. The behavior of 2 techniques of double-plate osteosynthesis for fractures of the adult distal humerus were examined using conventional reconstruction plates and locking compression plates.

Methods.—Forty fresh-frozen human distal humeri specimens were used in this experimental in vitro study. Four matched groups of 10 humeri each, with a median age of 74 years, were assembled by using similar bone mineral density values. Two standard configurations of double-plate synthesis—dorsal or 90° configuration—with either conventional reconstruction plates or locking compression plates were studied for biomechanical properties of the constructs.

A fracture model with a 5-mm supracondylar osteotomy gap simulating metaphyseal comminution (AO type 13-A3.3) was used. The main outcome measures were stiffness testing of the constructs in anterior/posterior bending, torsion, and axial compression loading. Alterations of the bone-implant interface and failure patterns under cyclic loading and strength testing were also evaluated.

Results.—Primary stiffness in anterior/posterior bending and torsional loading was found to be significantly increased by the use of locking compression plates in a 90° configuration as compared with dorsally applied plates. The differences between the different plate types are insignificant if they are applied in the same configuration.

None of the tested implants failed under cyclic loading within the number of cycles expected for 3 months of use. The bone-implant interface is less likely to fail during strength testing with locking compression plates.

Conclusion.—The biomechanical behavior of the osteosynthesis is dependent more on the configuration than on the type of plate. The advantages of locking compression plates are only significant in comparison with dorsal plate application techniques. Nevertheless, locking compression plates are helpful supplementary tools for obtaining primary stable fracture fixation. This finding may be of clinical significance for patients with diminished bone mineral quality or in the presence of metaphyseal comminution.

► This is one of several articles that has appeared in the recent literature assessing, in an experimental setting, the optimum orientation and type of place fixation for the difficult distal humeral fracture. Although the experimental design of these authors does demonstrate superiority of the 90° configuration, it should be noted that the model does not account for articular comminution. The practical difficulty of treating a noncomminuted fracture is much less than that posed by the comminuted C3 fracture. Nonetheless—at least with this experimental study and with the recon type of plate—the 90° plate orientation is demonstrated to be optimum.

B. F. Morrey, MD

Coronoid Process and Radial Head as Posterolateral Rotatory Stabilizers of the Elbow

Schneeberger AG, Sadowski MM, Jacob HAC (Univ of Zurich, Switzerland)

J Bone Joint Surg Am 86-A:975-982, 2004 10–7

Introduction.—In the complex injury known as the "terrible triad," an elbow dislocation is combined with fractures of the radial head and the coronoid process. Outcome is poor because of a relatively high risk of persistent instability and early osteoarthrosis. A cadaver study evaluated the function of the radial head and the coronoid process as posterolateral stabilizers of the elbow and analyzed the effects of various reconstructive procedures.

Methods.—Ten fresh-frozen upper extremities from cadavers with no evidence of pathologic changes at the elbow were used. Two were used for a pilot evaluation and 8 for measurements. Specimens were from 2 men and 3 women with a mean age of 82 years at the time of death.

The testing apparatus consisted of a specifically designed frame that allowed the posterolateral rotary displacement of the ulna to be measured after application of a valgus and supinating torque: (1) in 7 intact elbows, (2) after radial head excision, (3) after sequential resection of the coronoid process, (4) after subsequent insertion of each of 2 different types of medial head prostheses (a rigid implant and a bipolar implant with a floating cup), and (5) after subsequent reconstruction of the coronoid with each of 2 different techniques in the same cadaveric elbow.

Results.—The posterolateral rotatory laxity of the intact elbow averaged 5.4° at 60° of elbow flexion (Fig 6). Because laxities were usually greatest at 60° of flexion, results at 60° of elbow flexion were presented. With the surgical approach used, mean laxity increased insignificantly to 9°. After excision of the radial head in an elbow with intact collateral ligaments, the resulting mean posterolateral laxity was 18.6°.

Elbows were fully destabilized by additional removal of 30% of the height of the coronoid, and ulnohumeral dislocation always followed, even when ligaments were intact. The elbows were stabilized by implantation of a rigid radial head prosthesis, but a mean laxity of 16.9% persisted after a floating prosthesis was implanted. Elbows with a defect of 50% or 70% of the coronoid, loss of the radial head, and intact ligaments could not be stabilized by radial head replacement alone, but stability was restored by additional coronoid reconstruction.

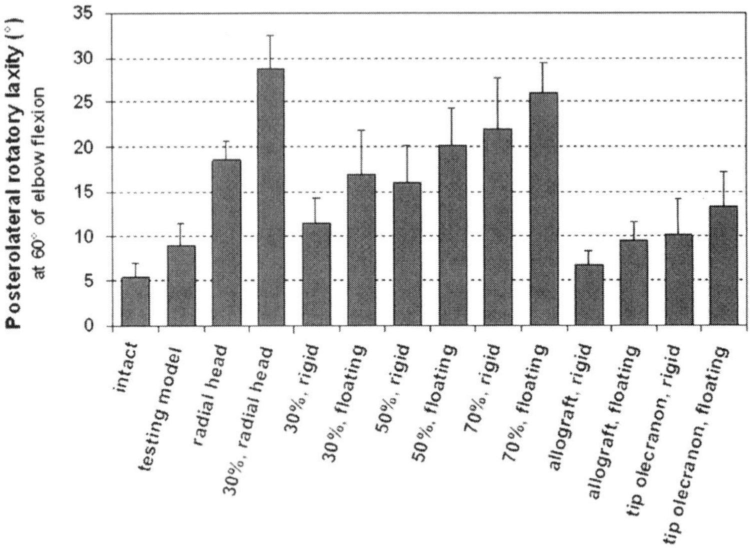

FIGURE 6.—Posterolateral rotatory laxities at 60° of elbow flexion, with the ligaments intact or reattached. *Radial head* indicates defect of the radial head; *30%, 50%, and 70%*, defect of 30%, 50%, and 70% of the height of the coronoid process; *rigid*, rigid radial head prosthesis; *floating*, floating radial head prosthesis; *allograft*, coronoid reconstruction with an allograft; and *tip olecranon*, coronoid reconstruction with the tip of the olecranon. (Republished with permission of the Journal of Bone and Joint Surgery, Inc, from Schneeberger AG, Sadowski MM, Jacob HAC: Coronoid process and radial head as posterolateral rotatory stabilizers of the elbow. *J Bone Joint Surg Am* 86-A:975-982, 2004. Reproduced by permission of the publisher via Copyright Clearance Center, Inc.)

Conclusion.—A rigid implant appears to restore stability better than a floating prosthesis when the radial head is replaced. Coronoid reconstruction and radial head replacement can be used to stabilize elbows with a defect of 50% of the coronoid or greater plus a radial head defect. Laxities measured in vitro may be greater than those in clinical practice.

► This is a very important investigation as it provides additional scientific support for the emerging treatment logic and approach for the so-called "terrible triad injury" of the elbow. The terrible triad consists of a fracture of the radial head, coronoid, and medial and lateral collateral ligaments. This study documents, in a laboratory setting, that which has been observed clinically; specifically: at least 50% of the coronoid must be present to provide an opportunity for restoration of elbow function. If the radial head has been fractured and is not repairable, a prosthetic radial head implant is essential to offer the necessary stability for such an injury.

B. F. Morrey, MD

11 Shoulder

Introduction

Shoulder surgery continues to emerge as a popular and growing subspecialty within our discipline. Insights referable to subtleties of implant replacement are emerging. The so-called reverse shoulder is discussed, as this does appear to be a viable concept with growing interest by shoulder surgeons involved in joint replacement arthroplasty. Insights with regard to various surgical techniques and long-term outcome of multidirectional instability are addressed. As might be expected, the value of arthroscopy is examined in several articles, with particular focus on instability and rotator cuff disease. Overall, the difficulty in this particular section was selecting those several articles that seemed to provide the best cross-section and insight into the current state-of-the-art of shoulder surgery.

Bernard F. Morrey, MD

Accuracy of the Speed's and Yergason's Tests in Detecting Biceps Pathology and SLAP Lesions: Comparison With Arthroscopic Findings

Holtby R, Razmjou H (Univ of Toronto; Sunnybrook & Women's College, Toronto)

Arthroscopy 20:231-236, 2004 11–1

Introduction.—The clinical usefulness of a shoulder test depends on properties such as reliability and validity and on its ability to aid the clinician in making a correct diagnosis. Yergason's test and Speed's test, both originally noted to be specific to bicipital tendinitis, were tested for their ability to predict biceps tendon pathology and SLAP lesions. Shoulder arthroscopy was used as the gold standard.

Methods.—Eligible patients were referred for shoulder assessment because of persistent pain and functional disability. Excluded were patients with previous shoulder surgery or upper extremity fractures. Of the 152 patients referred, 50 (16 women and 34 men) met criteria for surgery. The validity of Yergason's and Speed's tests was evaluated against surgical findings. Results of specific clinical tests were not available to the surgeon at arthroscopy.

A positive Speed's test results in pain in the anterior shoulder or glenohumeral joint when the examiner applies a downward pressure to the upper extremity with 90° of shoulder elevation, full supination, and with the elbow completely extended. With Yergason's test, pain occurs in the bicipital groove area or glenohumeral joint when the patient's elbow is flexed to 90° and stabilized against the thorax with the forearm pronated, and the examiner resists supination. In both tests, a true negative examination produces no symptoms.

Results.—Surgical findings of interest included 2 cases of bicipital tendinitis, both associated with significant rotator cuff pathology; 10 biceps with partial tears; and 2 complete ruptures. Fifteen patients had SLAP lesion type I, 12 had type II, and 1 had type IV. Yergason's test had a sensitivity of 43%, a specificity of 79%, a positive predictive value of 60%, and a negative predictive value of 65%. For Speed's test, these values were 32%, 75%, 50%, and 58%, respectively. Positive likelihood ratios were 1.28 for Speed's test and 2.05 for Yergason's test; negative likelihood ratios were, respectively, 0.91 and 0.72.

Conclusion.—Both Speed's test and Yergason's test are moderately specific but do not perform consistently and have variable predictive values. Sensitivity was low, indicating a high percentage of false-negative results, and the tests are unlikely to significantly change the pretest diagnosis.

▶ Prospective randomized studies—particularly those designed to evaluate the accuracy of commonly employed diagnoses, tests, or assumptions—are quite important and relevant to our ongoing educational processes. This article, therefore, is of particular interest since it does offer a very careful methodology. Unfortunately, it demonstrates the inaccuracy of 2 commonly performed studies to diagnose the so-called SLAP lesion. This does not negate the value of these studies, but it does emphasize the need for a careful clinical history and the further need to thoughtfully assemble and interpret all elements of the patient's evaluation before proceeding with arthroscopy.

B. F. Morrey, MD

Biomechanical Function of Surgical Procedures for Acromioclavicular Joint Dislocations

Jari R, Costic RS, Rodosky MW, et al (Univ of Pittsburgh, Pa)
Arthroscopy 20:237-245, 2004 11–2

Background.—Dislocation of the acromioclavicular (AC) joint is a common injury among the athletic population. Most often these injuries occur after a fall on the tip of the shoulder, which results in a direct blow to the lateral aspect of the shoulder with the arm in an adducted position. The result of this mechanism is an inferior and anterior dislocation of the acromion. Some studies have shown satisfactory outcomes with either nonsurgical or surgical treatments, but the management of type III injuries of the AC joint is controversial.

Surgical procedures for the treatment of AC joint dislocation replace the coracoclavicular (CC) ligaments to minimize motion, allow scarring, and increase the subsequent stability of the joint. Under evaluation was the biomechanical function of the surgically repaired or reconstructed AC joint after AC joint dislocation by 3 procedures: coracoclavicular suture fixation (the CC Sling), coracoclavicular screw fixation (the Rockwood Screw), and coracoclavicular suture fixation with a coracoacromial (CA) ligament transfer (CA Ligament Transfer Construct).

Methods.—The Robotic/UFS testing system was used to test 12 cadaveric shoulders. Three external loading conditions (anterior, posterior, or superior load of 70 N) were applied to intact and surgically repaired or reconstructed AC joints. The resulting kinematics of the AC joint and in situ forces in the CC ligaments or surgical constructs were then determined.

Results.—For the CC Sling, the anterior and posterior translation significantly increased by 110% and 330% in response to an anterior and posterior load, respectively. For the Rockwood Screw, the posterior translation significantly decreased by 60%. Anterior, posterior, and superior translation for the CA Ligament Transfer Construct significantly increased by 110%, 360%, and 100%, respectively.

There were also significant increases in the coupled translations for the CC Sling and CA Ligament Transfer Construct in response to all loading conditions. However, the coupled translation for the Rockwood Screw showed a tendency to decrease. In addition, the in situ forces increased significantly for all 3 surgical constructs compared with the intact CC ligaments in response to an anterior and posterior load.

Conclusion.—At time zero, increases in the primary and coupled motion for the CC Sling and CA Ligament Transfer Construct could comprise the initial healing period prescribed for dislocation of the AC joint. The Rockwood Screw provides a highly rigid fixation, and these findings may explain the complications frequently observed in clinical practice.

► There is relatively little information regarding the biomechanical effectiveness of AC joint stabilization. These studies show that the effectiveness of some of the commonly performed reconstructive procedures is not adequate to stabilize this joint. On the other hand, the use of a screw from the clavicle to the coronoid may result in too rigid fixation. Thus, the authors' conclusion seems logical that new reconstructive strategies might be considered to stabilize AC separations. The larger issue remains, however, under what circumstances does an AC separation require stabilization to begin with? Certainly, for high-grade lesions with muscle stripping, stabilization remains the treatment of choice. Controversy continues regarding the appropriate management for grade III separations.

B. F. Morrey, MD

Nonoperative Management for In-Season Athletes With Anterior Shoulder Instability

Buss DD, Lynch GP, Meyer CP, et al (Sports and Orthopaedic Specialists, Minneapolis; Johnson County Orthopaedics, Olathe, Kansas; Univ of Minnesota, Minneapolis)

Am J Sports Med 32:1430-1433, 2004 11–3

Introduction.—Acute or recurrent anterior shoulder instability is a common injury among in-season athletes. Treatment may include shoulder immobilization, rehabilitation, and shoulder stabilization surgery. The ability of adolescent in-season competitive athletes to return to competition quickly and effectively after nonoperative treatment for an anterior instability episode was examined.

Methods.—Athletes who experienced an anterior dislocation or subluxation during a 2-year evaluation period were enrolled. Nineteen of 30 athletes enrolled experienced anterior dislocations; 11 had subluxations. The average age of 24 males and 6 females was 16.5 years (range, 14-20 years). There were 10 ice hockey players, 9 football players, 5 wrestlers, 4 basketball players, 1 downhill skier, and 1 gymnast. All participants underwent treatment with physical therapy and, when appropriate, with a brace. The number of recurrent instability episodes, additional injuries, subjective ability to compete, and ability to compete in their season or seasons of choice were documented.

Results.—After nonoperative treatment of anterior shoulder instability, 26 athletes were able to return to their sports for the complete season at an average time missed of 10.2 days (range, 0-30 days). Ten athletes experienced sports-associated recurrent instability episodes. An average of 1.4 recurrent instability episodes (range, 0-8 episodes) per season per athlete were observed. No additional injuries were attributable to the shoulder instability. Sixteen athletes underwent surgery for shoulder stabilization during the subsequent off-season.

Conclusion.—Most athletes were able to return to their sport and complete the season after experiencing an episode of anterior shoulder instability; 37% had at least 1 additional episode of instability during the season.

▶ The authors offer an interesting perspective on shoulder instability by asking the practical question of whether athletes can effectively complete a season after an initial anterior shoulder dislocation. That approximately 90% of athletes can return to sport in less than 2 weeks is an interesting observation. It is not surprising that 10 of the 30 had recurrent episodes and that half required surgical stabilization at the end of the season. However, in no instance did additional pathologic conditions occur after the athletes were allowed to participate in their sport.

B. F. Morrey, MD

Effectiveness of Glenohumeral-Joint Stability Braces in Limiting Active and Passive Shoulder Range of Motion in Collegiate Football Players

Weise K, Sitler MR, Tierney R, et al (Temple Univ, Philadelphia)

J Athl Train 39:151-155, 2004 11–4

Introduction.—Glenohumeral-joint stability braces are used to protect the shoulder from recurrent dislocation by restricting glenohumeral abduction and external rotation. The effectiveness of glenohumeral stability braces in limiting active and passive shoulder abduction and external rotation in collegiate football players was determined with the use of a 2-factor, repeated-measures design.

Methods.—The brace condition and force application (active, passive) were evaluated with the use of the Denison and Duke Wyre harness or the Sawa shoulder brace in 15 National Collegiate Athletic Association Division 1 male college football players. The median participant age, height, and weight were 19.9 years, 183.2 cm, and 89.9 kg, respectively. Measurements of shoulder abduction (45° braced limit) and external-rotation angular displacement were obtained. The PEAK Motus motion analysis system was used to measure angular displacement.

Results.—Neither brace was capable of maintaining the arm position at the 45° braced limit during active or passive shoulder abduction (motion ranges, 56.8°-73.0°). A priori external rotation limits were not used; motion ranged between 71.6° and 93.9° with the braces. Repeated-measures multivariate analysis of variance showed no significant interaction effect (P = .41); main effects were significant for the brace condition and force application ($P < .001$). All the following differences were significant: for abduction, the Denison and Duke Wyre harness resulted in 12.3° (21%) greater angular displacement than did the Sawa shoulder brace; passive abduction resulted in 3.9° (6%) more angular displacement than did active abduction; for external rotation, the Denison and Duke Wyre harness resulted in 6.7° (9%) more angular displacement than did the Sawa brace; passive external rotation resulted in 15.6° (21%) more angular displacement than did active external rotation.

Conclusion.—Preset, braced abduction motion limits were not observed during active and passive physiologic loading of the glenohumeral joint. Protection against the vulnerable position at 90° of abduction and external rotation was possible at a preset braced limit of 45° of abduction (the exception was the Denison and Duke Wyre harness during passive external rotation). The Sawa shoulder brace performed best for this function.

► As a complement to the article by Buss et al (Abstract 11–3), these investigators from Temple University evaluated the effectiveness of different devices to protect the athlete who is playing with shoulder instability. Although the motion control was less than might be desirable, these devices were effective in protecting against the most vulnerable position of 90° of abduction. However, not all devices performed in a comparable manner. This study was performed on healthy athletes; thus, extrapolation to assume protection of athletes after an initial episode of shoulder instability cannot necessarily be drawn.

B. F. Morrey, MD

Thermal Capsular Shrinkage for Treatment of Multidirectional Instability of the Shoulder

Miniaci A, McBirnie J (Univ of Toronto)

J Bone Joint Surg Am 85-A:2283-2287, 2003 11–5

Background.—Various techniques have been developed to treat multidirectional instability of the shoulder, including both open and arthroscopic procedures. Capsular laxity is the major problem to be addressed, and thermal techniques to shrink capsular tissue are often used as treatment. The clinical results of thermal capsular shrinkage with the use of a radiofrequency device were evaluated in patients with multidirectional shoulder instability. Factors that were predictive of the final result were also sought.

Methods.—Thermal shrinkage was performed in 19 patients with multidirectional instability. Instability was involuntary in 15 patients and voluntary in four. The direction of the instability was primarily anteroinferior in 10, posterior in 5, and in multiple directions in 4. Follow-up lasted a minimum of 2 years, unless surgery failed or symptoms recurred. Slings were worn for 3 weeks postoperatively. Evaluations were carried out 3, 6, and 12 months after the procedure. Functioning, ROM, pain, and instability were the clinical outcome measures and were determined with the use of the Western Ontario Shoulder Instability Index.

Results.—Instability recurred at an average of 9 months postoperatively in 9 patients; these cases were considered surgical failures. The failures were found in 5 patients with predominantly posterior instability, in 2 with no predominant direction, and in 2 with predominantly anterior instability. Four failures occurred in cases of voluntary instability, 5 occurred in cases of involuntary instability, 4 occurred in traumatic cases, and 5 occurred in atraumatic cases. The revision operations were all open surgical procedures, and the capsular tissue was abnormal in all cases. Thickened and stiff shoulder capsules and capsular deficiencies were seen. Neurologic symptoms and stiffness or loss of ROM also developed after surgery. With a worst score of 2100 and a best score of 0, the clinical outcome scores improved from a preoperative average of 1780.3 to a postoperative average of 1099.8. Considering only the results in patients who did not have surgical failures, the preoperative average of 1717.2 was improved to a postoperative average of 424.2.

Conclusions.—The use of a thermal capsular shrinkage technique to treat multidirectional instability was accompanied by a high rate of surgical failure, postoperative complications, a recurrence of instability, stiffness, and neurologic symptoms. The thermal technique is, therefore, not advocated for patients with multidirectional instability, particularly when a posterior or voluntary component is involved.

Prospective Evaluation of Thermal Capsulorrhaphy for Shoulder Instability: Indications and Results, Two- to Five-Year Follow-up

D'Alessandro DF, Bradley JP, Fleischli JE, et al (Miller Orthopaedic Clinic, Charlotte, NC; Burke and Bradley Orthopaedics, Pittsburgh, Pa)

Am J Sports Med 32:21-33, 2004 11–6

Background.—Thermal shrinkage of capsular tissue has been used to manage the capsular redundancy that occurs with shoulder instability. The efficacy of arthroscopic electrothermal capsulorrhaphy to treat shoulder instability was evaluated prospectively.

Methods.—The indications and results of thermal capsulorrhaphy were evaluated in 84 shoulders over an average follow-up of 38 months. The patients were classified into 3 subgroups that exhibited the following: (1) traumatic acute or recurrent anterior dislocation, (2) recurrent anterior–inferior subluxation with no previous dislocation, and (3) multidirectional instability (MDI). After the initial assessment, radiographs, and at least 3 months of nonoperative rehabilitation, patients underwent arthroscopic thermal capsulorrhaphy. Measures included the presence of pain, recurrent instability, return to work and/or sports, and the American Shoulder and Elbow Surgeons (ASES) Shoulder Assessment score.

Results.—Thirty-nine percent of the patients had excellent results, 24% had satisfactory results, and 37% had unsatisfactory results. ASES scores improved from a preoperative average of 48.7 to a postoperative average of 82.8. The patient satisfaction level was 7.9 on a scale of 0 to 10. Eleven arthroscopic Bankart repairs, 9 type II superior labral AP lesion repairs, 9 partial-thickness cuff tear debridements, and 7 labral debridements were required. Patients with dislocations had the best results, improving from an average preoperative ASES score of 57.1 to an average postoperative score of 93.0. Fifty percent had excellent results, 25% had satisfactory results, and 24% had unsatisfactory results. The group with recurrent subluxation improved their average ASES scores from 51.7 to 80.7, and 37% had excellent outcomes, 31.5% had satisfactory outcomes, and 31.5% had unsatisfactory outcomes. The MDI group had an average preoperative ASES score of 45.9 that improved to 80.9 postoperatively. Thirty-eight percent had excellent results, 21% had satisfactory results, and 41% had unsatisfactory results. Clinical results in this last group deteriorated with longer follow-up. Postoperatively, 69% of all patients were able to participate in athletic activity without any or only minimal difficulty; the percentage involved in athletics before surgery was 84%. Sixty-five percent of the MDI athletes returned to athletic activities, but this group included a significant number of female swimmers, volleyball players, and softball players whose return to sports participation presented difficulties, even after open capsulorrhaphy procedures. Sensory changes that developed in patients resolved spontaneously and completely within 3 months of surgery. Further surgical interventions were needed in 12% of the shoulders because of recurrent instability, discomfort, and subjective dissatisfaction. Fifty percent of these were successful.

Conclusions.—Only 63% of the 84 shoulders achieved successful clinical results with the use of thermal capsulorrhaphy. Excellent results were obtained in 39%, and satisfactory results were obtained in 24%. Thirty-seven percent of the shoulders had unsatisfactory outcomes. Patients with traumatic shoulder dislocation benefited most from thermal capsulorrhaphy. In these patients, it was often combined with arthroscopic labral repairs to handle the capsular laxity component. Seventy-five percent of this subgroup of patients had excellent or satisfactory results, and none required revision stabilization procedures. Thermal treatment for shoulder instability should be used cautiously because of the high failure rate, especially in the MDI subset of patients.

▶ These 2 articles (Abstracts 11–5 and 11–6) serve to document a growing awareness of the deficiencies of thermal capsular shrinkage for the management of multidirectional instability of the shoulder. The failure rate, which seems to increase with time, is one important consideration emphasized by D'Alessandro et al (Abstract 11–6). The rather significant additional complications including stiffness and neurologic symptoms are additional causes for concern and were emphasized by Miniaci and McBirnie (Abstract 11–5). The conclusion remains, as has been stated in the past, that this technology must be embraced very cautiously; clearly, it is not a panacea, although it may still remain a reasonable adjunct under certain circumstances.

B. F. Morrey, MD

Atrophy of the Deltoid Muscle Following Rotator Cuff Surgery

Hata Y, Saitoh S, Murakami N, et al (Shinshu Univ, Matsumoto, Japan)

J Bone Joint Surg Am 86-A:1414-1419, 2004 11–7

Introduction.—In an attempt to make open rotator cuff repair less invasive, a mini-open, deltoid-splitting approach was introduced at the study institution in 1997. Patients treated with the conventional open method and those treated with mini-open repair were compared for changes in the thickness of the anterior deltoid fibers and clinical outcomes.

Methods.—The mini-open repair was performed by a single surgeon on 35 consecutive shoulders of 35 patients. Excluded from this procedure were patients with tears involving more than 3 tendons or with tendon retraction greater than 5 cm. The patient group included 21 men and 14 women with a mean age of 60.6 years. Four had a small tear (less than 1 cm), 15 a moderate tear (1 to 3 cm), and 16 a large tear (3 to 5 cm). The same surgeon had performed open repair for 43 consecutive patients between 1994 and 1997.

The 2 groups were similar in age, gender distribution, size of the tears, and mean preoperative University of California at Los Angeles score. Both groups followed an identical postoperative rehabilitation program. The mean follow-up was 30.6 months for the mini-open repair group and 61.6 months for the conventional open repair group.

Results.—The thickness of the anterior deltoid fibers did not change significantly after mini-open repair, whereas a significant decrease was observed in the open repair group at both 6 and 12 months postoperatively. At 3-month follow-up, the mean University of California score for active forward flexion in the patients treated with mini-open repair was significantly greater than that in patients who underwent conventional open repair (4.9 and 4.6 points, respectively).

Patients returned to work significantly sooner after mini-open repair than after conventional open repair (2.4 and 3.4 months, respectively). All patients in both groups were able to return to work or sports activities at preoperative levels by 12 months after surgery.

Conclusion.—Compared with patients who underwent conventional open rotator cuff repair, those treated with mini-open repair recovered more quickly and had less postoperative atrophy of the deltoid muscle. The more extensive dissection in open repair was thought to have produced more deltoid atrophy.

► Not all investigators have demonstrated a superiority in the mini-open repair. However, this study does offer some important insight with regard to the postoperative atrophy that is more evident in the conventional open rotator cuff repair than was demonstrated in the mini-open procedure. It would be important to ask a similar question for the arthroscopically treated rotator cuff–deficient shoulder.

B. F. Morrey, MD

Open Bankart Repair Versus Arthroscopic Repair With Transglenoid Sutures or Bioabsorbable Tacks for Recurrent Anterior Instability of the Shoulder: A Meta-analysis

Freedman KB, Smith AP, Romeo AA, et al (Loyolya Univ, Maywood, Ill; Rush Med College, Chicago)

Am J Sports Med 32:1520-1527, 2004 11–8

Introduction.—The low rates of recurrence achieved by open stabilization have established this technique as the gold standard for operative repair of the Bankart lesion. A meta-analysis was conducted to determine whether arthroscopic techniques of Bankart repair for anterior shoulder instability could achieve the success of open repair.

Methods.—Relevant publications were identified by means of a Medline search for the period January 1966 to May 2002. Additional articles were obtained from reviews and the references cited in publications. Articles eligible for analysis directly compared open and arthroscopic techniques for the treatment of traumatic, unidirectional, recurrent anterior instability of the shoulder. Data collected included patient demographics, surgical technique, complications of surgery, ROM, and Rowe score at the final follow-up.

Results.—The 6 studies that met all inclusion criteria had a total of 328 patients, 172 in the arthroscopic group and 156 in the open group. Demographic characteristics were similar in the 2 groups. Ninety patients with arthroscopic repair had transglenoid sutures, 77 had arthroscopic tacks, and 5 had suture anchors. Rates of recurrent dislocation differed significantly, with 3% in the open group and 13% in the arthroscopic group.

The rate of total recurrence (dislocation plus subluxation) was twice as high in the arthroscopic group (20% vs 10% in the open group), and this was true when either bioabsorbable tacks or transglenoid sutures were used. The postoperative Rowe score differed significantly as well: 88% in the open group versus 71% in the arthroscopic group had an excellent or good Rowe score. Five of 6 studies reported better external rotation after arthroscopic repair. Surgical complication rates were similar in the 2 groups.

Conclusion.—Arthroscopic techniques for anterior stabilization of the shoulder have gained in popularity, but the findings of this meta-analysis demonstrate the advantages of open Bankart repair: lower rates of recurrent dislocation and total recurrence and a higher percentage of patients with a good or excellent postoperative Rowe score.

► In contrast to the article by Fabbriciani (see Abstract 11–9), the investigation of Freedman et al emphasizes the need to properly select and appropriately define the surgical technique. Suture anchor fixation, as the authors point out, should provide a solution to the failures that were documented with the bioabsorbable tacks.

B. F. Morrey, MD

Arthroscopic Versus Open Treatment of Bankart Lesion of the Shoulder: A Prospective Randomized Study

Fabbriciani C, Milano G, Demontis A, et al (Univ of Sassari, Italy)
Arthroscopy 20:456-462, 2004 11–9

Introduction.—There is considerable controversy regarding the diagnosis and treatment of shoulder instability. Arthroscopic treatment has a number of advantages compared with an open procedure, but arthroscopically treated patients may lose some ROM and have an increased rate of recurrence. In addition, arthroscopic stabilization of the shoulder requires complex technical knowledge and expensive instrumentation. Patients randomly assigned to an open procedure or to arthroscopic repair of an isolated Bankart lesion were compared for outcomes.

Methods.—Eligible patients had trauma-related anterior shoulder instability, no previous symptoms or surgery to the injured shoulder, no more than 4 episodes of anterior shoulder dislocation, no clinical evidence of multidirectional instability, and loss of substance of the humeral head not exceeding 30%. Patients in both arthroscopic and open procedure groups had the lesion repaired with the use of metallic suture anchors carrying nonabsorbable braided sutures.

TABLE 3.—Follow-Up Results According to Rowe Score

	Function	Pain	Stability	ROM	Total
Arthroscopic					
Mean	45.5	8.5	27	10	91
SD	7.25	2.42	6.32	0.00	15.06
Open					
Mean	41.0	8.5	28.5	8.5	86.5
SD	7.75	2.42	4.74	2.42	12.92
P	.196	1.000	.556	.065	.482

Note: Figures are mean ± standard deviation.

(Reprinted from Fabbriciani C, Milano G, Demontis A, et al: Arthroscopic versus open treatment of Bankart lesion of the shoulder: A prospective randomized study. *Arthroscopy* 20:456-462, 2004. Copyright 2004, with permission from The Arthroscopy Association of North America.)

Results.—Thirty patients had an arthroscopic repair and 30 had an open procedure. The 2 groups were similar in age, gender, dominance, number of dislocations, time elapsed between the first dislocation and surgery, pathologic findings, and postoperative rehabilitation. There were no intraoperative or postoperative complications, and no recurrence of dislocation of an involved shoulder was reported during 2 years of follow-up. The mean value for ROM was significantly greater in the arthroscopic group, but the 2 groups were similar in Constant scores for pain, function, and strength. Rowe scores (Table 3) were also comparable after arthroscopic and open repair.

Conclusion.—Athroscopic repair with suture anchors was an effective surgical technique for the treatment of an isolated Bankart lesion. Advantages in postoperative stability and ROM cause this technique to be recommended over the open procedure. In addition, arthroscopic repair is more cost effective because the duration of hospitalization and the risk of complications are both reduced.

► The literature continues to question the relative value of the open versus the arthroscopic repair for shoulder instability. With improving technique and arthroscopic systems, the results of the arthroscopic intervention approaches that of the open surgical procedure. This study does offer 2-year follow-up and has reasonable patient numbers and offers a reliable methodology that would tend to substantiate the authors' conclusions.

B. F. Morrey, MD

Rotator Cuff Repair in Patients Fifty Years of Age and Younger

Sperling JW, Cofield RH, Schleck C (Mayo Clinic, Rochester, Minn)

J Bone Joint Surg Am 86-A:2212-2215, 2004 11–10

Background.—The outcomes of rotator cuff repair for older patients have been well-documented, but there is little information available to clinicians to guide their decision-making in the treatment of younger patients with rotator cuff tears. The results, the risk factors for an unsatisfactory outcome, and the rates of failure of rotator cuff repair in patients aged 50 years and younger were investigated.

Methods.—Repair of a full-thickness rotator cuff tear was performed for 32 patients (36 shoulders) aged 50 years or younger between 1976 and 1987. Of these patients, 7 died after less than 13 years of follow-up. The final analysis included the remaining 29 shoulders, which had been followed up for a minimum of 13 years or until revision surgery. The most recent follow-up was performed in the clinic (5 shoulders) or by questionnaire (24 shoulders).

Results.—There were 3 small, 15 medium, 6 large, and 5 massive tears. Rotator cuff repair was associated with significant long-term pain relief. However, no significant long-term improvement was observed in active abduction or external rotation. There were no significant differences in postoperative pain, active abduction, or external rotation according to gender, tear size, repair type, or whether a distal clavicular excision had been performed.

Results were excellent in 11 patients, satisfactory in 5 patients, and unsatisfactory in 13 patients. Additional surgery was performed in 7 shoulders, including 5 for recurrent tear, 1 for instability, and 1 for osteoarthritis. Three of the 5 repairs for recurrent tear were performed 10 years or more after the time of the index procedure.

Conclusion.—Rotator cuff repair can provide long-term relief of pain for young patients. However, this procedure is not associated with significant long-term improvement in motion, and for many patients, the long-term results are unsatisfactory. The results of rotator cuff repair in young patients appeared to be less favorable than outcomes in a mixed-age population.

▶ The authors address a question that is one of the most commonly confronted in the busy orthopedic practice, particularly regarding upper extremity sports injuries. The relatively large sample of patients satisfying strict selection criteria tends to enhance the validity of the authors' observations. The overall finding that this sample of patients did not tend to have a favorable long-term outcome is of particular relevance when discussing this intervention and the expected long-term functional implication with our patients.

B. F. Morrey, MD

Grammont Inverted Total Shoulder Arthroplasty in the Treatment of Glenohumeral Osteoarthritis With Massive Rupture of the Cuff: Results of a Multicentre Study of 80 Shoulders

Sirveaux F, Favard L, Oudet D, et al (Clinic of Traumatology and Orthopaedics, Nancy, France)

J Bone Joint Surg Br 86-B:388-395, 2004 11–11

Background.—Unconstrained total shoulder arthroplasty has been successful in the treatment of shoulder arthropathy in the presence of an intact rotator cuff. However, poor results have been obtained with this type of im-

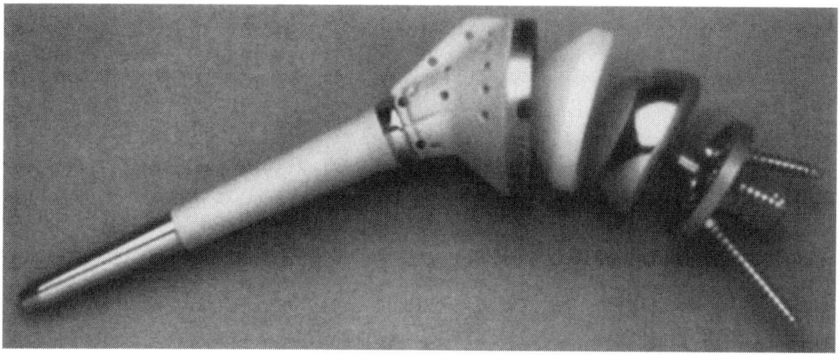

FIGURE 1.—Photograph showing components of the Grammont inverted prosthesis. (Courtesy of Sirveaux F, Favard L, Oudet D, et al: Grammont inverted total shoulder arthroplasty in the treatment of glenohumeral osteoarthritis with massive rupture of the cuff: Results of a multicentre study of 80 shoulders. *J Bone Joint Surg Br* 86-B:388-395, 2004.)

plant when the rotator cuff is torn or is nonfunctional. The Delta shoulder prosthesis (DePuy, France), which was developed in France by Grammont et al, is an inverted versions of the constrained designs for prostheses developed in the 1970s (Fig 1).

In this inverted design, the resultant force applied to the neck of the scapula limits the shear forces that are responsible for loosening of the glenoid. The midterm results of the use of the inverted prosthesis in the treatment of glenohumeral osteoarthritis in the presence of a massive rupture of the cuff was assessed and compared with previously published results from other techniques.

Methods.—A review was conducted of 80 shoulders of 77 patients with a mean follow-up of 44 months after insertion of a Grammont inverted shoulder prosthesis. Three implants had failed and had been revised.

Results.—There was an increase in the mean Constant score from 22.6 points preoperatively to 65.5 points. There was no pain or only minimal

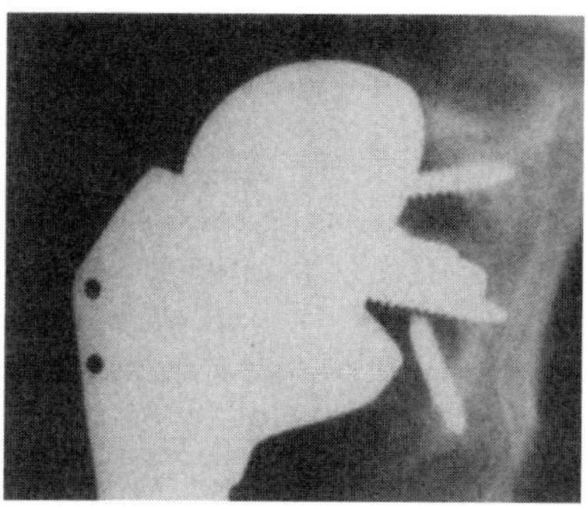

FIGURE 5.—Anteroposterior radiographs of 3 cases of glenoid loosening showing progressive unscrewing of the glenosphere associated with loosening of the baseplate. (Courtesy of Sirveaux F, Favard L, Oudet D, et al: Grammont inverted total shoulder arthroplasty in the treatment of glenohumeral osteoarthritis with massive rupture of the cuff: Results of a multicentre study of 80 shoulders. *J Bone Joint Surg Br* 86-B:388-395, 2004.)

pain in 96% of these shoulders. The mean active forward elevation was increased from 73° to 138°. The integrity of teres minor is essential for the recovery of external rotation and significantly influenced the Constant score. There were 5 cases of aseptic loosening of the glenoid and 7 of dissociation of the glenoid component (Fig 5).

Conclusion.—The promising early results obtained with the inverted prosthesis for treatment of a rotator cuff tear arthropathy were confirmed by this study. The use of this inverted total shoulder arthropathy should be considered in the treatment of osteoarthritis with a massive tear of the cuff but should only be used in elderly patients.

▶ This retrospective study of a reasonable number of patients introduces what to some is a new design concept in shoulder replacement. The so-called inverted total shoulder employs a ball in the glenoid and a cup to replace the humeral head. The important point is that this is considered a salvage option for those with deficient and irreparable rotator cuff lesions. The authors' indications of elderly patients with irreparable or massive rotator cuff pathology should be noted and emphasized. Because these prostheses do place a significant force at the glenoid, the long-term effect of this biomechanical alteration is yet to be clearly understood. There is also a considerable variation in implant designs that have applied this so-called "inverted" philosophy, and the implications of this are unclear.

B. F. Morrey, MD

Copeland Surface Replacement Arthroplasty of the Shoulder in Rheumatoid Arthritis

Levy O, Funk L, Sforza G, et al (Royal Berkshire Hosp, Reading, England)
J Bone Joint Surg Am 86-A:512-518, 2004 11–12

Background.—Glenohumeral arthroplasty is the treatment of choice for patients with symptomatic severe rheumatoid arthritis of the shoulder. The Copeland surface replacement arthroplasty was designed specifically for use in arthritic shoulders. Unlike stemmed shoulder prostheses, the Copeland cementless surface replacement arthroplasty is designed to replace only the damaged joint-bearing surfaces and to restore anatomy with minimal bone resection. Whether surface replacement is superior to stemmed prostheses in shoulders with rheumatoid arthritis was determined.

Methods.—Surface replacement arthroplasty was performed in 75 shoulders between 1986 and 1998 for the treatment of rheumatoid arthritis. Included in this series were 33 hemiarthroplasties and 42 shoulder arthroplasties. Outcomes were reviewed after an average follow-up of 6.5 years. The patients were assessed with the Constant score, a patient satisfaction score, and radiographs.

Results.—The average Constant score was 47.9 points (age- and sex-adjusted score, 71%) in the hemiarthroplasty group and 53.4 points (age- and sex-adjusted score, 76%) in the total shoulder replacement group. The mean range of active flexion improved from 50° to 101° in the hemiarthroplasty group and from 47° to 104° in the total shoulder replacement group. Of the 75 shoulders evaluated, 72 were considered by the patients to be better or much better at the time of review.

Of the 68 humeral implants that were evaluated radiographically, 56 (82%) showed no lucencies, 11 (16%) showed localized lucencies of less than 1 mm in width, and 1 was definitely loose (Fig 3). There were no lucencies evident adjacent to the hydroxyapatite-coated implants. Of the 68 humeral implants, 39 (57%) showed some degree of superior subluxation. Major reoperation was required for 3 patients, including 2 for loosening of both components and 1 because of pain at the site of a hemiarthroplasty. The latter patient underwent revision to a total shoulder arthroplasty to provide pain relief.

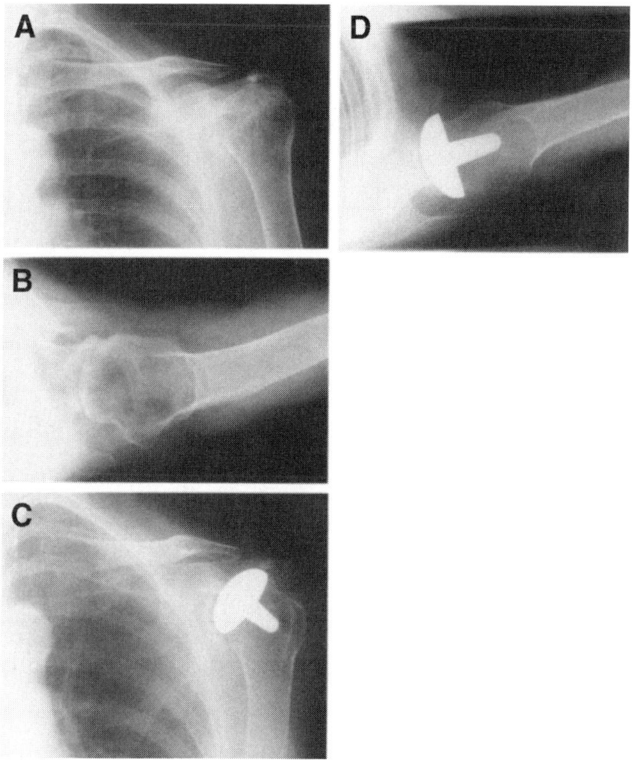

FIGURE 3.—**A**, AP radiograph demonstrating destructive rheumatoid arthritis of the shoulder with glenoid erosion but sufficient humeral head bone for surface replacement. **B**, Preoperative axillary radiograph. **C**, AP radiograph made 5 years after surgery. Only the diseased surface of the humeral head has been replaced, in the anatomical position. This implant has a hydroxyapatite coating. **D**, Postoperative axillary radiograph made 5 years after surgery. (Republished with permission of the Journal of Bone and Joint Surgery, Inc, from Levy O, Funk L, Sforza G, et al: Copeland surface replacement arthroplasty of the shoulder in rheumatoid arthritis. *J Bone Joint Surg Am* 86-A:512-518, 2004. Reproduced by permission of the publisher via Copyright Clearance Center, Inc.)

Conclusion.—Indications for the Copeland surface replacement arthroplasty of the shoulder for patients with rheumatoid arthritis are the same as those for the conventional stemmed prostheses. However, the surface replacement provides the advantage of bone preservation and avoids the complications associated with a long humeral stem in rheumatoid bone. The Copeland procedure is not appropriate for severely damaged joints in which the humeral head is insufficient or is too soft.

▶ The concept of a limited replacement only to the pathology involved is in general becoming more accepted for many applications including the knee, the elbow, ankle, and—as reported here—the shoulder. The readers should note that the senior author has employed this technique for almost 20 years. Thus, this experience is noteworthy as is the long-term follow-up and careful review of the large number of patients so treated.

The encouraging outcome of the novel approach to shoulder arthritis is encouraging. Importantly, the replication of this experience by those not involved in the design will be, as with other joints, critically important to fully assess its value in the routine practice of those dealing with shoulder reconstructive surgery.

B. F. Morrey, MD

12 Spine Surgery

Introduction

The 10 articles in the Spine Surgery chapter of the 2005 YEAR BOOK OF ORTHOPEDICS include 5 that address the evaluation and management of spondylolisthesis. The sixth article discusses optimization of the radiographic technique for the sagittal standing long cassette spine radiograph, which is a useful tool in assessing global sagittal balance in spinal deformity patients, including those who have spondylolisthesis. The seventh article deals with adult spinal reconstruction via total disk arthroplasty, and it presents data from the pivotal clinical trial that supported US Food and Drug Administration approval of total disk arthroplasty in 2004. I would also ask our spine surgical community to consider using the term "adult spinal reconstruction" to communicate our surgical care of patients with degenerative spine conditions, including degenerative disk disease and degenerative spondylolisthesis. This term would convey our care of these patients accurately, in a manner analogous to our hip and knee colleagues, whose care of patients with degenerative hip and knee arthritis is routinely called adult reconstruction, and who classify their post-residency training programs as adult reconstruction fellowships. The arrival of total disk arthroplasty has brought us an option to offer these patients reconstruction, when appropriate, in addition to the fusion option to which we have been limited.

The eighth and ninth articles deal with screw osteosynthesis of dens fractures and C1-C2 transarticular fixation. The authors of these articles provide information on indications, surgical technique, and outcome for both of these upper cervical spine applications. The tenth and final article is a Cochrane review regarding cervical mechanical pain treatment. The Cochrane Collaboration is an organization that provides cogent assessments of the literature to encourage evidence-based medicine management decisions, and the discussion that follows the article gives information to guide the clinician to this useful resource.

Finally, a note regarding 2 commonly used forms of a Greek-based English word that describes slipping of one vertebra on another: "olisthesis" and "listhesis." Both these words appear frequently in the first 5 articles of this chapter and refer to the same anatomic deformity. Consultation with an American colleague whose native language is Greek and several English-Greek dictionaries reveals that the Greek word for "slip," written in the English language alphabet, is "olisthesis."

The editors of the YEAR BOOK OF ORTHOPEDICS sincerely hope that the collection of articles selected for inclusion in this chapter will provide a concise summation of frequently encountered spine conditions. The authors of these studies are commended for their contributions toward the improvement of our collective decision making and treatment capabilities in the care of our patients.

Michael J. Yaszemski, MD, PhD

New Concepts on the Pathogenesis and Classification of Spondylolisthesis

Hammerberg KW (Rush Univ, Chicago)
Spine 30:S4-S11, 2005 12–1

Study Design.—A review of the literature in the English language pertaining to the pathogenesis and classification of spondylolisthesis.

Objective.—To review the morphology and biomechanics of the lumbosacral junction as it relates to spondylolisthesis. To present contemporary theories of the development and progression of spondylolisthesis and an etiology-based classification system.

Summary of Background Data.—The proper treatment of spondylolisthesis is dependent on recognizing the type of slip and its natural history. Although a number of clinical and radiographic features have been identified as risk factors, their role as primary causative factors or secondary adaptive changes is not clear. In particular, confusion persists over the classification of slips with "isthmic defects." The early identification of spondylolisthesis that will progress to a high grade without intervention remains elusive.

Methods.—A review of English language literature regarding the pathogenesis and classification of spondylolisthesis.

Results.—Current literature suggests that spinopelvic parameters, in addition to the morphology and biomechanics of the lumbosacral junction, play a causative role in the development of spondylolisthesis. Progression of developmental slips may be due to growth deficiencies of the anterosuperior sacrum, analogous to Blount's disease at the knee. The Marchetti-Bartolozzi classification system emphasizes the distinction between developmental dysplastic slips and acquired laminar stress fractures, both of which may have isthmic defects. These two types of spondylolisthesis have significantly different natural histories, suggesting the need for different treatment strategies. The Marchetti-Bartolozzi system also allows for the classification of postsurgical, pathologic, and degenerative forms of spondylolisthesis.

Conclusions.—The morphology of the lumbosacral junction resists high shear and compressive forces. The loss of the posterior restraint through an incompetent bony hook may result in the forward displacement of one vertebra on the subjacent vertebra. The spinopelvic parameters, such as pelvic incidence, may be greater determinants of development and progression than previously appreciated. The Marchetti-Bartolozzi classification system is applicable to all forms of lumbar spondylolisthesis, and seems to be clinically relevant in terms of treatment decisions. Their system emphasizes the distinction between developmental spondylolisthesis with lysis and acquired spondylitic spondylolisthesis, which have been included together in previous classification systems and caused confusion over natural history and treatment. Developmental slips have a greater propensity toward progression, which may be secondary to growth deficiencies of the upper sacrum. Further study is required to confirm these observations.

▶ This study summarizes the results of the Scoliosis Research Society's Workshop on spondylolisthesis, which occurred in October 2004. The workshop participants recommended the Marchetti-Bartolozzi etiology-based spondylolisthesis classification as the most appropriate system for communication regarding this condition.[1] The Marchetti-Bartolozzi system emphasizes the distinction between developmental and acquired forms of spondylolisthesis. This report suggests that use of the word "isthmic" be avoided, as dysplastic spondylolisthesis and spondylolisthesis based on acquired laminar stress fractures may both have isthmic defects, but differ significantly in their optimal management approaches. The report mentions that the pelvic incidence parameter is a fixed parameter, unique to each person, and that larger values of pelvic incidence are associated with increased shear forces at the lumbosacral junction.[2,3] The pelvic incidence is defined as the angle between the perpendicular to the sacral plate at its midpoint and a line that connects the midpoint of the sacral plate to the midpoint of a line connecting the femoral heads.

The Newman classification of spondylolisthesis into congenital, spondylolytic, traumatic, degenerative, and pathologic includes 3 descriptors that have been retained in the acquired category of the Marchetti-Bartolozzi system (traumatic, degenerative, and pathologic).[4] The elimination of the term "congenital" that occurred in the Newman system, and the appearance of the term "developmental" in the Marchetti-Bartolozzi system, parallel an evolution in thinking by our hip colleagues, who have transitioned to the term "developmental dysplasia of the hip" from the earlier "congenital dislocation of the hip." The suspicion of a developmental etiology for spondylolisthesis is evident in Newman's 1963 study, even though he chose the word "congenital" in his classification system. In that study, there was mention that no evidence of spondylolisthesis had ever been found in a fetus or newborn infant, and that the process occurred under the effects of a forward shear force acting on L5 relative to S1 after the onset of walking.

The author indicates that an effective means of communicating the nature of a particular person's spondylolisthesis is a combination of the Marchetti-Bartolozzi description and an indication of the extent of translation, using the familiar Meyerding system of grades I to V.[5]

M. J. Yaszemski, MD, PhD

References

1. Marchetti PG, Bartolozzi P: Classification of spondylolisthesis as a guideline for treatment, in *The Textbook for Spinal Surgery*, vol 2. Philadelphia, Lippincott Raven, 1997, pp 1211-1254.
2. Legaye J, Duval-Beaupere G, Hecquet J, et al: Pelvic incidence: A fundamental pelvic parameter for three-dimensional regulation of spinal sagittal curves. *Eur Spine J* 7:99-103, 1998.
3. Hanson DS, Bridwell KH, Rhee JM, et al: Correlation of pelvic incidence with low- and high-grade isthmic spondylolisthesis. *Spine* 27:26-29, 2002.
4. Newman PH, Stone KH: The etiology of spondylolisthesis. *J Bone Joint Surg [Br]* 45:39-59, 1963.
5. Meyerding HW: Spondylolisthesis. *Surg Gynecol Obstet* 54:371-377, 1932.

Adult Low-Grade Acquired Spondylolytic Spondylolisthesis: Evaluation and Management

Kwon BK, Albert TJ (Univ of British Columbia, Vancouver, Canada; Thomas Jefferson Univ, Philadelphia)

Spine 30:S35-S41, 2005 12–2

Study Design.—Literature review.

Objective.—To discuss the presentation and evaluation of adult patients with acquired spondylolytic spondylolisthesis of low-grade severity and to review surgical treatment options.

Summary of Background Data.—Low-grade adult acquired spondylolytic spondylolisthesis is one of the most common forms of spondylolisthesis.

Methods.—Literature review.

Results.—Adults with symptomatic low-grade spondylolytic spondylolisthesis are treated predominantly nonoperatively, with activity modification, physiotherapy, nonsteroidal anti-inflammatory agents, and local injections. Surgical treatment is reserved for individuals with intractable back pain and/or radicular symptoms. A number of surgical options exist, including direct pars repair, and fusion with or without decompression. Fusion can be achieved by providing anterior column support alone, posterior support alone, or a combined circumferential approach; the optimal method by which fusion should be achieved has not been established.

Conclusions.—The management of low-grade acquired spondylolytic spondylolisthesis requires a thoughtful and individualized approach, recognizing the frequently benign natural history of the deformity and the potentially good clinical outcomes from surgery in those select patients with intolerable back and leg pain. While fusion is the mainstay of surgical management, a prospective randomized study would be extremely useful to delineate the optimal fusion technique.

▶ Kwon and Albert provide a framework for the clinician to approach this condition that, among the types of spondylolisthesis, is seen frequently in a spine surgical practice They point out that low-grade (Meyerding I or II) acquired spondylolisthesis in the adult can often be managed nonoperatively. Those patients who have persistent, intractable radicular or low back pain despite an appropriate nonoperative management plan are candidates for surgical treatment. The wide variety of presenting symptoms and patient comorbidities necessitates individualization of the surgical approach for those patients who might be best helped by surgery. The selection of decompression, fusion, instrumentation, and anterior, posterior, or combined approaches is best made for that particular patient's constellation of symptomatology and pathologic anatomy, so that appropriate counseling for reasonable treatment expectations can be done.

The authors also discuss the role of indirect decompression by deformity reduction and fusion to mitigate dynamic nerve root compression. Surgeons should consider both fixed compressive contributions to neural injury and dynamic contributions from instability, using whatever system to define instability with which the surgeon is comfortable. This study conveys a description of spondylolisthesis in a manner identical to that recommended by Hammerberg in Abstract 12–1 of this chapter. That is, Kwon and Albert use a combination of the Marchetti-Bartolozzi etiologic classification and the Meyerding severity of translation classification.

We should also note that adult patients with low-grade acquired spondylolisthesis often present differently than adults with high-grade (Meyerding III, IV, and V) slips. The high-grade slips, if they have not been associated with symptoms before adulthood, occasionally have a benign course. When these high-grade slips do become symptomatic in adult years, the treatment strategy is different from that for the adult-acquired low-grade slips. DeWald et al[1] provide a good discussion of the decision-making strategy for high-grade adult spondylolisthesis.

M. J. Yaszemski, MD, PhD

Reference

1. DeWald CJ, Vartabedian JE, Rodts MF, et al: Evaluation and management of high-grade spondylolisthesis in adults. *Spine* 30:S49-S59, 2005.

Degenerative Spondylolisthesis: Review of Current Trends and Controversies

Sengupta DK, Herkowitz HN (Dartmouth-Hitchcock Med Ctr, Lebanon, NH; William Beaumont Hosp, Royal Oak, Mich)

Spine 30:S71-S81, 2005 12–3

Study Design.—A literature-based review.

Objectives.—To review management and controversies and to present authors recommendations.

Summary of Background Data.—There is considerable controversy regarding indication for surgery, role for decompression alone, and decompression with fusion with or without instrumentation.

Methods.—Review of English language medical literature.

Results.—The condition may stabilize itself with the collapse of the disc spaces and osteophytes but may continue to progress in nearly a third of the cases. It may cause predominantly back pain due to segmental instability, or radicular pain/neurogenic claudication secondary to root entrapment or spinal stenosis. When conservative treatment fails, the mainstay of surgical treatment is decompressive laminectomy and fusion, with or without instrumentation.

Conclusions.—Decompression primarily relieves radicular symptoms and neurogenic claudication whereas fusion primarily relieves back pain by elimination of instability. The goals for instrumentation are to promote fusion and to correct deformity. Fusion has a better long-term outcome than decompression alone. There is evidence that instrumentation improves fusion rate but does not improve clinical outcome in a relatively short-term follow-up. However, outcome of pseudarthrosis cases deteriorates over time and solid fusion produces better long-term outcome. The benefit of instrumentation comes with a price of higher postoperative morbidity and complication rate. Bone morphogenetic proteins are being tried to increase the rate of fusion, without increasing the complication rate, but the cost is prohibitive. More recently, dynamic stabilization with instrumentation but without fusion has been introduced as an alternative treatment. The current trends of surgical treatment and controversies are discussed.

▶ This study provides a framework within which to evaluate and manage patients who have degenerative spondylolisthesis. Sengupta and Herkowitz remind us that the degenerative changes in the disk and facet joints may eventually reach a point at which the condition stabilizes itself. However, patients may have progression of their symptoms and will present with low back pain, radicular symptoms, neurogenic claudication, or some combination of these symptoms. The authors review some of the distinguishing features of neurogenic claudication as opposed to those of vascular claudication. One example is the potential for relief of neurogenic claudication symptoms by flexing the spine while continuing to walk, whereas vascular claudication symptoms require rest from walking to bring relief. Likewise, neurogenic claudication symptoms can start after prolonged standing erect without walking, whereas vascular claudication symptoms usually appear after a period of walking.

The indications to transition from nonoperative management to surgical management include persistent back or leg pain, neurogenic claudication, a progressive neurologic deficit, and bowel or bladder dysfunction. The authors review preoperative and intraoperative factors that enter into the decision to add deformity reduction, fusion, and instrumentation to the decompression. They emphasize that the decompression is the mainstay of surgical treatment, and that the factors to consider when deciding whether to add a fusion, with or without instrumentation, and with or without deformity reduction, include the preoperative disk height, the degree of kyphosis, the presence of degenerative scoliosis, the degree of instability, the degree of olisthesis, the presence of a previous laminectomy, and the status of adjacent spinal segments. The intraoperative factors involved in this decision include the extent of the decompression procedure, the nature of any olisthesis correction, and the available bone stock for fusion. They note that, in patients with multilevel neural compression, if only 1 level has an olisthesis, then they will consider a "selective fusion." That is, the decision to fuse will be made independently for each level decompressed and will take into account the presence of any scoliosis. Finally, they clarify the bone stock issue by noting that a patient with adequate bone for transplantation and appropriate-sized transverse processes for fusion does not necessarily require opening and bone grafting of the facets at the spondylolytic level. Thus, a patient whose facets have not been removed in whole or in part during the decompression may receive a posterolateral fusion, and the intact facets can provide some stability if the surgeon elects to perform a noninstrumented fusion. If the facets are partially or completely removed, either as part of the decompression or because the surgeon chooses to add a facet fusion, then there exists a greater indication to add instrumentation.

Finally, the authors remind us that the 1991 prospective study by Herkowitz and Kurz showed that patients who received both a decompression and a fusion had better outcomes than those who received only a decompression. However, over the short term (the average follow-up time was 3 years), there was no improvement in outcome based on the achievement of a solid fusion. Those patients who had a pseudarthrosis did well in the short term and did better than those patients who had a decompression alone. However, a later follow-up report showed that the patients with a solid fusion had better long-term outcomes than did those who had a pseudarthrosis.[1] This issue, whether the goal of achieving a solid fusion warrants the addition of instrumentation in a degenerative spondylolisthesis surgical patient, will be addressed in the next 2 studies in this chapter (Abstracts 12–4 and 12–5). In these reports, Phillips et al will argue the position for a noninstrumented fusion in these patients, and Fischgrund et al will argue the position for the addition of instrumentation.

M. J. Yaszemski, MD, PhD

Reference

1. Kornblum MB, Fischgrund JS, Herkowitz HN, et al: Degenerative lumbar spondylolisthesis with spinal stenosis: A prospective long-term study comparing fusion and pseudarthrosis. *Spine* 29:726-732, 2004.

The Argument for Noninstrumental Posterolateral Fusion for Patients With Spinal Stenosis and Degenerative Spondylolisthesis

Phillips FM (Rush Univ, Chicago)
Spine 29:170-172, 2004 12–4

Background.—Surgical intervention is recommended for spinal stenosis with degenerative spondylolisthesis. The primary goal of this surgery is decompression of the neural elements to relieve symptoms of neurogenic claudication. Concomitant posterolateral arthrodesis has been recommended for prevention of progression of spondylolisthesis after decompression, which may reduce postoperative back pain. In recent years, there has been an increase in the supplementation of the arthrodesis with instrumentation. Instrumentation has been shown to improve fusion rates, but the use of instrumentation in the treatment of degenerative spondylolisthesis has not been shown to provide clinical benefits.

Overview.—A review of the literature has not identified compelling data to support the view that instrumentation provides any clinical advantage in the treatment of degenerative spondylolisthesis. The improved fusion rate achieved with instrumentation has been associated with some adverse effects, including longer surgical time, greater blood loss, more medical complications, and a higher rate of reoperation than noninstrumented arthrodesis. A review of the cost-effectiveness of arthrodesis with and without instrumentation for patients with degenerative spondylolisthesis and spinal stenosis found that the cost effectiveness of laminectomy with noninstrumented fusion compared favorably with other surgical procedures; however, instrumented fusion was quite expensive in light of the small gain in health outcome.

Conclusions.—The advantage of routine instrumentation in the treatment of degenerative spinal stenosis with spondylolisthesis must be more convincingly demonstrated. It must be recognized that doing less and creating less esthetic radiographs may be in the best interests of the patient.

► This manuscript mentions the 1991 Herkowitz and Kurz prospective study of 50 patients that showed better outcomes at the 3-year point for the 25 patients who had a fusion in addition to their decompression. Nine of those 25 patients had a pseudarthrosis. Five of those 9 patients had an excellent outcome, and 4 had a good outcome at the 3-year follow-up point. Fischgrund reported a prospective randomized study of 68 patients in 1997 who had undergone decompression and posterolateral fusion for spinal stenosis with degenerative spondylolisthesis. These patients were randomized into receiving either instrumented or noninstrumented fusions. At the 2-year follow-up point, the fusion rate in the instrumented group was 82%, compared with 45% in the noninstrumented group. There was, however, no improvement in clinical outcome based on the presence of instrumentation. Eighty-three percent of the noninstrumented patients in Fischgrund's study (15 of 18 patients) had good and excellent clinical outcomes, despite having a pseudarthrosis rate of 55%. By comparison, good and excellent outcomes occurred in 76% of the instrumented patients.

Dr Phillips notes that a survey of North American Spine Society members showed that 67% of respondents favored an instrumented fusion for their patients undergoing decompression and fusion for degenerative spondylolisthesis, while only 9% would recommend a noninstrumented fusion in the same clinical situation. He cautions that this position does not have the support of evidence-based medicine, because no Cochrane review exists that shows a benefit for instrumentation in this patient group. Since there is added risk to the patient when instrumentation is included in a fusion procedure, he reminds us that the burden of proof must be to show that this added risk carries with it a demonstrable added benefit to the patient.

M. J. Yaszemski, MD, PhD

The Argument for Instrumental Decompressive Posterolateral Fusion for Patients With Degenerative Spondylolisthesis and Spinal Stenosis
Fischgrund JS (Southfield, Md)
Spine 29:173-174, 2004 12–5

Background.—There has been debate in the past several decades regarding the role of arthrodesis in the operative management of lumbar spinal stenosis with associated degenerative spondylolisthesis. There have been some reports of clinical success after decompression alone, but the majority of reports have recommended concomitant posterolateral fusion for the patient in need of decompression for spinal stenosis with associated degenerative spondylolisthesis. Several studies have shown that patients undergoing decompression for spinal stenosis and degenerative spondylolisthesis have an improved clinical outcome when arthrodesis is included in the procedure. The increasing use of spinal instrumentation, beginning in the early 1990s, prompted questions concerning the outcome in these patients when instrumentation was performed at the same time of arthrodesis. Would the fusion rate improve with this procedure? Would the clinical outcome be improved? And what are the prospects for these patients in the long term?

Overview.—A review of studies over the past 2 decades have shown that patients who have at least an attempt at arthrodesis will have better outcomes than patients who have no attempt at arthrodesis. This fibrous union may benefit patients in the short term, but long-term results deteriorate in patients who do not have a solid fusion. It is also clear that patients who have an instrumentation procedure at the same time as arthrodesis will have a higher fusion rate. Further studies are ongoing as to the use of local bone graft for posterolateral fusion, and at one center the use of local bone graft with the addition of pedicle screw instrumentation has provided promising early results.

Conclusions.—The recommendation in this report is that patients undergoing surgical decompression for spinal stenosis with degenerative spondylolisthesis also undergo an instrumented fusion at the time of the initial surgical procedure.

► Dr Fischgrund and his colleagues published the 1997 prospective study that showed no improvement in clinical outcome at the 2-year postoperative point from adding instrumentation to a degenerative spondylolisthesis decompression and fusion, even though the solid fusion rate was increased in the patients who had instrumentation. A recent follow-up study[1] that included a subset of those patients and a subset of the patients from the 1991 Herkowitz and Kurz study reviewed those patients from both studies who had a noninstrumented fusion. Recall that the 2 groups in the 1991 Herkowitz and Kurz study were decompression without fusion and decompression with fusion. All of the 25 fusion patients in that study were noninstrumented. Recall also that the 1997 study by Fischgrund and colleagues had 68 patients, all of whom had a decompression and a fusion. Half of them received an instrumented fusion, and half received a noninstrumented fusion. The 25 fusion patients from the 1991 study and the 34 noninstrumented fusion patients from the 1997 study constituted the study group for this long-term follow-up study by Kornblum and colleagues. The patients for the follow-up study were classified as having either a solid fusion or a pseudarthrosis based on the last radiograph they had at the conclusion of their respective first study, and they answered a questionnaire regarding their current status. Forty-seven of the initial patients were included in this follow-up study. The combined pseudarthrosis rate for the patients from the 2 contributing studies was 53%. The average follow-up interval for the study by Kornblum et al was just under 8 years. Good and excellent outcomes were present in 86% of those patients who had a solid fusion and in 56% of those patients who had a pseudarthrosis. The authors conclude that a fibrous pseudarthrosis provides good short-term results (2-3 years) relative to a decompression without a fusion, but that the long-term results (slightly less than 8 years) deteriorate in those patients who do not achieve a solid fusion.

In the point-of-view commentary that follows the Kornblum et al article,[2] Dr Katz notes the the Kornblum study included neither the 1991 study patients who had no fusion nor the 1997 patients who had instrumentation. The importance of this statement is that a decision to include instrumentation for a spinal stenosis decompression and fusion based on these data must be speculative. That is, the data from the 2004 Kornblum study show a decline over an 8-year interval of results for those patients who had a pseudarthrosis, and the 1997 data from the Fischgrund et al study show an increase in the solid fusion rate for those patients who had an instrumented fusion. The inference is that the addition of instrumentation, and hence an increased fusion rate, will improve long-term outcome. This has not been shown directly from these data, and Dr Katz mentions that the authors could have done so by including the remaining patients from the 1991 and 1997 studies (ie, the decompression without fusion patients from 1991 and the instrumented fusion patients from 1997) in the long-term follow-up study. He also mentions that we should be sensitive to the costs associated with our surgical decisions, and cites the Kuntz et al study[3] from 2000, which shows that the cost of a decompression with an instrumented fusion, expressed as dollars per quality-adjusted life year, is 6 times that of a decompression with a noninstrumented fusion.

M. J. Yaszemski, MD, PhD

References

1. Kornblum MB, Fischgrund JS, Herkowitz HN, et al: Degenerative lumbar spondylolisthesis with spinal stenosis: A prospective long-term study comparing fusion and pseudarthrosis. *Spine* 29:726-732, 2004.
2. Katz JN: Point of view. *Spine* 29:726-734, 2004.
3. Kuntz KM, Snider R, Weinstein J, et al: Cost-effectiveness of fusion with and without instrumentation for patients with degenerative spondylolisthesis and spinal stenosis. *Spine* 25:1132-1139, 2000.

Is There an Optimal Patient Stance for Obtaining a Lateral 36" Radiograph? A Critical Comparison of Three Techniques

Horton WC, Brown CW, Bridwell KH, et al (Emory Univ, Atlanta, Ga; Panorama Orthopaedics, Golden, Colo; Washington Univ, St Louis; et al)

Spine 30:427-433, 2005 12–6

Study Design.—Scoliosis patients were prospectively x-rayed in three positions with independent analysis.

Objectives.—To determine if one positioning technique provides superior visualization of critical landmarks (C7, T2, T12, L5–S1) and to determine any position dependent variations in regional measures or sagittal balance.

Summary of Background Data.—Different techniques for positioning patient's arms are used for 36" lateral radiograph with no data on relative effects.

Methods.—A total of 25 scoliosis patients were prospectively studied with 36" lateral radiographs in three positions varying arm location (straight out, partially flexed, and the "clavicle" position). Films were analyzed independently by three surgeons. Vertebral landmarks were scored for clarity; and lordosis, kyphosis, and global balance were analyzed. Statistical analysis was done with a General Estimating Equations model.

Results.—The overall visualization score for the clavicle position was superior to either the 60° or 90° positions (clavicle *vs.* 60°, $P < 0.0001$; clavicle *vs.* 90°, $P < 0.0003$). Analysis of vertebral landmarks showed significantly better visualization of T2 with clavicle *versus* 90° ($P < 0.047$), better visualization of T12 with clavicle *versus* either 60° ($P < 0.006$) or 90° ($P < 0.049$), and better visualization of L5-S1 with clavicle *versus* 90° ($P < 0.02$). Regional measures showed no differences, but sagittal balance was significantly more positive in the 60° position than either clavicle ($P < 0.04$) or 90° ($P < 0.015$).

Conclusions.—The clavicle position for obtaining lateral 36" radiographs produces significantly better overall visualization of critical vertebral landmarks. Regional measures do not differ between the three positions, but global balance is more positive with the 60° position. Clinically, the clavicle position may result in more accurate radiographic measures and may minimize repeated radiograph exposures.

▶ The prior articles in this section of the YEAR BOOK describe spondylolisthesis evaluation and management issues. The authors of this study remind us that the imaging of spinal deformities is becoming more critical as we increase our appreciation of the importance of global sagittal balance in all deformities, including scoliosis, kyphosis, fractures, and spondylolisthesis. We get important sagittal balance information from the standing lateral long cassette spine radiograph. Horton et al ask in this study whether the commonly used techniques to obtain this standing lateral radiograph differ in their ability to show the key vertebral landmarks (C7, T2, T12, and L5-S1), and whether they cause differences in regional lordosis and kyphosis measurements or in the global sagittal balance assessment. The 3 positions tested were the 60°, the 90°, and the clavicle position. The 60° and 90° positions require an external support, often an IV pole. In the 60° position, the patient's forearms are parallel to the floor, the hands grasp the IV pole, and the arms are forward flexed at the shoulders so that the olecranon lies just anterior to the sternum. In the 90° position, the arms and forearms are straight out in front of the body with the elbows fully extended, and the hands grasp the IV pole at shoulder level. The clavicle position has the arms flexed forward at the shoulders, the elbows fully flexed, and the hands in the supraclavicular fossae. In all 3 positions, the patient is asked to assume the body position in which they feel most relaxed and in which they feel they have their most "normal" posture. The standing lateral spinal radiograph is not taken with the patient in the ideal sagittal balance assessment position, that of standing with the arms at the sides, because this would obliterate all the key vertebral landmarks.

The results show that none of the 3 positions causes a change in regional lordosis (L1-S1) or kyphosis (T2-T12). The 60° and 90° positions cause reproducible changes in global balance: the 60° position causes a forward movement of the C7 plumb line, and the 90° position causes a rearward movement of the C7 plumb line.

The clavicle position provided the best combination of visualization of the key vertebrae, together with the least effect on the global sagittal balance assessment. The rising popularity of 3-dimensional CT and MRI reconstructions may soon provide adjunctive data for the assessment of coronal and sagittal global balance, and the open, standing MRI instruments may allow these data to be gathered while the patient stands relaxed with her or his arms at the sides.

M. J. Yaszemski, MD, PhD

Prospective Randomized Study of the Charité Artificial Disc: Data From Two Investigational Centers

Guyer RD, McAfee PC, Hochschuler SH, et al (Texas Back Inst, Plano, Tex; St Joseph's Hosp, Towson, Md)

Spine J 4:252S-259S, 2004 12–7

Background Context.—For decades there has been a desire to restore motion of a painful degenerated spinal segment. Artificial discs have been used in Europe for almost 20 years. In the few reports available in the literature, the results have been promising. However, there have been no prospective randomized studies comparing artificial discs with spinal fusion.

Purpose.—The purpose of this study was to determine if patients with symptomatic degenerative disc disease treated with Charité artificial disc (DePuy Spine, Raynham, MA) arthroplasty would show significant improvement in functional outcome measures and to compare these results to fusion.

Study Design/Setting.—This was a prospective randomized clinical trial comparing total disc replacement with anterior lumbar interbody fusion using cages. The data reported were collected from two spine specialty centers participating in a Food and Drug Administration regulated trial.

Methods.—A consecutive series of 144 patients were randomized using a 2:1 ratio of Charité versus BAK (Zimmer Spine, Minneapolis, MN). All patients were being treated for single-level discogenic pain confirmed by plain radiography, magnetic resonance imaging and provocative discography. Data were collected at designated follow-up periods for up to 24 months.

Results.—The mean age was 40.1 years (range, 21 to 56 years). Forty-four cases had BAK anterior interbody fusion, and 100 cases were randomized to Charité disc replacement. The mean operating time was 76.2 minutes (range, 54 to 137 minutes) for the Charité cases. The mean estimated blood loss was 196.2 cc (range, 50 to 1,800 cc). Most patients were discharged in 1 to 2 days with a soft corset and returned to normal activities within 3 weeks if they underwent the disc replacement. The mean Oswestry Disability Index score for the BAK group was 69.6±12.8 preoperatively and 27.5±26.4 at 24-month follow up ($p<.001$). The corresponding mean Oswestry score for the Charité disc patients was 70.9 preoperatively and 30.0 at 24-month follow-up ($p<.001$).

Conclusions.—In this prospective randomized study, both surgical groups improved significantly. Complications of total disc replacement were similar to those encountered with anterior lumbar interbody fusion. Total disc replacement appears to be a viable alternative to fusion for the treatment of single-level symptomatic disc degeneration unresponsive to nonoperative management.

► The ability to offer motion-retaining reconstruction as an option to a patient with a condition that affects the functional spinal unit now exists. This study describes the prospective, randomized clinical trial comparing total disk replacement to anterior lumbar interbody fusion for symptomatic degenerative disk disease. These data were part of the multicenter study that supported the Food and Drug Administration approval for total disk arthroplasty in the United States. The study design was a 2:1 randomization of total disk arthroplasty to anterior lumbar interbody fusion in 144 patients (100 total disk arthroplasties, 44 fusions) with a 2-year follow-up period. The mean patient age was just under 41 years. This emphasizes the fact that the total disk arthroplasty patient population is younger than the THA and TKA patient population, and the required service life for the total disk prosthesis will be longer than that for a THA or TKA prosthesis. The design parameters of the Charité prosthesis include an ultra–high molecular weight polyethylene on Co-Cr-Mo bearing surface, a mobile as opposed to a fixed bearing articulation, a porous ingrowth surface, and maximal preservation of vertebral bone stock. The patient inclusion criteria for the study were single-level degenerative disk disease at either L4-L5 or L5-S1, a positive discogram, and a minimum of 6 months of nonoperative treatment. Exclusion criteria were a previous fusion attempt anywhere in the thoracolumbar spine, osteoporosis, objective evidence of nerve root compression, spinal fracture, spinal tumor, facet arthrosis, scoliosis, spondylolysis, spondylolisthesis, and body weight more than 1 standard deviation above the mean.

The authors emphasize the following surgical points: (1) complete discectomy is required, (2) the lateral annulus must be preserved bilaterally, (3) the anterior vertebral midline must be confirmed intraoperatively with imaging and then marked on the vertebra, (4) the disk height must be restored, and (5) there must be coverage of as much of the cross-sectional area of the endplates as possible. The ideal prosthesis position on the anteroposterior x-ray is such that the center of the prosthesis is at the center of the vertebra. The ideal prosthesis position on the lateral x-ray is such that the center of the prosthesis is 2 mm posterior to the vertebral midline on the lateral image.

The patients in both the fusion group and the total disk arthroplasty group improved significantly at the 2-year follow-up point compared with their preoperative status. The surgical complications were similar in type and frequency in both groups. The authors emphasize that the most significant predictor of good result is appropriate patient selection. Finally, note that the surgeons who participated in the study did 5 cases to mitigate any learning curve effect before enrolling the first patient who would be part of the study. These authors have emphasized that surgeons who feel that total disk arthroplasty will be a treatment option that they offer to their patients should consider 2 preparatory actions: (1) attend a total disk arthroplasty surgical technique course, and (2) visit a surgeon who has already acquired experience with the technique and perform several cases together with her or him. The availability of this reconstructive option for our low back pain patients offers an additional treatment modality that will be appropriate for a subset of those patients.

M. J. Yaszemski, MD, PhD

Atlantoaxial Transarticular Screw Fixation: A Review of Surgical Indications, Fusion Rate, Complications, and Lessons Learned in 191 Adult Patients

Gluf WM, Schmidt MH, Apfelbaum RI (Univ of Utah, Salt Lake City)

J Neurosurg: Spine 2:155-163, 2005 12–8

Object.—In this, the first of two articles regarding C1–2 transarticular screw fixation, the authors assessed the rate of fusion, surgery-related complications, and lessons learned after C1–2 transarticular screw fixation in an adult patient series.

Methods.—The authors retrospectively reviewed 191 consecutive patients (107 women and 84 men; mean age 49.7 years, range 17–90 years) in whom at least one C1–2 transarticular screw was placed. Overall 353 transarticular screws were placed for trauma (85 patients), rheumatoid arthritis (63 patients), congenital anomaly (26 patients), os odontoideum (four patients), neoplasm (eight patients), and chronic cervical instability (five patients). Among these, 67 transarticular screws were placed in 36 patients as part of an occipitocervical construct. Seventeen patients had undergone 24 posterior C1–2 fusion attempts prior to referral. The mean follow-up period was 15.2 months (range 0.1–106.3 months). Fusion was achieved in 98% of cases followed to commencement of fusion or for at least 24 months. The mean duration until fusion was 9.5 months (range 3–48 months). Complications occurred in 32 patients. Most were minor; however, five patients suffered vertebral artery (VA) injury. One bilateral VA injury resulted in patient death. The others did not result in any permanent neurological sequelae.

Conclusions.—Based on this series, the authors have learned important lessons that can improve outcomes and safety. These include techniques to improve screw-related patient positioning, development of optimal instrumentation, improved screw materials and design, and defining the role for stereotactic navigation. Atlantoaxial transarticular screw fixation is highly effective in achieving fusion, and the complication rate is low when performed by properly trained surgeons.

► Gluf et al present their C1-C2 posterior fusion experience with transarticular fixation by the Magerl technique. They present their indications, fusion rate, the nature and rate of complications, and surgical technique that includes critical intraoperative decision criteria gleaned from 191 cases. In a companion article, Gluf and Brockmeyer[1] present these same issues as they apply to pediatric C1-C2 fusion patients.

The adult patients included 107 women and 84 men, whose mean age was 49.7 years. Indications for posterior C1-C2 fusion included trauma, rheumatoid arthritis, congenital anomaly, os odontoideum, neoplasia, and chronic cervical instability. Fusion occurred in 98% of the patients. The mean duration to fusion was 9.5 months. There were 32 complications in the 191 patients. All were minor except 5 vertebral artery injuries, one of which was bilateral and resulted in the patient's death. There were no permanent neurologic sequelae in the other 4 patients who had a vertebral artery injury.

The key preoperative and intraoperative surgical points that the authors emphasize include the performance of a sagittal and axial formatted CT scan along the screw trajectory to ensure that a safe path for the screws exists. Twenty percent of people have a vertebral artery foramen that lies in the optimal screw path. If a safe path does not exist, then no screw can be placed on that side. In such cases, the surgical choices include using only 1 screw and an additional method of C1-C2 fixation, or choosing the combination of C1 lateral mass screws, C2 pars interarticularis screws, and rods as the fixation method. In the same issue of the *Journal of Neurosurgery: Spine*, Hott et al[2] provide cadaver data that compare the strength of several C1-C2 instrumentation constructs. The C1 lateral mass screws and C2 pars interarticularis screws with connecting rods performed in a similar mechanical manner to 2 transarticular screws, with the exception of being less effective in resisting extension. The difference in resistance to extension loading disappeared when an adjunct structural graft and cable construct was placed between the posterior arch of C1 and the posterior aspect (lamina and spinous process) of C2.

Several additional technical points can be clarified. First, postoperative immobilization is not used routinely, but is selectively chosen in patients who have poor bone quality. Second, after patient positioning, but before beginning the surgical approach, a long Steinmann pin is placed alongside the patient's neck, and over her or his back, to demonstrate by a lateral fluoroscope image that the positioning is appropriate to permit passage of the drill, tap, and screw along the appropriate trajectory. The optimal aiming point for the screw is at the upper half of the lateral image of the C1 anterior arch. Third, the axial CT image of C1 should be studied, and the relationship of the screw's intended target point on the anterior C1 arch to the anterior C1 tubercle assessed. Then, an estimate of how far this point lies behind the anterior C1 tubercle should be made. The drill, tap, and screw should all stop at this distance behind the C1 tubercle when viewed on the lateral C-arm image during their respective insertions. Note that if, on the lateral image, the screw tip is as far forward as the anterior C1 tubercle, then the screw has likely extended past the anterior cortex of the C1 anterior arch. In this position, it may be near the internal carotid artery. A preoperative CT scan with contrast to identify the location of the internal carotid artery will permit the surgeon to assess the risk to the artery when planning the screw trajectory.[3]

The surgical exposure is made from occiput to C3, and the C2-C3 interspinous and supraspinous ligaments remain intact. Screw placement should begin on the side that has the best bony path on the preoperative imaging. Thus, the chance of injuring a vertebral artery during the first screw placement will be minimized. If arterial bleeding occurs on preparation of the first screw hole, a screw should be placed in the hole, as this is the best method to control the bleeding, and arterial repair is not feasible from this approach. If this situation occurs, the second screw should not be placed, and adjunct posterior fixation or a postoperative halo vest should be used.

The authors' pediatric experience is similar. They reviewed 67 patients aged 16 and younger (average age was 9 years). All 67 patients achieved a solid fusion, and there were complications in 7 patients. Two of those complications were vertebral artery injuries.

This large series of Magerl transarticular C1-C2 instrumentation for atlantoaxial fusion shows the technique to be effective in achieving fusion and demonstrates that the risk-benefit ratio is appropriate for those patients whose condition warrants surgery for a C1-C2 fusion.

M. J. Yaszemski, MD, PhD

References

1. Gluf WM, Brockmeyer DL: Atlantoaxial transarticular screw fixation: A review of surgical indications, fusion rate, complications, and lessons learned in 67 pediatric patients. *J Neurosurg Spine* 2:164-169, 2005.
2. Hott JS, Lynch JJ, Chamberlain RH, et al: Biomechanical comparison of C1-2 posterior fixation techniques. *J Neurosurg Spine* 2:175-181, 2005.
3. Todd LT, Yaszemski MJ, Maus TP, et al: Relationship of the internal carotid artery to the anterior aspect of the C1 vertebra: Implications for C1-2 transarticular and C1 lateral mass screw fixation. *Spine* 2005. In press.

Results of Long-term Follow-up in Patients Undergoing Anterior Screw Fixation for Type II and Rostral Type III Odontoid Fractures

Fountas KN, Kapsalaki EZ, Karampelas I, et al (Mercer Univ, Macon, Ga; Med College of Georgia, Augusta)

Spine 30:661-669, 2005 12–9

Study Design.—Retrospective analysis of the fusion rate of a group of 38 patients having undergone anterior screw fixation for type II and "shallow" type III odontoid fractures.

Objective.—To determine primarily the long-term fusion rate after anterior screw fixation and to study the clinical characteristics of patients that have a statistically significant or nonsignificant influence on successful outcome.

Summary of Background Data.—Long-term outcome of anterior screw fixation for odontoid fractures has been evaluated in very few studies. This information should be critical for further establishing this technique as a major therapeutic strategy for these cases.

Methods.—Thirty-eight patients, 25 males and 13 females (with mean age 48.4 ± 0.4 years), with type II and rostral type III odontoid fractures, underwent anterior cannulated screw fixation during a 62-month period. Radiologic examination of the cervical spine with plain radiographs was performed at 6 weeks, and 2, 6, 12, and 24 months, while computerized tomography of the upper cervical spine (C1–C3) was obtained at 6 months after surgery. Follow-up was available for 31 patients, and the follow-up time ranged from 39 to 87 months (mean 58.4).

Results.—Radiographic evaluation of the follow-up group showed satisfactory bony fusion and no evidence of abnormal movement at the fracture site in 27 (87.1%) patients. Pseudarthrosis developed in 4 (12.9%) patients; however, 3 (9.6%) of them without instability and 1 (3.2%) with instability. One (3.2%) patient had an instrumentation failure without instability.

Conclusions.—In our series, anterior odontoid screw fixation comprised a safe therapeutic modality with high stability and low mechanical failure rates during short-term and long-term follow-up.

▶ Fountas et al present their results in 38 patients who had type II or high type III dens fractures treated with anterior screw fixation. There were 31 patients for whom follow-up was available. The average follow-up interval was approximately 59 months. Twenty-seven of the 31 fractures healed. Of the remaining 4 patients who had a nonunion, 3 had a stable pseudarthrosis. The average time to fusion in this series was 11 months. The authors review other series of surgically treated dens fractures and note that their results are similar to others in the literature, which demonstrate fusion rates from 84% to 100%, and time to fusion from 3.5 to 11 months.

Early patients in this series (n = 11) received 2 screws, and later patients (n = 26) had a single screw. This paralleled the trend from 2 screws to 1 screw in the peer-reviewed literature. There was no statistical difference in fusion rate between the 1- and 2-screw patients, also in agreement with other studies in the literature. There was no effect of patient age or sex on the fusion rate. This contrasts with the 1985 multicenter study by Clark and White[1] in which increasing age did have a negative effect on fusion rate in type II fractures that were treated in a halo. The authors note that the high fusion rate in surgically treated patients, compared with nonoperative treatment of these fractures and coupled with the low incidence of complications, should cause spine surgeons to carefully assess whether surgical treatment might become the major therapeutic strategy for these injuries.

M. J. Yaszemski, MD, PhD

Reference

1. Clark CR, White AA III: Fractures of the dens. A multicenter study. *J Bone Joint Surg [Am]* 67-A:1340-1348, 1985.

A Cochrane Review of Manipulation and Mobilization for Mechanical Neck Disorders

Gross AR, and the Cervical Overview Group (McMaster Univ, Hamilton, Ont, Canada; St Joseph's Healthcare, Hamilton, Ont, Canada; Monash Univ, Melbourne, Australia; et al)

Spine 29:1541-1548, 2004 12–10

Study Design and Objectives.—Our systematic review of randomized trials assessed whether manipulation and mobilization relieve pain or improve function/disability, patient satisfaction, and global perceived effect in adults with mechanical neck disorders.

Summary of Background Data.—Neck disorders are common, disabling, and costly.

Methods.—Computerized bibliographic databases were searched up to March 2002. Two independent reviewers conducted study selection, data abstraction, and methodologic quality assessment. Relative risk and standardized mean differences were calculated. In the absence of heterogeneity, pooled effect measures were calculated using a random effects model.

Results.—Of the 33 selected trials, 42% were high quality trials. Single or multiple (3–11) sessions of manipulation or mobilization showed no benefit in pain relief when assessed against placebo, control groups, or other treatments for acute/subacute/chronic mechanical neck disorders with or without headache. There was strong evidence of benefit favoring multimodal care (mobilization and/or manipulation plus exercise) over a waiting list control for pain reduction [pooled standardized mean differences −0.85 (95% CI: −1.20 to −0.50)], improvement in function [pooled SMD −0.57 (95% CI: −0.94 to −0.21)] and global perceived effect [standardized mean differences −2.73 (95% CI: −3.30 to −2.16)] for subacute/chronic mechanical neck disorders with or without headache.

Conclusions.—Mobilization and/or manipulation when used with exercise are beneficial for persistent mechanical neck disorders with or without headache. Done alone, manipulation and/or mobilization were not beneficial; when compared to one another, neither was superior. There was insufficient evidence available to draw conclusions for neck disorder with radicular findings. Factorial design would help determine the active agent(s) within a treatment mix.

▶ This study is a review by the Cochrane Collaboration of 33 randomized clinical trials that assessed manipulation and mobilization as treatments for mechanical neck pain. These trials were identified from the published literature on treatment for mechanical neck pain, abstracted, and subjected to methodologic quality assessment. Forty-two percent of the studies were determined to be high-quality trials.

These studies showed a substantial benefit of manipulation, mobilization, and exercise done together for acute, subacute, and chronic mechanical neck disorders with or without headache. There was no benefit for either manipulation or mobilization done alone or with other modalities. The benefits of the multimodal treatment regimen of manipulation, mobilization, and exercise were in pain relief, functional improvement, and global perceived effect.

The Cochrane Collaboration provides a description of its organization and purpose on its Web site (www.cochrane.org). It is an international, nonprofit, and independent organization dedicated to making up-to-date, accurate information about the effects of health care readily available worldwide. It produces and disseminates systematic reviews of health care interventions and promotes the search for evidence in the form of clinical trials and other studies of interventions. The Cochrane Collaboration was founded in 1993 and named for the British epidemiologist Archie Cochrane. The major product of the Collaboration is the Cochrane Database of Systematic Reviews, which is published quarterly as part of The Cochrane Library. The Cochrane Collaborative Back Review Group (www.cochrane.iwh.on.ca) is a useful source for spine care physicians and surgeons to keep informed of studies that may be pertinent to their practices.

M. J. Yaszemski, MD, PhD

13 Orthopedic Oncology

Introduction

The tumor selections this year comprise a wide variety of orthopedic pathologic entities. I have divided this section into reconstructive techniques, tumors in general—benign, malignant, and metastatic—and orthopedic infections.

We continue to evaluate the results of various reconstructive techniques. I have selected a number of interesting articles detailing the results of endoprosthetic reconstructions as well as some innovative uses for allografts, both osteoarticular and intercalary.

The tumor selections represent a wide variety of benign and soft tissue, benign and malignant bone, and soft tissue tumors. I have selected an article (Abstract 13–24) detailing the early experience with bisphosphonates and giant cell tumors. I have also selected 5 articles from the Massachusetts General Hospital (Abstracts 13–32, 13–34, 13–35, 13–36, and 13–37). These are important studies that detail a very long and extensive experience with the aplasia.

Finally, I have included a small selection of articles relating to orthopedic infection, highlighting the successful treatment of infected failed joint arthroplasty.

Christopher P. Beauchamp, MD

Tumor Reconstruction

Custom Cross-Pin Fixation of 32 Tumor Endoprostheses Stems

Cannon CP, Eckardt JJ, Kabo JM, et al (Madigan Army Med Ctr, Ft Lewis, Wash; Univ of California, Los Angeles)

Clin Orthop 417:285-293, 2003 13–1

Introduction.—The main cause of mechanical failure of primary and revision cemented tumor endoprosthetic stems is aseptic loosening. The placement of custom designed pins through the bone, the cement, and the stem can create a bone-cement-prosthesis composite that resists the rotatory stresses that lead to aseptic loosening. At risk situations include large primary reconstructions where the residual short metaphyseal articular segments lack sufficient length and cortical contact to provide lasting fixation, and revision prostheses that are to be recemented into straight diaphyseal segments that already have experienced aseptic loosening. Current modular tumor endoprosthetic systems have improved availability and allow for some intraoperative flexibility, but they do not provide solutions for these at risk scenarios. Additional customization is necessary. We report on the 16-year experience with 32 custom cross-pin stems at the University of California, Los Angeles (UCLA). Twenty of these patients have been followed up for more than 2 years. There were three mechanical failures, three patients were lost to follow-up, and five patients died of disease. There have been no cases of aseptic loosening in this series. Cross-pin fixation has been effective when used in carefully selected cases.

► The greatest problem that we face with distal femoral modular endoprosthetic replacements is related to loosening of the femoral component. The authors share their results of dealing with this particular problem in patients who have very small segments of proximal femur remaining. These are patients whose proximal femur really precludes simply recementing an implant. The authors have designed a custom stem that is fixed with a locking device similar to a reconstruction nail with the device also fixed with methylmethacrylate. They have reported quite satisfactory results with this method of reconstruction in an otherwise very difficult situation that in some instances would necessitate a total femoral replacement.

Hopefully, with the newer generation cementless stems with biologic fixation, many of these issues of loosening of cemented devices can be avoided.

C. P. Beauchamp, MD

Survivorship Analysis of 141 Modular Metallic Endoprostheses at Early Followup

Zeegen EN, Aponte-Tinao LA, Hornicek FJ, et al (Massachusetts Gen Hosp, Boston; Children's Hosp, Boston)

Clin Orthop 420:239-250, 2004 13–2

Introduction.—Although our institution historically has been known for its use of osteoarticular allografts in limb salvage surgery for tumors, during the last 8 years there has been an increase in the use of metallic modular endoprostheses. A retrospective review of 141 patients in whom a modular endoprosthesis was implanted in the past 8 years was done, and survival data were compiled using Kaplan-Meier survival analysis, clinical score was determined using a previously described system, and a multivariate regression analysis was done to identify independent risk factors. There were 13 failures (defined as need for revision of the majority of the prosthetic components, excluding cases of local recurrence) yielding an overall implant survival of 91%. Based on Kaplan-Meier estimates, the endoprosthetic survival rate was 88% at 3 years and 76% at 5 years; per location, it was 100% for the proximal humerus, 100% for the proximal femur, 87% for modular knees, and 53% for total femoral implants at 3 years. The clinical scores were good to excellent in 74% of the patients. Multivariate analysis showed that only location and infection were independent risk factors for prosthesis failure. Loosening, infection, and dislocation were independently predictive of a fair or poor clinical score. Age, gender, diagnosis, length of implant, dislocation, nor failed prior allograft had an independent effect on implant survival or clinical outcome. The proximal humeral and proximal femoral implants had greater survival rates than modular knee and total femoral implants. Conversion of failed allografts to modular endoprostheses had a trend for a higher failure rate, but after a multivariate analysis, did not prove to be an independent risk factor for failure. We think that our experience is similar to other endoprosthesis survivorship reports in the literature with short-term followup.

► Osteoarticular allograft reconstruction for musculoskeletal tumor defects has largely given way to prosthetic or allograft prosthetic reconstructive options. There still remain a number of centers who still have a large volume of osteoarticular allograft reconstructions. The group at Massachusetts General Hospital has also seen a shift toward using endoprosthetic reconstructions for some selected situations. They report their results of a large group retrospectively reviewed. Their results are similar to other reports and indicate in the absence of significant complications that these patients will do well. The main problem associated with these implants, which were largely cemented in place, has been loosening and those sites that typically have low rates of loosening, such as the humerus and proximal femur, have a much better result and their overall results certainly confirm this. Hopefully, when we begin to get some long-term results of the newer generation implants, in which cement can be avoided, we will see a more significant improvement in the long-term performance of modular metallic endoprosthetic reconstructions for these defects.

C. P. Beauchamp, MD

Allografts About the Knee in Young Patients With High-Grade Sarcoma

Brigman BE, Hornicek FJ, Gebhardt MC, et al (Duke Univ, Durham, NC; Massachusetts Gen Hosp, Boston; Children's Hosp, Boston)

Clin Orthop 421:232-239, 2004 13–3

Introduction.—Reconstruction after resections for high-grade sarcomas about the knee in children and adolescents is a challenging problem because of the large soft tissue and skeletal defects, the effects of adjuvant therapy, and the potential for long-term use of the limb. One hundred sixteen patients, all 18 years or younger, with osteosarcoma or Ewing's sarcoma located between the middle femur and middle tibia, were treated with chemotherapy, resection, and allograft reconstruction. One hundred three patients with osteosarcoma and 13 patients with Ewing's sarcoma had 105 Stage II and 11 Stage III tumors. There were 72 osteoarticular grafts (39 femur, 33 tibia), 28 intercalary grafts (19 femur), seven allograft-prosthetic composites (all femur,) and nine allograft-arthrodeses (seven femur, two tibia). At latest followup, 49% of all of the allograft reconstructions were rated good or excellent, 14% were rated as fair, and 37% were failures. Sixteen percent had an infection develop. Twenty-seven percent of patients had a fracture, 34% had a nonunion, and 14 patients eventually required amputation. Reconstruction of large bone defects about the knee in young patients who are being treated with chemotherapy is difficult. Although complications significantly affect outcome, allografts are a viable option for reconstruction in children with high-grade sarcomas about the knee.

▶ The authors share their experience with a large number of patients treated with allografts for skeletal defects after resection of musculoskeletal tumors. This method of reconstruction certainly does carry some advantages in some circumstances. Limb salvage surgery in patients who are growing provide significant reconstructive challenges. Until lately, we have not had very many satisfactory options in terms of growing prostheses. There are certainly advantages to reconstructing missing bone with a biologic substitute, but we are still left with the issue of dealing with limb lengthening qualities. They have demonstrated that in select circumstances and in the absence of complications, an allograft certainly does provide significant advantages, particularly in intercalary reconstructions. The negative effects of chemotherapy in this patient group are somewhat offset by the better outcome in improved healing capacity of allografts in children.

C. P. Beauchamp, MD

The Use of Cement in Osteoarticular Allografts for Proximal Humeral Bone Tumors

DeGroot H III, Donati D, Di Liddo M, et al (Univ of Massachusetts, Worcester; First Univ, Bologna, Italy)

Clin Orthop 427:190-197, 2004 13–4

Introduction.—In a proximal humerus resection for a bone tumor, the use of an osteoarticular allograft is considered the best restoration of shoulder function. We retrospectively reviewed the outcomes of 31 patients who had an intraarticular resection of the proximal humerus for a bone tumor. Twenty-three of the allografts were filled with cement. The average followup was 5.3 years. Of the 31 patients with more than 24 months followup, seven had revision surgery or removal of the allograft. Kaplan-Meier analysis showed that the probability of survival of the reconstruction was 78% at 5 years. Fracture was the main complication in 11 patients (37%) of whom seven were in the noncemented group. Four of these patients had successful surgery for conversion to an allograft-prosthetic composite, whereas one patient had a new allograft. Allografts that were filled with cement had four fractures (18%); three were subchondral fractures discovered by routine CT scans. None of these patients had pain or needed revision surgery. Osteochondral allograft in proximal humerus replacement is a reliable reconstructive technique if the allograft is augmented by filling the intramedullary space with cement. Moreover, cement augmented allografts are less expensive and technically easier than allograft-prosthetic composites.

▶ One of the significant complications that plagues the use of osteoarticular allografts for bone tumor reconstruction is the problem of allograft fracture and dissolution. Allograft prosthetic composites have largely resolved this issue mainly because the allograft is structurally strengthened by the use of metal and cement. Graft resorption is a contributor to allograft fracture, and by using methylmethacrylate to fill the intramedullary canal, the authors have demonstrated a significant reduction in the risk of fracture associated with allografts. This is a useful method that we have used for many years, particularly in intercalary grafts and in particular, grafts that are fixed with plate fixation. It does, however, create a potential problem for the subsequent conversion of an osteoarticular graft to a prosthesis if the other complication of degenerative osteoarthritis or subchondral collapse occurs.

C. P. Beauchamp, MD

Technique of Forequarter (Interscapulothoracic) Amputation

Ferrario T, Palmer P, Karakousis CP (State Univ of New York, Buffalo; VA Med Ctr, Buffalo, NY)

Clin Orthop 423:191-195, 2004 13–5

Introduction.—In the anterior approach to forequarter amputation, a segment of clavicle is removed and early dissection and division of the subclavian vessels are done. In the posterior approach after division of the trapezius and muscles attached to the vertebral border of the scapula, the trunks of the brachial plexus and the subclavian vessels are serially ligated and divided, while the pectoral muscles are intact. In both approaches, the dissection around the subclavian vessels can be slow and tedious to avoid bleeding, which could be difficult to control because the vessels have not been cleared circumferentially for application of a vascular clamp. Our technique combines an anterior and a posterior approach, which rapidly divides all the relevant muscles and clavicle, and leaves at the end the division of the nerves and subclavian vessels as the extremity is gently supported to avoid undue traction on the vessels. The trunks of the brachial plexus are divided posteriorly and the subclavian vessels at the thoracic inlet, allowing a greater proximal margin than that achieved by the anterior or posterior approach. When extra skin has to be removed from the axilla because of tumor involvement, a fasciocutaneous deltoid flap may provide coverage of the defect.

▶ The authors provide a technical description of a modification for patients undergoing forequarter amputation to facilitate the resection and, particularly, the ease of control of the neurovascular structures. This provides a simpler technique than those described previously.

C. P. Beauchamp, MD

Imaging of Vascularized Fibula Autograft Placed Inside a Massive Allograft in Reconstruction of Lower Limb Bone Tumors

Manfrini M, Vanel D, De Paolis M, et al (Istituto Ortopedico Rizzoli, Bologna, Italy; Centro Traumatologico Ortopedico, Firenze, Italy)
AJR 182:963-970, 2004 13–6

Objective.—Bone allografts and vascularized fibula autografts were combined (the fibula inside the massive allograft) for skeletal reconstruction in a homogeneous group of patients. To verify the biologic behavior of the grafts, we followed the series using conventional radiography and CT analysis.

Materials and Methods.—Twenty-four patients with bone tumors had intercalary segments of tibia or femur reconstructed and were followed up for 36-120 months. Sequential radiographs and CT scans were analyzed.

Results.—Three types of behavior were observed. In 13 patients, the allograft maintained its architecture without fracture, although a regular enlargement of the inlaid fibula led to progressive integration with the allograft. A dense line on allograft endosteum was the first sign of bone bridges heralding fusion of the two grafts (Fig 4). In eight patients, fracture or nonunion of the allograft occurred, and the autograft reacted with rapid appearance of dense hypertrophy that again induced bridges to the allograft. In three patients, no changes in autograft size and density were followed by fracture with no callus formation. This behavior was interpreted as unsuccessful vascularization of the autograft.

Conclusion.—Sequential radiography and CT analysis enabled us to understand the changes in a combined graft offering an original way to revascularize bone allografts.

► The use of a vascularized fibula in conjunction with an allograft has been pioneered by the group in Bologna. The authors have extensive experience with this technique and have shared with us their radiographic methodology for evaluating graft healing and incorporation. The results of this method of reconstruction are quite striking, and this certainly is a very useful technique in the management of patients with musculoskeletal defects.

C. P. Beauchamp, MD

FIGURE 4.—12-year-old boy with intercalary reconstruction of proximal tibia because of osteosarcoma. *Dotted line* on radiographs corresponds to level of CT images (see Fig 4 E-H, page 969 in original article). A, Postoperative anteroposterior radiograph shows fibula autograft (*solid arrow*) and massive allograft (*dotted arrow*). B, Anteroposterior radiograph at 1 year shows patient wearing partial weight-bearing brace. Decrease in cortex density of fibula and complete fusion of osteotomies (*arrows*) are evident. C, Anteroposterior radiograph at 3 years in patient who had been walking for 18 months with no support shows further remodeling of implant. Transverse fusion of transplanted fibula to allograft is noted. D, Anteroposterior radiograph at 6 years shows displaced fracture (*arrow*) (healed in cast) of distal portion of implant. (Courtesy of Manfrini M, Vanel D, De Paolis M, et al: Imaging of vascularized fibula autograft placed inside a massive allograft in reconstruction of lower limb bone tumors. *AJR* 182:963-970, 2004. Reprinted with permission from the *American Journal of Roentgenology*.)

FIGURE 4

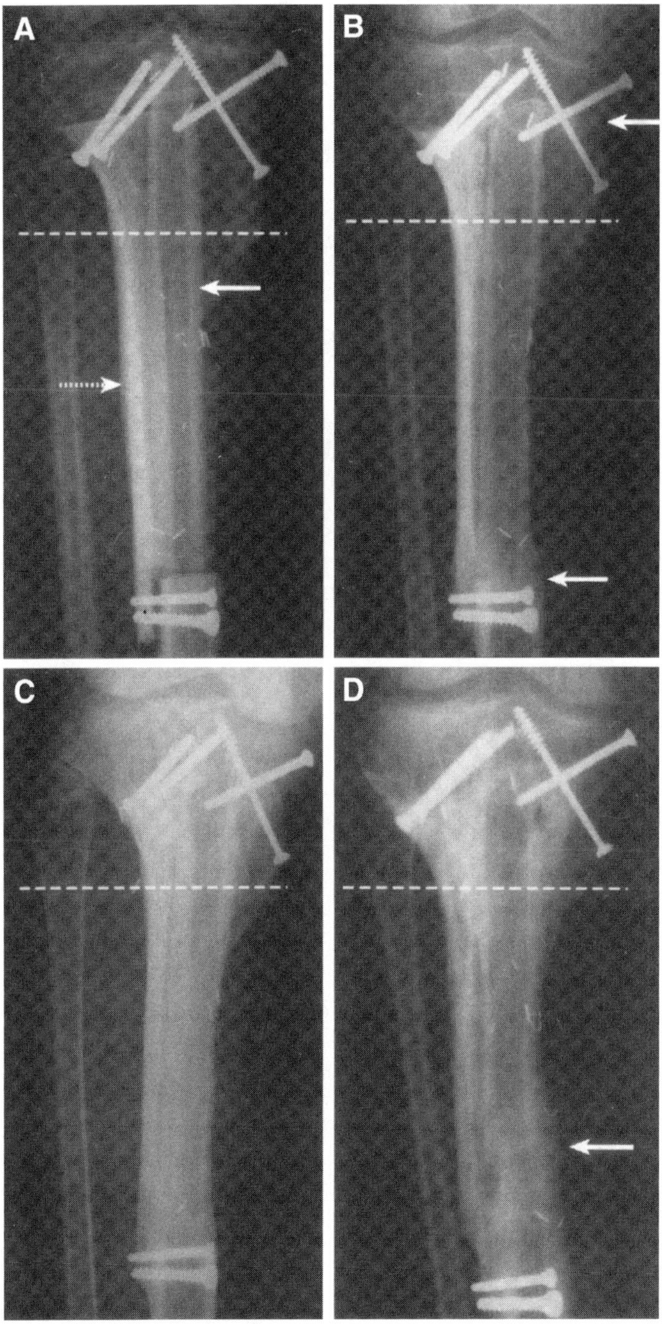

Segmental Femur Reconstruction Using an Intercalary Allograft With an Intramedullary Vascularized Fibula Bone Flap

Chang DW, Weber KL (MD Anderson Cancer Ctr, Houston)

J Reconstr Microsurg 20:195-199, 2004 13–7

Introduction.—The use of intercalary allografts has been an important innovation for use in limb-salvage surgery. However, the principal disadvantage of intercalary allografts is a high incidence of nonunion, fracture, and infection. With a recent trend toward higher doses of chemotherapy, an increased incidence of nonunion and healing problems can be anticipated with the use of allografts.

In this article, the authors report two cases in which a vascularized fibula bone flap was used with an intercalary allograft, utilising an intramedullary approach, for immediate femur reconstruction following sarcoma resection. The rationale for this approach is to combine the mechanical strength of an allograft with the biologic activity of a vascularized bone flap. The allograft provides bone stock and early stability, while the addition of the vascularized bone flap substantially facilitates the host-allograft union.

▶ The use of an allograft with a vascularized autograft has been recommended to try to reduce some of the complications associated with allograft-only reconstructions, namely, nonunion graft fracture, etc. The authors describe a novel technical modification to the combination of an allograft and a vascularized fibula. This being an alternative to a simple onlay vascularized graft.

C. P. Beauchamp, MD

Treatment of Advanced Metastatic Lesions of the Acetabulum Using the Saddle Prosthesis

Benevenia J, Cyran FP, Biermann JS, et al (Univ of Medicine and Dentistry of New Jersey, Newark; Northeastern Ohio College of Medicine, Akron; Univ of Michigan, Ann Arbor)

Clin Orthop 426:23-31, 2004 13–8

Introduction.—Current methods of treating advanced patients with metastatic periacetabular disease are complex and result in high complication rates. The purpose of this study was to show whether the implantation of the saddle prosthesis would serve as an additional tool to help treat metastatic disease in these patients. From 1991 to 2003, 20 patients with advanced metastatic periacetabular lesions (Harrington Class III) were treated using the saddle prosthesis. Goals of surgery were a decrease in pain, functional restoration, and ambulation. The mean age was 61 years. Average length of followup was 20 months. Postoperatively, ambulation was achieved in 16 of 20 patients. There were four postoperative complications (20%) in three patients. Surgical goals were met in 18 of 20 patients. The MSTS-ISOLS emotional score was 2.9 of 5. The average total MSTS-ISOLS score was 16.6 of

30 (55%). Using the Allan scoring system consisting of analgesia, independence and ambulation, and mobility, all scores had significant improvements postoperatively. Careful surgical indications and technique should result in a stable, functional reconstruction allowing patients the ability to ambulate outside the house with a cane. Patients can expect to be emotionally satisfied with the procedure while using nonnarcotic analgesia and can expect an improved quality of life despite bone metastasis.

▶ The management of periacetabular lesions secondary to metastatic disease can be challenging. Patients with massive bone loss are often treated with a resection arthroplasty. The authors have shown that many of these patients could be treated with a saddle prosthesis which would provide potentially a better function. Functional scores provided in the paper are encouraging but need to be compared with a similar group who have been treated with a resection arthroplasty before further recommendations can be made using this very expensive prosthesis.

C. P. Beauchamp, MD

Segmental Amputation for Recurrent Malignant Bone Tumors of the Distal Femur

Chen C-Y, Chien S-H, Lin G-T, et al (Yuan's Gen Hosp, Taiwan; Kaohsiung Med Univ, Taiwan)

Clin Orthop 426:239-243, 2004 13–9

Introduction.—We describe an alternative method for lengthening a short femoral stump after wide amputation of a malignant bone tumor of the distal femur in two patients. The method consists of two procedures during the operation. The first procedure is amputation of the affected cylindrical segment of the involved limb. The second procedure is elongation of the amputation stump using the tumor-free segment of the ipsilateral lower leg as a free composite osseous myocutaneous graft. Both patients had good function and were satisfied with the results with no complications or tumor recurrence 4 years postoperatively. We think the segmental amputation is a good procedure that results in a longer functional stump in patients who have above-knee amputation.

▶ The authors have described a variant of rotationplasty, which truly is an amputation-sparing procedure. While a rotationplasty has been shown to provide superior functional results, this may be an alternative to consider in patients who are very uncomfortable with the cosmetic appearance of a rotationplasty. This is also a useful procedure to consider in patients having a very high amputation. It is important to evaluate the remaining portion of the limb to determine if any of it can be salvaged to improve the functional results of an amputation.

C. P. Beauchamp, MD

Use of a Smooth Press-Fit Stem Preserves Physeal Growth After Tumor Resection

Neel MD, Heck R, Britton L, et al (St Jude Children's Research Hosp, Memphis, Tenn)
Clin Orthop 426:125-128, 2004 13–10

Introduction.—We conducted this study to determine whether the small-diameter, press-fit stem of a novel, noninvasive expandable endoprosthetic device implanted in the limbs of 6 pediatric patients with Stage IIB osteosarcoma affected the growth of the physis through which the stem was inserted. Local control of the tumor necessitated resection of the involved growth plate, and implantation of the device required penetration of the adjacent uninvolved bone, through the growth plate, by the stem of the device. We measured longitudinal growth and the rate of growth of the adjacent uninvolved bone in the salvaged limb and of the equivalent bone in the unoperated contralateral limb. In all cases but one (in which the patient's growth in the contralateral limb appeared complete), longitudinal growth continued in the limb into which the device was implanted: the adjacent uninvolved bone in the salvaged limb grew by an average of 2.4 cm, and the equivalent bone in the unoperated contralateral limb grew by an average of 2.3 cm. We conclude that implantation of a smooth, press-fit stem through the central portion of the uninvolved adjacent physis does not result in growth retardation or arrest.

▶ Preservation of growth potential in immature patients undergoing resections and reconstructions for neoplasms is critical for the success of growing implants. Around the knee, the standard form of reconstruction involves a component that passes through the physis and into the metaphysis of the retained bone. The use of a smooth rod inserted relatively atraumatically through the physis has been shown by the authors to not affect growth. The downside of using a smooth portion of the component is that this can be a source of discomfort, as fixation into the residual tibia or femur is not entirely rigid and the patients develop micromotion at the bone prosthesis interface.

C. P. Beauchamp, MD

Intercalary Femur and Tibia Segmental Allografts Provide an Acceptable Alternative in Reconstructing Tumor Resections

Muscolo DL, Ayerza MA, Aponte-Tinao L, et al (Italian Hosp of Buenos Aires, Argentina)
Clin Orthop 426:97-102, 2004 13–11

Introduction.—Intercalary femur and tibia segmental allografts were implanted in 59 consecutive patients after segmental resection—52 for malignant and seven for benign aggressive bone tumors. The patients were followed up for an average of 5 years. Allograft survival was determined with the Kaplan-Meier method. Infection, fracture, and nonunion rates were determined. The overall 5-year survivorship for the 59 intercalary allografts was 79%, and we found no significant differences between allograft survival in patients receiving or not receiving adjuvant chemotherapy. Infection and fracture rates were 5% and 7% respectively. From 118 host-donor junctions, 11 did not initially heal (9%). The nonunion rate (10 of 69 osteotomies) for diaphyseal junctions was higher than the rate (one of 49 osteotomies) for metaphyseal junctions. Although some patients required reoperations because of allograft complications, it seems that the use of intercalary allograft clearly has a place in the reconstruction of a segmental defect created by the resection of a tumor in the diaphyseal and/or metaphyseal portion of the femur or tibia.

► Without question, patients reconstructed with allografts for musculoskeletal defects do very well in the absence of complications. Intercalary allograft reconstructions have the advantage of not having any of the complications associated with joint reconstruction; namely, degenerative osteoarthritis, ligament instability, etc. The risks of infection and nonunion and graft dissolution still remain, however, and contribute to the failures of these implants. This group has a very long history of experience with allograft reconstructions, and their results demonstrate again the excellent results obtained with intercalary allograft reconstructions. Typically, an increased risk of complications is seen in patients receiving chemotherapy. This was not noted in this large series.

C. P. Beauchamp, MD

Equal Quality of Life After Limb-sparing or Ablative Surgery for Lower Extremity Sarcomas

Zahlten-Hinguranage A, Bernd L, Ewerbeck V, et al (Univ of Heidelberg, Germany)

Br J Cancer 91:1012-1014, 2004 13–12

Introduction.—Limb-salvage surgery (LSS), compared to amputation, is often correlated with better quality of life (QOL) since it is less disfiguring and has a better potential functional outcome. Little data is available concerning patients with orthopedic cancer. Previous QOL data in orthopedic oncology was assessed by analyzing QOL separately for functional psychological, social, and health factors. The QOL and function of 124 patients with lower extremity sarcoma who underwent either amputation or LSS were evaluated to determine the potential differences in subjective treatment outcome.

Methods.—The EORTC QLQ-C30 core instrument in its standard German version 3.0 was used to assess disease-specific QOL. Functional assessment was performed using the Musculoskeletal Tumor Society Score. The Life Satisfaction Questionnaire was used to evaluate QOL. All psychometric tests were performed by an experienced observer not otherwise involved in patients' medical treatment. The cancer registry was used to obtain demographic, clinical, and oncological data. The treating physician assessed functional outcome within the context of follow-up.

Results.—Results were similar in measures of disease-specific and global QOL after LSS or amputation (LSS mean score, 67.9; amputation, 68.2). Overall functional scores were slightly higher among patients treated with ablative surgery (74.0 vs 77.7). The symptoms index was similar (12.3 vs 13.4). Global QOL evaluation showed a mean score of 268.8 for patients who underwent amputation versus 263.8 for those who underwent LSS (this corresponds to a response of "rather satisfied"). Descriptive data showed a better physical performance status after LSS versus amputation. Discriminant analysis revealed physical function regarding unrestricted level of activity, independent of assistive devices, unlimited walking ability, normal gait pattern, emotional acceptance, followed by favorable economic conditions and recreational activity were the most discriminating items ($P < 0.05$) in the LSS group (85% accurate classification rate). The abilities of physical and cognitive functioning and enjoyment of good food, maintaining social and sexual relationships, and low level of pain were linked with a positive QOL in patients with amputation (73% accurate classification rate).

Conclusion.—No benefit in overall measures of QOL was observed for LSS versus amputation. At an average of 5 years after the procedure, patients who underwent LSS or amputation reported an acceptable functional outcome and similar QOL. Compared with patients who underwent LSS, in those who underwent amputation QOL was strongly linked in terms of high physical status with social acceptability and good self-reported health.

► This is an important study investigating the QOL and function of patients with lower extremity sarcoma treated either with amputation or limb salvage surgery. There was no question that the functional outcome was improved following limb salvage surgery, however, the amputee group had a high level of QOL. This demonstrates the resiliency of the patient in adapting to an amputation. It again emphasizes the ability of the patient to adapt to an amputation. The difficulty is that a limb sparing surgical procedure is highly attractive to patients who are facing an amputation.

C. P. Beauchamp, MD

Complications Following Operative Treatment of Primary Malignant Bone Tumours in the Pelvis

Zeifang F, Buchner M, Zahlten-Hinguranage A, et al (Orthopaedic Univ Hosp of Heidelberg, Germany)

Eur J Surg Oncol 30:893-899, 2004 13–13

Aim.—To report the complication rates of limb-salvage reconstruction in the pelvis. Detailed analyses about the type, treatment and outcome of postoperative complications, various reconstruction options are presented.

Methods.—Factors that might influence the occurrence of complications were evaluated of 50 consecutive surgically treated patients.

Results.—The mean follow-up was 57 months. Limb-salvage procedures were used in 42/50 patients, amputations in 8/50 patients. After limb-salvage procedures complications occurred in 32/42 patients, after hemipelvectomy in 6/8 patients. The 1 and 5-year overall survival rate was 92 and 68%, respectively.

Conclusion.—There is a high complication rate in reconstructive techniques using hemipelvic autografts and/or allografts. These procedures are appropriate only in well selected patients. The complication rates following endoprosthetic reconstruction are comparably low.

▶ The authors again emphasize the extremely high complication rate in patients who undergo limb salvage surgery for pelvic neoplasia. They emphasize the importance of patient selection in determination of what types of reconstruction are appropriate for a given patient.

C. P. Beauchamp, MD

Contained Femoral Defects: Biomechanical Analysis of Pin Augmentation in Cement

Murray PJ, Damron TA, Green JK, et al (State Univ of New York, Syracuse; George Washington Univ, DC; Univ of Washington, Seattle)

Clin Orthop 420:251-256, 2004 13–14

Introduction.—Although in the proximal tibia the need for pin augmentation of cemented giant cell tumor defects depends on whether the defect is contained, there is controversy regarding the role for pins in the distal femur. The current study investigated whether Steinmann pin augmentation offers biomechanical advantages in cement reconstruction of contained defects of the lateral femoral condyle. Twelve pairs of human femurs were used. They were tested either with the bone intact, with a standardized contained defect in the lateral condyle, with a defect repaired with cement alone, and with a defect repaired with pins in the cement. Intact specimens had significantly higher load to failure than specimens with a defect. In the repaired specimens there were no significant differences in stiffness, peak load to failure, and energy to failure between the specimens repaired with just cement or augmented with pins. This study did not show any significant biomechanical advantage of this configuration of Steinmann pin reinforcement in cement for contained defects of the lateral femoral condyle.

▶ Cementation for the management of giant cell tumor has provided a very useful method in the reconstruction of large skeletal defects created during curettage of benign giant cell tumors. Various reconstructive adjuvants to this method of reconstruction have been recommended, including the use of pin augmentation. This biomechanical study failed to show any significant biomechanical advantage to the addition of Steinmann pins. Rather, these provide a significant barrier to removal of the cement if the patient has a local recurrence or if for any reason the cement is needed to be removed in the future.

C. P. Beauchamp, MD

Complications and Results of Arthroplasty for Salvage of Failed Treatment of Malignant Pathologic Fractures of the Hip

Jacofsky DJ, Haidukewych GJ, Zhang H, et al (Mayo Clinic, Rochester, Minn)

Clin Orthop 427:52-56, 2004 13–15

Introduction.—The purpose of this study was to evaluate the results and complications of hip arthroplasty done for salvage of failed treatment of pathologic proximal femoral fractures secondary to malignancy. Between 1980 and 2000, 42 patients with a mean age of 63 years were treated with hip arthroplasty to salvage failed treatment of a pathologic proximal femoral fracture. Total hip arthroplasty was done in 16 patients (3 uncemented, 2 hybrid, 11 cemented), and bipolar hemiarthroplasty in 26 (2 uncemented, 24 cemented). A modular, proximal femoral replacement construct was used in 15 patients. Patients were followed a mean of 5.8 years (range, 15 days-20 years). Four hips required reoperation, all for deep infection. Harris Hip score improved from an average of 42 points (range, 17-76 points) preoperatively to an average of 83 points (range, 52-100 points) postoperatively. Most recent radiographs showed femoral component loosening in only one patient. Implant survivorship free of revision for any reason at 5 years was 90% (range, 65-96%) and free of revision for aseptic failure or radiographic failure was 97% (range, 64-99%). Hip arthroplasty is an effective treatment for salvage of failed treatment of pathologic proximal femoral fractures. Modular proximal femoral replacements were often required. The most concerning complication was deep prosthetic infection, which occurred in nearly 10% of this patient population, and in 21% of patients with prior irradiation.

▶ The prime objective of the management of patients with proximal femoral fractures secondary to metastatic disease is to obtain an immediate sound reconstruction that will allow the patient to immediately ambulate and fully weight bear. Unfortunately, in a significant number of individuals, this surgical objective is not achieved and the patients linger with protected weight bearing and ultimate failure of the reconstruction consuming very valuable time in the limited amount of remaining life expectancy of these patients. It is extremely important to carefully evaluate patients with proximal femoral fractures to ensure that they do not undergo a surgical procedure that is doomed to failure. Nonetheless, when this does occur, the subsequent conversion to a joint arthroplasty is an effective method of treatment of failed fixation of proximal femoral fractures. A wide array of different components is necessary to deal with all the potential problems of bone deficiencies in these individuals.

C. P. Beauchamp, MD

Inferior Vena Cava Filters Prevent Pulmonary Emboli in Patients With Metastatic Pathologic Fractures of the Lower Extremity

Benevenia J, Bibbo C, Patel DV, et al (Univ of Medicine and Dentistry of New Jersey, Newark; Marshfield Clinic, Wis; New Jersey Health Care System, East Orange; et al)

Clin Orthop 426:87-91, 2004 13–16

Introduction.—The records of 47 consecutive patients with metastatic pathologic fractures of the lower extremity were analyzed with respect to thromboembolic complications. All patients were unable to receive pharmacologic deep venous thrombosis prophylaxis, and were stratified into two groups, based on use of an inferior vena cava filter. Group I (n = 24) consisted of patients who had an inferior vena cava filter plus mechanical deep venous thrombosis prophylaxis (compression stockings and sequential compression boots); Group II (n = 23) consisted of a group of patients receiving only mechanical deep venous thrombosis prophylaxis. All patients had routine lower extremity venous duplex imaging preoperatively, postoperatively, and before hospital discharge. At final followup, patients were examined for deep venous thrombosis and reviewed for thromboembolic events. At a mean followup of 11.5 months, Group I had two detectable deep venous thromboses and no pulmonary emboli; Group II had one detectable deep venous thrombosis and five pulmonary embolisms. In Group II, 40% (two of five) of pulmonary embolisms were fatal, yielding an 8.7% (two of 23) group mortality rate. Overall, the entire group had an approximately 17% deep venous thrombosis rate. Only 6.4% (three of 47) of deep venous thromboses were detectable by standard duplex imaging. The majority of deep venous thromboses (five of eight, 62.5%) were nondetectable by duplex imaging. Overall, a 4.3% (two of 47) death rate was attributable to pulmonary embolism. In contrast, an 8.6% (four of 47) mortality rate occurred in Group II alone. All pulmonary embolisms occurred in patients who did not receive an inferior vena cava filter. The majority of venous thromboses (62.5%) were not detectable on duplex scanning, therefore were thought to arise from the pelvic venous system. Complications related to inferior vena cava filter insertion were minimal. For patients with metastatic pathologic fractures of the lower extremities who are unable to receive pharmacologic deep venous thrombosis prophylaxis, the use of inferior vena cava filters, in conjunction with standard mechanical deep venous thrombosis prophylaxis, is a procedure that has a low risk and is useful adjunct to prevent fatal pulmonary embolisms.

► Patients with malignant neoplasms have an increased risk of thromboembolic disease. Patients who have undergone resection of musculoskeletal tumors or treatment for metastatic bone disease are at significant risk for complications associated with anticoagulation. The authors share with us their experience of using prophylactic inferior vena cava filters in patients who are at high risk for prophylactic anticoagulation. They have demonstrated a reduction in fatal pulmonary emboli in patients who received prophylactic vena cava filters and have justifiably advocated their use in patients who are at high risk for thromboembolic disease and who are not candidates for prophylactic anticoagulation.

C. P. Beauchamp, MD

Comparative Analysis of Risk Factors for Pathological Fracture With Femoral Metastases: Results Based On a Randomised Trial of Radiotherapy

Van der Linden YM, Dijkstra PDS, Kroon HM, et al (Leiden Univ, The Netherlands; St Radboud Univ, Nijmegen, The Netherlands)

J Bone Joint Surg Br 86-B:566-573, 2004 13–17

Introduction.—Several risk factors, based primarily upon retrospective surgical data, have been formulated to identify impending pathological fractures of the femur from low-risk metastases. A large series of patients participating in a randomized trial of radiotherapy were prospectively assessed to determine whether these factors were effective in predicting fractures.

Findings.—Between March 1996 and September 1998, 1157 patients with painful bone metastases from solid tumors were randomized to treatment with either a single fraction of 8 Gy or 6 fractions of 4 Gy. Fourteen fractures occurred during follow-up in 102 patients with 110 femoral lesions. There were no significant between-group differences in age, gender, Karnofsky Performance Scale, initial pain score, or primary tumor among patients who fractured and those who did not experience fractures. All fractures occurred at a median of 8.5 weeks (2-36 weeks) after baseline; 909% occurred within 6 months. There were no significant differences in survival among patients who did and did not experience fractures. The median patient survival was 38 weeks (95% confidence interval, 29-47 weeks). No prophylactic internal fixation was necessary for increased pain or to prevent a pathological fracture. Of 110 lesions identified on conventional radiographs, CT, MRI, and/or bone scintigrams, 10 were unmeasurable and were invisible on conventional radiographs; ultimately, 100 were measured and 110 were scored radiographically. Increased pain during the weeks preceding fracture did not occur in all 14 patients who fractured. The median Mirel's scoring for lesions with fractures was 11 (9.12) among patients with fracture versus 10 (7-12) for those without fracture ($P = .36$). Shifting the cut-off point did not enhance outcome. With the cut-off point between 9 and 10, 61 lesions without fracture scored as high-risk; the specificity rose to 36%. Yet, 3 fractures would have been missed, lowering sensitivity to 79%. Only axial cortical involvement above 30 mm ($P = .01$) and circumferential cortical involvement above 50% ($P = .03$) were predictive of fracture.

Discussion/Conclusion.—There is a need for the evaluation of relatively simple and objective risk factors for predicting an impending fracture. Most conventional risk factors overestimate the actual occurrence of pathological fractures of the femur. In this cohort, the only risk factor that met this criteria was the axial cortical involvement; it is a simple, objective tool that can be used to ascertain which treatment is appropriate.

▶ We have long struggled with the issue of the impending fracture. Attempts have been made to more precisely define who is at increased risk for fracture. The authors have evaluated a large group of patients with metastatic femoral disease trying to apply current methodology to predicting pathologic fracture. They were able to only note that axial cortical involvement and circumferential cortical involvement were predictors of fracture. This provides yet another useful tool in the decision making for recommendation of prophylactic internal fixation for pathologic fractures.

C. P. Beauchamp, MD

Bone and Soft Tissue Tumors

Clinical Relevance of Calcaneal Bone Cysts: A Study of 50 Cysts in 47 Patients

Pogoda P, Priemel M, Linhart W, et al (Hamburg Univ, Germany)

Clin Orthop 424:202-210, 2004 13–18

Introduction.—The clinical relevance and nature of calcaneal cysts is controversial. The risk of pathologic fracture is undefined and diagnostic criteria to differentiate between cysts in patients who can be treated nonoperatively and patients who require surgical intervention are not available. To address these questions, 50 calcaneal bone cysts in 47 patients were evaluated. The majority of cysts (40 of 50) were asymptomatic and were treated nonoperatively. Cysts reaching a critical size, defined as 100% intracalcaneal cross section in the coronary plane and at least 30% in the sagittal plane, are at risk for becoming symptomatic and at risk for fracture. Fracture is a significant complication and occurred in four of 47 patients, three of whom were treated by open reduction internal fixation and bone grafting. In addition, six patients with symptomatic critical size cysts without apparent fracture were treated by curettage and subsequent autogenous bone grafting or calcium-phosphate cement filling, and there were no recurrences. We report one of the largest series of cysts in the calcaneus. The results suggest that calcaneal cysts are clinically relevant because of the potential risk of fracture and that size is a significant factor in terms of the treatment of the cyst.

▶ This is a large group of patients with calcaneal bone cysts. Patients presenting with an asymptomatic calcaneal bone cyst present a difficult therapeutic challenge. The authors provide some guidance as to when the patient is at risk for fracture and when should surgical intervention be considered.

C. P. Beauchamp, MD

Multicentric Osteoid Osteoma

Zmurko MG, Mott MP, Lucas DR, et al (Wayne State Univ, Detroit; Karmanos Cancer Inst, Detroit)

Orthopedics 27:1294-1296, 2004 13–19

Introduction.—Osteoid osteoma is a benign primary bone tumor responsible for about 11% of benign tumors. Most are monofocal with a single nidus. Reported is an osteoid osteoma with a single nidus that progressed to a multicentric osteoid osteoma.

Case Report.—Man, 19, was seen with a 2-year history of right thigh and knee pain. He had no history of right thigh tumor and denied fever, chills, night sweats, weight loss, or other constitutional symptoms. His discomfort was most pronounced during the night and occasionally during the early hours of morning. Physical examination was normal and a presumptive diagnosis of osteoid osteoma was given. An MRI study performed 2 years previously showed a solitary lesion in the right medial mid-diaphyseal femur with a single nidus. Treatment with nonsteroidal anti-inflammatory (NSAID) medications was initiated with good initial relief of pain. Several months later, even in the presence of continued NSAID use, he experienced recurrence of the right thigh and knee pain. A second MRI revealed a second nidus located close to the initial lesion. Treatment with NSAIDs was continued and he was sent for further evaluation. The patient ambulated with a normal reciprocal gait pattern. Assessment of the right lower extremity demonstrated atrophy of the quadriceps musculature. The right and left mid-thigh circumferences were 40 cm and 44.5 cm, respectively. Radiographs of the right femur demonstrated increased sclerosis of the medial mid-diaphysis of the right femur with 2 distinct nidi (lesions were about 1 cm in diameter); the 2 nidi were also observed on CT and technetium-phosphate bone scan. Open biopsy was performed; location was verified via fluoroscopic assistance. The lesions were curetted and burred; removal was complete. There was no communication between the 2 lesions during surgery. Pathology showed osteoid osteoma and reactive bone. The patient was placed in a knee immobilizer postoperatively; weight bearing was increased to full weight bearing over 6 weeks. There were no recurrence or patient complaints at 1-year follow-up.

Conclusion.—Progression of a single nidus to multicentric nidus has not been reported previously. Periodic imaging of osteoid osteoma appears to be worthwhile if the lesion is being treated conservatively or does not respond to medical management.

► The authors provide an unusual report of multicentric osteoid osteoma. The radiographic images presented show clear evidence of a progression from a single to a double nidus. This patient underwent surgical procedure for removal of this and radiofrequency ablation today could deal with this nicely with low patient morbidity.

C. P. Beauchamp, MD

Osteoid Osteoma: Factors for Increased Risk of Unsuccessful Thermal Coagulation

Vanderschueren GM, Taminiau AHM, Obermann WR, et al (Leiden Univ, The Netherlands)

Radiology 233:757-762, 2004 13–20

Purpose.—To retrospectively identify risk factors that may impede a favorable clinical outcome after thermocoagulation for osteoid osteoma.

Materials and Methods.—Informed consent (permission for the procedure and permission to use patient data for analysis) was obtained from all patients who met study criteria, and institutional review board did not require approval. Analysis included age, sex, size and location of osteoid osteoma, presence of calcified nidus, number of needle positions used for coagulation, coagulation time, accuracy of needle position, learning curve of radiologist, and previous treatment in 95 consecutive patients with osteoid osteoma treated with thermocoagulation. With χ^2 analysis, Fisher exact test, or unpaired Student t test and logistic regression analysis, 23 unsuccessfully treated patients were compared with 72 successfully (pain-free) treated patients.

Results.—Parameters associated with decreased risk for treatment failure were advanced age (mean age, 24 years in treatment success group vs 20 years in treatment failure group) and increased number of needle positions during thermocoagulation. Estimated odds ratios were, respectively, 0.93 (95% confidence interval: 0.88, 0.99) and 0.10 (95% confidence interval: 0.02, 0.41). Patients with a lesion of 10 mm or larger seemed at risk for treatment failure (odds ratio = 2.68), but the 95% confidence interval of 0.84 to 8.52 included the 1.00 value. Needle position was inaccurate in nine of 23 patients with treatment failure; only one needle position was used in eight of these nine patients. Lesion location, calcification, sex, coagulation time, radiologist's learning curve, and previous treatment were not risk factors.

Conclusion.—Multiple needle positions reduce the risk of treatment failure in all patients and should especially, but not exclusively, be used in large (≥10-mm) lesions or lesions that are difficult to engage to reduce the risk for unsuccessful treatment.

► Percutaneous radio frequency oblation of osteoid osteomas has become the accepted, preferred method of management for patients with osteoid osteomas. Fortunately, we have significantly improved our ability to eradicate this benign disease but there still exists a number of patients who have persistent symptoms after radio frequency oblation. The authors share with us their experience of percutaneous radio frequency oblation and have outlined their recommendations to try to reduce the risk of persistent symptoms after treatment. In particular, multiple oblations and needle positions are noted to reduce the risk of treatment failure especially in patients with relatively large lesions.

C. P. Beauchamp, MD

Soft Tissue Aneurysmal Bone Cyst

Wang XL, Gielen JL, Salgado R, et al (Univ of Antwerp, Edegem, Belgium)

Skeletal Radiol 33:477-480, 2004 13–21

Introduction.—A soft tissue aneurysmal bone cyst located in the right gluteus medius of a 21-year-old man is reported. On conventional radiography, the lesion demonstrated a spherically trabeculated mass with a calcific rim. On CT scan, it showed a well-organized peripheral calcification resembling a myositis ossificans. On MRI, it presented as a multilocular, cystic lesion with fluid-fluid levels. The lesion had no solid components except for intralesional septa. Although findings on imaging and histology were identical to those described in classical aneurysmal bone cyst, diagnosis was delayed because of lack of knowledge of this entity and its resemblance to the more familiar post-traumatic heterotopic ossification (myositis ossificans).

► The authors describe an unusual diagnosis of a soft tissue aneurysmal bone cyst. This lesion initially had the radiographic appearance highly suggestive of myositis ossificans, but had the typical MRI appearance of an aneurysmal bone cyst. Although it may have reassuring radiographic features suggestive of an aneurysmal bone cyst, the approach should still be an incisional biopsy frozen section to exclude an unusual soft tissue osteosarcoma.

C. P. Beauchamp, MD

Giant Cell Tumor of the Pelvis and Sacrum: 17 Cases and Analysis of the Literature

Leggon RE, Zlotecki R, Reith J, et al (Marshfield Clinic, Wis; Univ of Florida, Gainesville)

Clin Orthop 423:196-207, 2004 13–22

Introduction.—The optimal treatment of giant cell tumors of the pelvis and sacrum is controversial. Our current patient series was combined with cases identified in a review of the literature published in the past 50 years, yielding a combined group of 239 lesions for study. Recurrence rates were 49% for patients who had radiation therapy alone, 47% for patients who had surgery with intralesional margins, 46% for patients who had surgery with intralesional margins and radiation therapy, and 0% for patients who had surgery with wide margins. Six percent of patients had benign lung metastases develop, 2% of patients had secondary malignancies, 2% of patients died in the perioperative period, and less than 1% of patients had multicentricity. Radiation-induced sarcoma developed in 11% of patients who received radiation for primary or recurrent lesions. Larger doses of radiation therapy did not decrease the rate of local recurrence. Recurrence after surgery and radiation was not lower than after either treatment alone. Local recurrence was more likely in the patients with sacral tumors (48%) than in the patients with pelvic tumors (34%). Disease status was worse in the patients with sacral lesions (23% died of disease) than in the patients with pelvic lesions (6% died of disease).

▶ Giant cell tumor of the pelvis and sacrum presents a challenge to the oncologic surgeon. This tumor has a significant propensity for local recurrence largely due to the fact that intralesional treatment results in an incomplete resection. The authors have noted that the addition of radiation therapy did not improve the local recurrence rate. Whenever possible, wide excision in this location is the preferred treatment of choice; however, this is seldom possible to do without significant morbidity. The authors conclude that radiation therapy is best reserved for large sacral lesions, and the combination of surgery with intralesional margins and radiation therapy is not supported by this review.

C. P. Beauchamp, MD

Spontaneous Malignant Transformation of Conventional Giant Cell Tumor

Grote HJ, Braun M, Kalinski T, et al (Heinrich Heine Univ, Düsseldorf, Germany; Univ of Witten/Herdecke, Wetter (Ruhr), Germany; Otto von Guericke Univ, Magdeburg, Germany; et al)

Skeletal Radiol 33:169-175, 2004 13–23

Introduction.—Spontaneous malignant transformation of conventional giant cell tumor (GCT) of bone is exceedingly rare. We report on a case of GCT of the iliac crest in a 35-year-old woman with malignant change into a high-grade osteosarcoma 10 years after the first appearance of GCT on a radiograph. Since the patient refused therapy for personal reasons the tumor remained untreated until sarcomatous transformation occurred. Image cytometry showed DNA aneuploidy and a suspiciously high 2c deviation index (2cDI) in the primary bone lesion. A thorough review of the world literature revealed only seven fully documented cases of secondary malignant GCT which matched the definition of a "sarcomatous growth that occurs at the site of a previously documented benign giant cell tumor" and not treated by radiotherapy. These cases as well as the current one suggest that a spontaneous secondary malignant GCT presents as a frankly sarcomatous tumor in the form of an osteosarcoma or malignant fibrous histiocytoma. It usually appears at sites of typical GCTs—often without any recurrent intermediate state—and is diagnosed 3 or more years after the primary bone lesion. The prognosis is poor.

► This case report describes a patient with an untreated GCT biopsy proven to be benign that subsequently went on to develop spontaneous malignant transformation. If one accepts the concept that patients with secondary malignant GCTs have a persistent GCT that becomes malignant, I believe this tumor still falls into the category of a secondary GCT. The only difference is that this patient did not have any of the tumor excised before malignant transformation. It provides an interesting view to the biology of this neoplastic process.

C. P. Beauchamp, MD

Bisphosphonates May Reduce Recurrence in Giant Cell Tumor by Inducing Apoptosis

Chang SS, Suratwala SJ, Jung KM, et al (Columbia Univ, New York)

Clin Orthop 426:103-109, 2004 13–24

Introduction.—Giant cell tumor of bone is an aggressive tumor characterized by extensive bone destruction and high recurrence rates. This tumor consists of stromal cells and hematopoietic cells that interact in an autocrine manner to produce tumoral osteoclastogenesis and bone resorption. This autocrine regulation may be disrupted by novel therapeutic agents. Nonspecific local adjuvant therapies such as phenol or liquid nitrogen have been used in the treatment of giant cell tumor, but specific adjuvant therapies have not been described. The bisphosphonates pamidronate and zoledronate can induce apoptosis in giant cell tumor culture in a dose-dependent manner. We established giant cell tumor cultures from patients with extensive destruction of bone. One of the four cultures formed osteoclastlike giant cells in vitro after more than six passages without exogenous receptor activator of NF-kappaB ligand or macrophage colony stimulating factor. Annexin V staining, presence of active cleaved form of caspase-3, and disappearance of poly (ADP-ribose) polymerase on Western blotting indicated activation of apoptosis by bisphosphonates in giant cell tumor. These results indicate that topical or systemic use of pamidronate or zoledronate can be a novel adjuvant therapy for giant cell tumor by targeting osteoclastlike giant cells, mononuclear giant cell precursor cells, and the autocrine loop of tumor osteoclastogenesis.

► Giant cell tumor of bone continues to have a high risk of local recurrence despite improvements in the physical treatment of this tumor. The use of bisphosphonates for this neoplasm has been on the horizon for some time, and the authors have provided some support for the topical or systemic use of pamidronate or zoledronate as an adjuvant agent. I have on an empirical basis been using bisphosphonates in patients who either are at high risk for local recurrence or have sustained a local recurrence in giant cell tumor.

C. P. Beauchamp, MD

Giant-Cell Tumor of the Distal Forearm

Harness NG, Mankin HJ (Harvard Med School, Boston)

J Hand Surg [Am] 29A:188-193, 2004 13–25

Purpose.—Many authorities express concern that giant-cell tumors of the distal forearm are more frequently recurrent and difficult to treat chiefly because of the proximity to the carpus and the resultant diminished range of motion in the hand and forearm. We have studied the results from our institution for 49 patients with giant-cell tumors of the distal forearm treated from 2 to 28 years (mean, 14 ± 7 years) and compared the results for different methods of treatment.

Methods.—Through the computer database 49 patients with giant-cell tumors of the distal forearm (46 of the radius, 3 of the ulna) were identified. By using material from patient visits, chart review, and when necessary telephone interviews it was possible to gather demographic and outcome data for the 49 patients. For the radial lesions, 15 of the patients had a marginal resection of the distal radius along with the periosteum and ligamentous structures and implantation of cadaveric allografts. Twenty-six patients had intralesional curettage and insertion of polymethylmethacrylate (PMMA) and 5 had curettage and autograft insertion. The 3 patients with ulnar lesions were treated with Darrach resections.

Results.—There were no deaths, infections, metastases, or amputations. In addition to the 49 original surgeries, the patients required 41 additional surgical procedures, 17 of which were for recurrent disease. The greatest numbers of recurrences were in the patients who underwent curettage with autograft or PMMA implantation. Only 2 recurrences were in patients who had a marginal resection and implantation of cadaveric allografts. The overall results for the patients showed that many had mostly minor complaints referable to function or pain and that only 18 of the 49 patients were asymptomatic.

Conclusions.—Although the patients with distal forearm giant-cell tumors have had a difficult course in terms of local recurrence and subsequent surgeries required for treatment failures, the ultimate outcomes for both allograft transplantation and curettage and insertion of PMMA are satisfactory. The patients with complete distal radial allografts had a better record for prevention of recurrence than the patients treated with curettage and PMMA insertion but the percentages of currently asymptomatic patients are approximately the same for both series (40% [6/15], 35% [9/26]). These data support the concept that marginal resection and complete distal radial allograft implantation should be used for patients with tumors that have destroyed much of the bone and have extensive soft tissue components and that curettage and PMMA insertion should be reserved for patients where the structural alteration of the bone is minimal.

▶ Giant-cell tumors of the distal radius have a more ominous reputation than at other sites with a reported increased risk of local recurrence and metastatic disease. The authors' study of a large group of patients somewhat dispels that myth, especially in the fact that none of the patients had metastatic disease develop. They have confirmed that those treated with more aggressive surgery, that is a resection as opposed to an intralesional curettage, had a better risk of local recurrence. The group as a whole, though, did confirm that many of these patients will require more than 1 surgical intervention.

C. P. Beauchamp, MD

Severity of Disease and Risk of Malignant Change in Hereditary Multiple Exostoses: A Genotype-Phenotype Study

Porter DE, Lonie L, Fraser M, et al (Edinburgh Univ, England; Henry Wellcome Building for Genomic Medicine, Oxford, England; Univ of Oxford, England)
J Bone Joint Surg Br 86-B:1041-1045, 2004 13–26

Introduction.—We performed a prospective genotype-phenotype study using molecular screening and clinical assessment to compare the severity of disease and the risk of sarcoma in 172 individuals (78 families) with hereditary multiple exostoses. We calculated the severity of disease including stature, number of exostoses, number of surgical procedures that were necessary, deformity and functional parameters and used molecular techniques to identify the genetic mutations in affected individuals. Each arm of the genotype-phenotype study was blind to the outcome of the other. Mutations *EXT1* and *EXT2* were almost equally common, and were identified in 83% of individuals. Non-parametric statistical tests were used.

There was a wide variation in the severity of disease. Children under ten years of age had fewer exostoses, consistent with the known age-related penetrance of this condition. The severity of the disease did not differ significantly with gender and was very variable within any given family. The sites of mutation affected the severity of disease with patients with *EXT1* mutations having a significantly worse condition than those with *EXT2* mutations in three of five parameters of severity (stature, deformity and functional parameters). A single sarcoma developed in an *EXT2* mutation carrier, compared with seven in *EXT1* mutation carriers. There was no evidence that sarcomas arose more commonly in families in whom the disease was more severe.

The sarcoma risk in *EXT1* carriers is similar to the risk of breast cancer in an older population subjected to breast-screening, suggesting that a role for regular screening in patients with hereditary multiple exostoses is justifiable.

► The issue of screening and follow-up with patients with multiple hereditary exostoses is controversial. This is primarily because there is such a wide variation of severity of the disease. The authors have shown that patients with *EXT1* mutations had an increased risk of sarcoma development. This suggests the patients with *EXT1* mutations should be considered for regular screening. At the very least, patients with multiple hereditary exostoses need to be well educated in their disease and the patients need to be aware of the signs and symptoms of malignant degeneration.

C. P. Beauchamp, MD

Scapular Chondrosarcomas Have High Rates of Local Recurrence and Metastasis

Schneiderbauer MM, Blanchard C, Gullerud R, et al (Mayo Clinic College of Medicine, Rochester, Minn)

Clin Orthop 426:232-238, 2004 13–27

Introduction.—This is the first report of a large series of patients with scapular chondrosarcomas. The grade distributions, locations of the tumors in the scapula, surgical techniques, status of margins, chondrosarcoma subtypes, Enneking stages, adjuvant therapies, local recurrence rates, metastasis rates, and survival prognoses of patients with scapular chondrosarcoma were evaluated. Forty-seven patients treated between 1921 and 1999 were analyzed retrospectively. Grade 3 disease was significantly associated with a poorer survival prognosis when compared with Grades 1 or 2 disease. Patients with tumors smaller than 5 cm were treated mainly with partial scapulectomy, and patients with tumors larger than 5 cm often were treated with total scapulectomy. The survival prognoses of patients with intralesional resections at initial surgery showed a tendency toward poorer survival when compared with patients with wide resections at initial surgery. Metastasis and local recurrence (21.3% and 40.4%) were higher in scapular chondrosarcomas than rates reported for patients with general chondrosarcomas, and local recurrence or metastasis was associated with limited survival. The 5- and 15-year survival probabilities subsequent to diagnosis were 79% and 53%, respectively. The high rates of local recurrence and metastasis likely were caused by the difficult anatomic relationships encountered during scapular resections. This study shows the importance of wide margins which must be achieved to provide local disease control.

► This study reports the results of patients with scapular chondrosarcomas treated surgically. The authors report a rather alarmingly high risk of metastatic disease and local recurrence. They reemphasize the importance of obtaining a wide resection. The anatomic peculiarities of the scapula with the concomitant imaging difficulties make the risk in an intralesional procedure slightly higher in this location.

C. P. Beauchamp, MD

Radiographic Differentiation of Enchondroma From Low-Grade Chondrosarcoma in the Fibula

Kendell SD, Collins MS, Adkins MC, et al (Duke Univ, Durham, NC; Mayo Clinic, Rochester, Minn)

Skeletal Radiol 33:458-466, 2004 13–28

Introduction.—To evaluate demographic and radiographic features that may differentiate between enchondroma and low-grade chondrosarcoma of the fibula. The radiographs of ninety-three histologically-confirmed cartilaginous tumors of the fibula were retrospectively reviewed along with demographic information as to patient age and gender. Fifty-four enchondromas and thirty-nine low-grade chondrosarcomas were included in the study. Multiple previously-established radiographic features distinguishing enchondroma from chondrosarcoma were evaluated in each fibular tumor in a consensus manner by two experienced, board-certified and fellowship-trained musculoskeletal radiologists. Five radiographic features were shown to statistically favor chondrosarcoma over enchondroma in the fibula. These were soft-tissue mass ($p<0.0001$), periosteal reaction ($p=0.008$), cortical disruption in the juxta-articular fibula ($p=0.0133$), cortical thickening ($p=0.032$), and tumor size greater than 4 cm ($p=0.0046$). No statistically-significant demographic differences were found between patients with enchondroma and chondrosarcoma of the fibula (Table 2). When two or more of the identified features of malignancy are identified in the same patient, chondrosarcoma is 2.4 times more likely than in those patients exhibiting none of the features of malignancy. Soft-tissue mass, periosteal reaction, cortical disruption in the juxta-articular fibula, cortical thickening, and tumor size greater than 4 cm indicate chondrosarcoma over enchondroma of the fibula. Radiographs demonstrating more than one of the identified malignant features are more likely to be due to chondrosarcoma than radiographs

TABLE 2.—Statistically-Significant Versus Not-Statistically-Significant Features Favoring Chondrosarcoma Over Enchondroma of the Fibula (*P*-Values Less Than 0.05 are Considered Significant)

Statistically-Significant Features	Not-Statistically-Significant Features
Lesion size	Patient age
Cortical disruption	Patient gender
	Lesion location (epiphysis, metaphysis,
Periosteal reaction	diaphysis)
	Fraction of cortical scalloping in
Soft-tissue mass	diaphysis
Cortical thickening	Margin definition
	Fraction of mineralized matrix
	Appearance of mineralized matrix
	Pathologic fracture
	Expansile lesion

(Courtesy of Kendell SD, Collins MS, Adkins MC, et al: Radiographic differentiation of enchondroma from low-grade chondrosarcoma in the fibula. *Skeletal Radiol* 33:458-466, 2004.)

demonstrating none or only one of the identified features. No unique malignant features of chondrosarcoma in the fibula were observed when compared to previous descriptions of these tumors in the long and short tubular bones of the appendicular skeleton.

▶ Benign enchondromas and low-grade chondrosarcomas can be difficult to distinguish radiographically. There are radiographic features that we rely upon to help guide us toward one diagnosis or the other. The proximal fibula, however, presents some unusual anatomic features that make the distinction between these 2 entities even more challenging. The authors have reviewed their experience in this particular location and have provided some helpful guidance to suggest that those factors, which in this particular site, are more important to consider. These include the size of the lesion, the presence of cortical destruction, periosteal reaction, which seldom occurs elsewhere, the presence of a soft tissue mass and cortical thickening. These features tend to point toward the diagnosis of chondrosarcoma. This is helpful information that can guide treatment either toward consideration of some form of incisional or excisional biopsy.

C. P. Beauchamp, MD

Dedifferentiated Chondrosarcoma: Use of MRI to Guide Needle Biopsy

Saifuddin A, Mann BS, Mahroof S, et al (Royal Natl Orthopaedic Hosp NHS Trust, Stanmore, Middlesex, England; London Bone and Soft-Tissue Tumour Unit)

Clin Radiol 59:268-272, 2004 13–29

Aim.—To describe the use of MRI to identify and biopsy areas of dedifferentiation in patients with a suspected diagnosis of dedifferentiated chondrosarcoma.

Materials and Methods.—Low-grade chondrosarcoma is characterized at magnetic resonance imaging (MRI) as having a lobulate, hyperintense appearance on T2-weighted spin-echo sequences. T2-weighted MR images were assessed in 15 patients with a final pathological diagnosis of dedifferentiated chondrosarcoma for regions of atypical reduced signal intensity. Information regarding the site of ultrasound or computed tomography (CT)-guided biopsy was available in 10 cases.

Results.—Nine patients were male and six female with a mean age of 60 years (range 25-77 years). The sites involved were the distal femur (n = 4), pelvis (n = 3), proximal femur (n = 4), femoral diaphysis (n = 1), proximal humerus (n = 2) and proximal tibia (n = 1). The dedifferentiated component consisted of osteosarcoma (n = 5), malignant fibrous histiocytoma (n = 6), spindle cell sarcoma (n = 1), leiomyosarcoma (n = 1) and pleomorphic sarcoma (n = 1). In 14 of the 15 cases, areas of lower signal intensity lacking in lobulation were identified. In nine of the 10 cases, biopsy site included such areas and yielded high-grade sarcoma.

Conclusions.—Dedifferentiation within chondrosarcoma may be identified on T2-weighted MRI as areas of reduced signal intensity. These areas should be the preferred site of biopsy.

▶ Dedifferentiated chondrosarcoma can be difficult to diagnose accurately if a sampling error is made. The misdiagnosis of a low-grade chondrosarcoma, when in fact the patient has a dedifferentiated chondrosarcoma, can make a huge difference in patient management. The authors emphasize the utilization of radiographic information to select the most appropriate area of biopsy, and indicated that the T2-weighted MRI will show an area of reduced signal intensity in the dedifferentiated area. This area should therefore be the preferred site of radiographic-guided biopsy.

C. P. Beauchamp, MD

Dedifferentiated Chondrosarcoma: The Role of Chemotherapy With Updated Outcomes

Dickey ID, Rose PS, Fuchs B, et al (Mayo Clinic, Rochester, Minn)

J Bone Joint Surg Am 86-A:2412-2418, 2004 13–30

Background.—There are very few published data on the survival of patients with dedifferentiated chondrosarcoma, or, more specifically, on the efficacy and role of chemotherapy, especially in the era of modern diagnostic and treatment modalities. The current study examines the influence of advancements in imaging and chemotherapy on outcome and serves as an extension to a previous study published in 1986.

Methods.—Forty-two patients with dedifferentiated chondrosarcoma who had presented to our institution between 1986 and 2000 were identified, and a retrospective chart review was performed. The study group included twenty-four men and eighteen women with an average age of sixty-six years. The diagnosis of dedifferentiated chondrosarcoma was verified histologically, and data on treatment, adjuvant therapy, and survival were obtained from the medical records of all patients. All patients had been followed for a minimum of twenty-four months.

Results.—The tumors were classified, according to the system of the Musculoskeletal Tumor Society, as grade IIA (five), grade IIB (twenty-six), and grade III (eleven). Three patients underwent biopsy only, eighteen had a limb-sacrificing procedure, and twenty-one had a limb-sparing procedure. In the group of patients who underwent resection, the surgical margins were classified as intralesional in three, marginal in two, wide in nineteen, and radical in fifteen. Twenty-seven patients received neoadjuvant therapy; of these, twenty-three received chemotherapy only, two received radiotherapy only, and two received combined therapy. The median survival time was 7.5 months, and the five-year rate of disease-free survival was 7.1%(Fig 3). With the numbers available, there was no significant difference in the rate of disease-free survival with respect to the use of chemotherapy ($p = 0.54$), the location of surgical margins ($p = 0.14$), the histological subtype ($p = 0.87$),

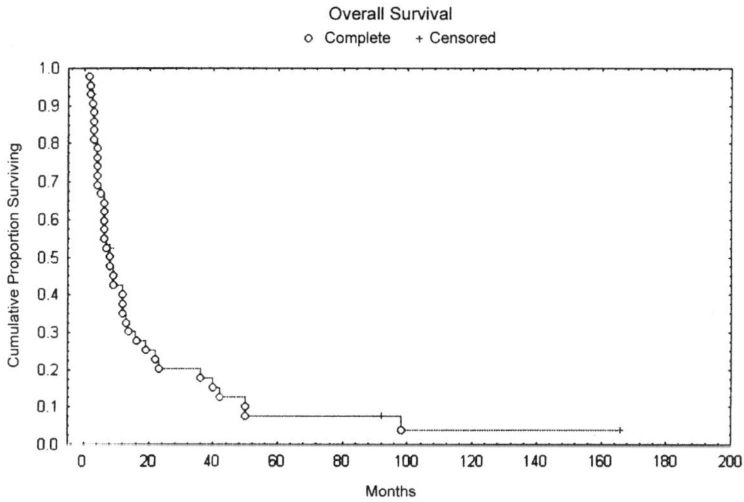

FIGURE 3.—Kaplan-Meier survival curve showing the overall five-year survival rate of 7.1%, with a median survival time of 7.5 months. (Republished with permission from the Journal of Bone and Joint Surgery, Inc, from Dickey ID, Rose PS, Fuchs B, et al: Dedifferentiated chondrosarcoma: The Role of chemotherapy with updated outcomes. *J Bone Joint Surg Am* 86-A:2412-2418, 2004. Reprinted with permission of the publisher via Copyright Clearance Center, Inc.)

the tumor stage at the time of diagnosis ($p = 0.43$), the tumor size ($p = 0.79$), or the performance of limb-sparing as opposed to limb-sacrificing procedures ($p = 0.42$).

Conclusions.—Despite advances in diagnostic modalities and adjuvant therapies, dedifferentiated chondrosarcoma continues to carry a poor prognosis. While local control is achieved in the majority of cases, distant disease remains the greatest clinical challenge, developing in 90% of patients. Efforts are needed to continue to encourage earlier diagnosis and to develop effective adjuvant therapies for the control of distant disease. The routine use of current adjuvant chemotherapy and its inherent risks in this population should be reconsidered.

► This study shares with us disappointing results for the treatment of dedifferentiated chondrosarcoma with patients treated with aggressive chemotherapy. Local control is not a problem, but distant disease remains the greatest challenge in these individuals with more than 90% of them having metastatic disease develop. This remains a deadly disease with an extremely poor outcome and continued efforts need to be made at trying to devise some form of systemic treatment for these patients.

C. P. Beauchamp, MD

Prognostic Factors in Ewing's Sarcoma of the Foot

Casadei R, Magnani M, Biagini R, et al (Rizzoli Inst, Bologna, Italy; Univ of Bologna, Italy)

Clin Orthop 420:230-238, 2004 13–31

Introduction.—The outcome of treatment and prognostic factors were reviewed in 36 patients who had Ewing's sarcoma of the foot. The tumor was most common in the calcaneus (19 patients) and metatarsals (15 patients). Age, levels of lactate dehydrogenase, degree of anemia, tumor volume, type of surgery, and radiotherapy were not related to prognosis. Females with pain for less than 6 months, fever, high levels of erythrocyte sedimentation rate, and high levels of alkaline phosphatase showed a tendency for a poorer prognosis. The only observed prognostic factors are tumor site and treatment. Patients treated with four-drug neoadjuvant chemotherapy had the best survival. Four patients with metastatic disease at diagnosis died. Fourteen of 32 patients (44%) with localized Ewing's sarcoma were continuously disease-free at an average followup of 7 years.

► It is generally believed that Ewing's sarcoma of the foot has a better prognosis than extremity surgery, but this is not demonstrated in this study, which consists of a large group of patients numbering 36 with Ewing's sarcoma of the foot. They noted a worse prognosis in patients treated with a below-knee amputation, but again, as with Ewing's sarcoma more surgery generally means more advanced disease at the time of surgery. They do reiterate that the best results are obtained with a combination of surgery, chemotherapy and radiation therapy.

C. P. Beauchamp, MD

Distal Lower Extremity Sarcomas: Frequency of Occurrence and Patient Survival Rate

Zeytoonjian T, Mankin HJ, Gebhardt MC, et al (Massachusetts Gen Hosp, Boston)

Foot Ankle Int 25:325-330, 2004 13–32

Background.—Primary sarcomas in the distal leg, tibia, fibula, ankle, and foot are uncommon and are believed to be less malignant than those that arise in other sites, but only limited information is available to support this contention.

Methods.—Using a computerized system containing extensive information regarding over 14,000 patients, mostly with tumors treated by our center over a 25-year period, 175 sarcomatous lesions with MSTS stage I, II, and III were located in the distal lower extremity. These were compared with 2367 lesions of similar diagnoses in other body parts. The principal studies included diagnostic distribution and outcome (recorded as death as a result of disease). Data were compared for diagnosis, gender, age, Musculoskeletal

TABLE 3.—Statistics for Both Series

Parameter	Leg-Ankle-Foot No. of Patients	Leg-Ankle-Foot No. of Deaths (%)	Other Sites No. of Patients	Other Sites No. of Deaths (%)
Gender				
Male	94	13 (14%)	1424	363 (25.5%)
Female	81	5 (6%)	1142	268 (23.5%)
Stage[a]				
Stage I	32	1 (3%)	423	46 (11%)
Stage II	134	16 (12%)	1571	394 (25%)
Stage III	9	1 (13%)	253	110 (43%)
Age[a]				
<20	52	6 (12%)	660	103 (16%)
20-40	57	6 (11%)	747	152 (20%)
40-60	46	2 (4%)	603	147 (24%)
>60	20	4 (20%)	594	234 (39%)
Operative Procedures[a]				
Amputation	40	0 (0%)	67	15 (22%)
Allograft	21	4 (19%)	484	47 (10%)
Other	118	14 (12%)	1816	568 (31%)
Site[b]				
Tibia	63	12 (19%)		
Fibula	7	0 (0%)		
Ankle	26	0 (0%)		
Foot	79	6 (8%)		

[a]For gender, stage, age, and operative procedures data, the differences between the "leg-ankle-foot," group and the "other sites" are highly significant (P is at least <.0001).

$P < .03$.

(Courtesy of Zeytoonjian T, Mankin HJ, Gebhardt MC, et al: Distal lower extremity sarcomas: Frequency of occurrence and patient survival rate. *Foot Ankle Int* 25:325-330, 2004. Copyright 2004 by the American Orthopaedic Foot and Ankle Society. Reproduced with permission.)

Tumor Society (MSTS) stage, anatomic site, and treatment methods and evaluated statistically by chi-square methods.

Results.—The most frequent distal lower limb tumors were synovial cell sarcoma, osteosarcoma, and Ewing's tumor and the percentage distribution of the various tumors for that site as compared with the rest of the body was quite different. Of even more importance was the remarkable difference in outcome with the death rate for the lower limb tumors set at 10%, while the same tumors at other sites had a death rate of 27% ($p < .000002$). Furthermore, gender, stage, age, and the type of operative procedure showed highly significant differences between the tumors of the lower leg and those of the remainder of the body (Table 3).

Conclusions.—On the basis of these data, it is evident that far fewer sarcomas occur in the lower leg, tibia, fibula, ankle, and foot than in other body sites and that their diagnostic distribution is different. Of perhaps greater interest is the fact that the rate of metastasis and death is markedly reduced for this site as compared with others. The authors speculate on the causes of this remarkable alteration in numbers and outcome.

► The data used in this study are gathered from a retrospective database. The study group consists of patients with sarcomas affecting the distal lower extremity. The results obtained in this review are somewhat striking in that the authors observed a much lower rate of metastatic disease and death in this particular location. Whether there was something specific about this anatomic location or whether it is merely that the lesions are identified at an earlier rate, or more likely to be treated by an ablative procedure is discussed in detail in this article and it provides some interesting ideas to consider.

C. P. Beauchamp, MD

Osteosarcoma of the Pelvis

Donati D, Giacomini S, Gozzi E, et al (Istituto Ortopedico Rizzoli, Bologna, Italy; City Hosp Ravenna, Italy; Univ of Massachusetts, Worcester)
Eur J Surg Oncol 30:332-340, 2004 13–33

Aims.—To describe the outcomes of a large number of patients with pelvic osteosarcoma, and to define the guidelines for appropriate treatment.

Methods.—We reviewed 60 consecutive patients with primary pelvic high-grade osteosarcoma. The tumour involved the whole hemipelvis in 15 cases, while the most common location was the iliac wing in 29 cases (48.3%): 25 of these adjacent to or passing the sacroiliac joint.

Results.—Thirty patients underwent surgery; there were 16 hindquarter amputations and 14 internal hemipelvectomies. All the patients who presented with metastasis died of their disease (Fig 1). In 18 cases wide margins

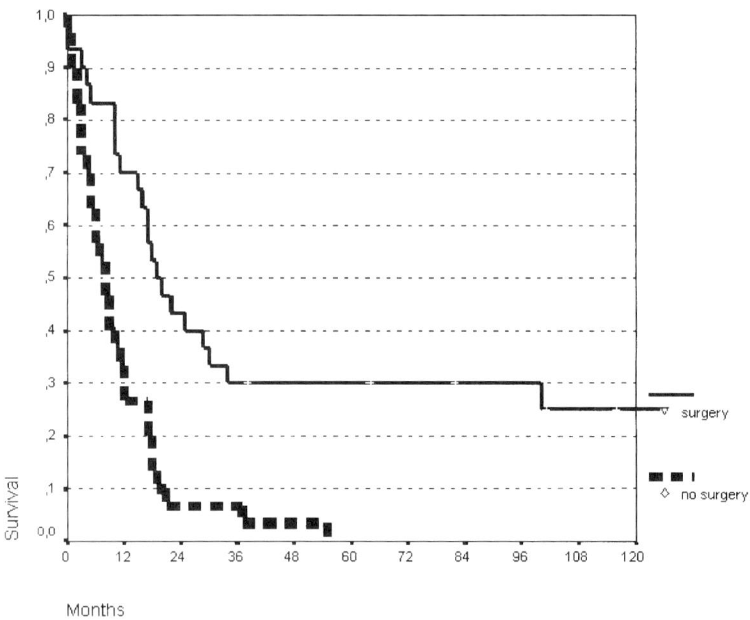

FIGURE 1.—Kaplan-Meier survival curve (Breslow) of the two groups operated and nonoperated patients ($P < 0.000$). (Courtesy of Donati D, Giacomini S, Gozzi E, et al: Osteosarcoma of the pelvis. *Eur J Surg Oncol* 30:332-340, 2004.)

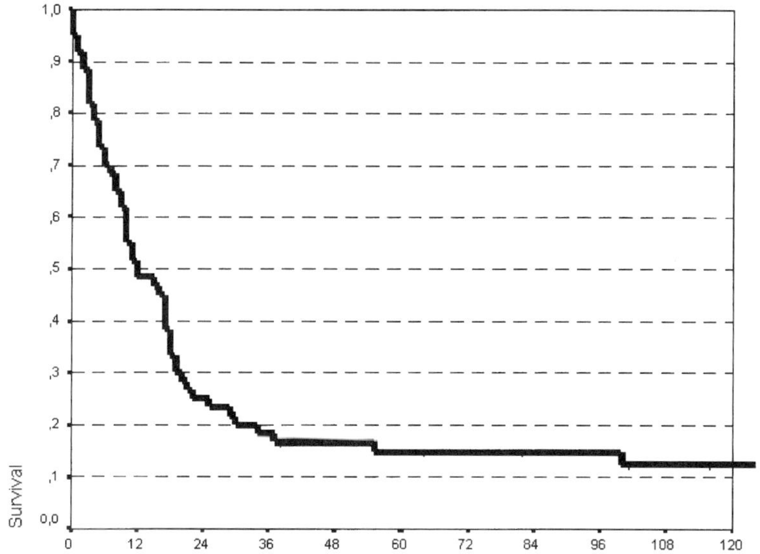

FIGURE 3.—Kaplan-Meier survival curve (Breslow) of all patients. (Courtesy of Donati D, Giacomini S, Gozzi E, et al: Osteosarcoma of the pelvis. *Eur J Surg Oncol* 30:332-340, 2004.)

were achieved, however, eight patients experienced local recurrence. Of the series, only eight patients are still alive (Fig 3).

Conclusion.—The use of intense chemotherapy and surgical wide margin, hardly seems to achieve local control, however, tumour necrosis was correlated with positive prognosis. When internal hemipelvectomy it is not safe enough, amputation must be considered, particularly for cases with sacrifice of the sciatic nerve roots or for older patients where a shorter surgical procedure can be less risky.

▶ This study comprises 60 consecutive patients with primary pelvic high-grade osteosarcoma. This is from a very skilled and accomplished group, and of note, only 30 patients subsequently underwent surgery and the majority of these patients were treated with a hemipelvectomy. The disappointing result from this group is that only 8 patients are still living. This emphasizes the grave prognosis that comes with the diagnosis of osteosarcoma involving the pelvis. It thoroughly underscores the need for adequate surgery even in those patients in whom a wide margin was achieved; almost 50% of them experienced a local recurrence. Patient selection therefore is extremely important in choosing the surgical management. The situation that we want to avoid is a high morbidity surgical procedure in someone whose prognosis is very poor. Hopefully, with the improvements in adjuvant chemotherapy, we will be able to improve results in the management of patients with pelvic osteosarcomas.

C. P. Beauchamp, MD

Survival Data for Patients With Malignant Schwannoma

Cashen DV, Parisien RC, Raskin K, et al (Harvard Med School, Boston)

Clin Orthop 426:69-73, 2004 13–34

Introduction.—Malignant schwannomas are uncommon sarcomas that arise from the sheath of Schwann surrounding peripheral nerve fibers. These tumors may arise spontaneously in adult patients or may occur with reportedly increased frequency in patients with neurofibromatosis Type I. The tumors have had a reputation for malignancy with rapid metastasis, especially when they arise in relation to neurofibromatosis. We have reviewed the experience of the connective tissue oncology unit with patients with these tumors during the past 25 years. There were 80 malignant schwannomas identified in 41 females and 39 males with a mean age of 36 ± 17 years. The largest numbers of tumors were seen in the thigh, shoulder, and pelvis but they also occurred in more central (abdomen and thorax) and distal (forearm, hand and foot) locations. The Musculoskeletal Tumor Society stages showed that the majority of the patients had Stage II (high grade but not metastasized) tumors; however, additionally, 10 of the patients had metastases at outset (Stage III). Patient gender was not a factor but stage was a notable determinant of survival. Anatomic location also had a significant effect. Overall, the entire series of patients had a survival of 85% at 11 ± 5 years and even more remarkable was the fact that there was no difference between the numbers and outcome statistics for tumors arising spontaneously and those occurring in patients with neurofibromatosis.

► The authors report on a large series of 80 patients with malignant schwannomas. Typically, this diagnosis carries with it a reputation for rapid metastases. The prognosis for this neoplasm is generally poor. The authors report rather surprising results with an overall survival of 85% at 11 years. Typically, patients with malignant schwannomas associated with neurofibromatosis have an even worse prognosis, but this was not demonstrated in this particular series.

C. P. Beauchamp, MD

Synovial Sarcoma: The Importance of Size and Location for Survival

Deshmukh R, Mankin HJ, Singer S (Harvard Med School, Boston)

Clin Orthop 419:155-161, 2004 13–35

Introduction.—A retrospective analysis was done on 135 consecutive patients with extremity and truncal synovial sarcomas seen at our institutions between 1961 and 1996. Ninety-nine patients (73%) presented with a newly diagnosed localized primary sarcoma, nine patients (7%) presented with a locally recurrent sarcoma previously treated at another institution, and 27 patients (20%) presented with metastatic disease. The median followup for surviving patients was 78 months (range, 20-420 months). The overall survival for patients with localized primary and locally recurrent synovial sarcoma was 51% at 10 years. Patients with localized synovial sarcomas less than 5 cm in longest diameter had a survival at 10 years of 88% compared with a 10-year survival of 38% and 8% for patients with sarcomas 5 to 10 cm and greater than 10 cm in longest diameter, respectively. Distal location (hands and feet) and histologic grade also were statistically significant predictors of patient survival for localized synovial sarcoma on univariate analysis. On multivariate analysis size greater than 10 cm and size 5 to 10 cm were associated with an 18-fold and a 3.1-fold increased risk of death compared with tumors smaller than 5 cm. Grade and location were not found to be independent predictors of survival on multivariate analysis. Primary tumor size and initial status at presentation were prognostic for survival and patients with synovial sarcomas larger than 5 cm or locally recurrent at presentation should be considered for more aggressive surgical and adjunctive radiotherapy or chemotherapy.

► This is a large group of synovial sarcomas managed at a tertiary tumor center. This study confirms the importance of size and location in patients with synovial sarcoma and noted a significantly poor survival rate for patients who had tumors greater than 5 cm in diameter. It also reaffirms the knowledge that patients with distal lesions have better survival quite possibly because these are diagnosed earlier and therefore tend to be smaller.

C. P. Beauchamp, MD

Long-term Effects of Connective Tissue Cancer Treatment
Mankin HJ, Gunnoe J, Farid Y, et al (Harvard Med School, Boston)
Clin Orthop 426:74-86, 2004 13–36

Introduction.—In 1999, we began a study to assess the long-term effect of connective tissue cancer treatment on clinical, social, and psychologic aspects of the lives of surviving patients. A specially designed computer program generated an 85-item questionnaire, which was sent to more than 2000 patients with malignant bone and soft tissue neoplasms. Twelve hundred forty-four patients responded. The data were entered into a computer system and were correlated with the clinical information already contained in the system for the individual patients. Although there are many possible uses for these data, we chose to do a study comparing the lifestyle and physical and sociologic problems for 144 patients treated with chemotherapy and surgery for high-grade osteosarcoma against a control population consisting of 61 patients treated surgically for benign giant cell tumors of bone. The data show a remarkable degree of compensation on the part of the patients with the malignant tumors in terms of some problems but some significant differences particularly in physical status and functional limitations.

► This is an excellent report on the clinical, social, and psychologic aspects of patient's lives who have survived treatment for soft tissue and bone sarcoma. The authors compared patients with high-grade sarcoma versus those treated for benign musculoskeletal condition. The differences between the 2 groups was surprisingly little that I think reflects the adaptability of the human psyche to adversity. The differences between the 2 groups related mainly to function.

C. P. Beauchamp, MD

Leiomyosarcoma of Somatic Soft Tissues

Mankin HJ, Casas-Genem J, Kim J-I, et al (Harvard Med School, Boston)
Clin Orthop 421:225-231, 2004 13–37

Introduction.—Leiomyosarcoma is a rare, aggressively malignant connective tissue tumor of mature adults, which arises from smooth muscle. It occurs most frequently in the uterus, bowel, vascular tissues, and less commonly in somatic soft tissue or bone. The tumor when it arises in soft tissue has distinctive histologic features which somewhat resemble malignant fibrous histiocytoma (otherwise known as myxofibrosarcoma). The Orthopaedic Oncology Service at our institution has treated 66 patients with these lesions and thus far, ½ of the patients have died of disease at a mean of 3 years after discovery. Factors that increase the death rate include size of the tumor, Musculoskeletal Tumor Society Stage of disease, and to a lesser extent particularly in the lower extremities, anatomic site. Radiation and chemotherapy had little direct effect on the outcome but patients treated with surgery and adjunctive agents seemed to live longer than their cohorts treated with surgery alone. The purpose of this study is a general review of the clinical and prognostic features of this cancer.

► This is a rare soft tissue sarcoma and this study represents a large collection of patients treated at 1 institution. In a detailed review of these patients, the authors describe an unusually high incidence of poor results with this disease suggesting that this subgroup of sarcomas has a particularly low rate of survival.

C. P. Beauchamp, MD

Lymph Node Metastasis in Soft Tissue Sarcoma in an Extremity

Riad S, Griffin AM, Liberman B, et al (Univ of Toronto, Canada)
Clin Orthop 426:129-134, 2004 13–38

Introduction.—For patients with soft tissue sarcoma in an extremity, the outcome is thought to be poor if lymph node metastasis develops. The purpose of this study was to examine the impact of lymphatic involvement from soft tissue sarcoma on patient survival. Thirty-nine (3.7%) of 1066 patients who had surgery for soft tissue sarcoma in an extremity had lymph node metastases develop. Three (20%) of 15 patients with epithelioid sarcoma, four (19%) of 21 patients with rhabdomyosarcoma, two (11.1%) of 18 patients with clear cell sarcoma, and two (11.1%) of 18 patients with angiosarcoma had lymphatic involvement. Thirty patients who had resection of involved lymph nodes had an estimated 5-year survival of 57%, whereas nine patients treated without surgery all died within 30 months. An estimated 4-year survival of 71% for patients with isolated lymph node metastases was significantly better than 21% for patients with synchronous systemic and lymph node involvement. There was no difference in outcome for patients with isolated lymphatic involvement compared with patients with American Joint Committee on Cancer Stage III extremity sarcomas. These results suggest that long-term survival is possible after surgical resection of lymphatic metastases from soft tissue sarcoma. The American Joint Committee on Cancer should consider separating isolated nodal metastases from systemic involvement in patients with Stage IV sarcoma.

▶ It is rare for patients to have metastatic disease to lymph nodes develop. When it does occur, it is believed to represent an ominous prognosis. In a large group of patients with soft tissue sarcomas, those with metastatic disease to local lymph nodes were evaluated and those patients who were treated with aggressive surgical treatment as well as adjuvant treatment had a better survival rate than one would consider for those patients who had metastatic disease develop elsewhere. These patients need to be treated with aggressive surgical treatment as their prognosis is not as poor as once was thought.

C. P. Beauchamp, MD

Imaging of Periosteal Osteosarcoma: Radiologic-Pathologic Comparison

Murphey MD, Jelinek JS, Temple HT, et al (Armed Forces Inst of Pathology, Washington, DC; Uniformed Services Univ of the Health Sciences, Bethesda, Md; Univ of Maryland, Baltimore; et al)

Radiology 233:129-138, 2004 13–39

Purpose.—To review the imaging appearance of periosteal osteosarcoma, with pathologic comparison.

Materials and Methods.—Data for 40 pathologically confirmed periosteal osteosarcomas were retrospectively reviewed. Patient demographic data were recorded, and radiographs (n = 40), bone scintigrams (n = 10), angiograms (n = 2), and computed tomographic (CT) (n = 11) and magnetic resonance (MR) (n = 12) images were evaluated for lesion location and size, cortical changes, marrow involvement, and intrinsic characteristics by two musculoskeletal radiologists, with agreement by consensus. Pathology reports were reviewed for presence and predominance of histologic components (fibrous, chondroid, and osteoid), tumor grade, and marrow involvement.

Results.—There were 25 male (62%) and 15 female (38%) patients with an age range of 10-37 years (average age, 20 years). The most frequent lesion locations were the diaphysis of the tibia (16 patients) or of the femur (15 patients). Radiographs showed a broad-based soft-tissue mass that was attached to the cortex (all patients) and showed cortical thickening (33 patients), cortical scalloping/erosion (37 patients), and/or perpendicular periosteal reaction (38 patients) extending into the soft-tissue mass. Soft-tissue masses were well defined in 91%-100% of cases and surrounded a median of 50%-55% of the cortex. Lesions commonly showed low attenuation at CT (10 patients) and high signal intensity on T2-weighted MR images (10 patients), reflecting the high water content of these largely chondroblastic lesions. Focal areas of adjacent marrow replacement were common at MR imaging (nine patients) but represented reactive changes unless they were in direct continuity with the overlying soft-tissue mass (this was rare, occurring in only one patient, and represented marrow invasion). Review of pathology reports revealed that all lesions contained chondroid tissue, which predominated in 34 patients.

Conclusion.—The radiologic appearance of periosteal osteosarcoma is a broad-based surface soft-tissue mass causing extrinsic erosion of thickened underlying diaphyseal cortex and perpendicular periosteal reaction extending into the soft-tissue component. Reactive marrow changes are commonly seen at MR imaging, but true marrow invasion is rare.

► The authors provide a very nice overview of the various radiographic appearances of periosteal osteosarcomas, a surface-based malignancy. This has a rather characteristic radiographic appearance and seldom involves the marrow canal.

C. P. Beauchamp, MD

Imaging of Ancient Schwannoma

Isobe K, Shimizu T, Akahane T, et al (Shinshu Univ, Nagano, Japan)

AJR 183:331-336, 2004 13–40

Objective.—We surveyed the clinical symptoms and radiologic features of ancient schwannoma, a rare variant of schwannoma characterized by degenerative changes.

Materials and Methods.—We present the clinical, radiologic, and pathologic features in seven patients with ancient schwannoma (mean age, 62 years; range, 45-80 years) treated at our department between 1998 and 2003.

Results.—The most characteristic clinical features were a sign like Tinel's sign and a long interval between the onset of symptoms and surgery (mean interval, 8.3 years). Ancient schwannomas can grow large; the biggest tumor seen in our study was 14 cm long. The highly accurate radiologic assessment made possible with contrast-enhanced MRI and CT scanning showed enhancement at a peridegenerative area and sometimes at a capsule. These findings differ from those of the typical schwannoma and neurofibroma patterns reported to date. Furthermore, bone scintigraphy showed uptake in the tumor, but no accumulation was seen on gallium-67 citrate scintigraphy.

Conclusion.—The characteristic clinical and radiologic findings of ancient schwannoma should make it possible to differentiate it from malignant tumors.

► This lesion can have bizarre radiographic appearance secondary to the degeneration that occurs with time. This results in a rather unusual but fairly characteristic appearance on magnetic scanning.

C. P. Beauchamp, MD

Surgery for Lung Metastases in Ewing's Sarcoma of Bone

Briccoli A, Rocca M, Ferrari S, et al (Istituto Ortopedico Rizzoli, Bologna, Italy)

Eur J Surg Oncol 30:63-67, 2004 13–41

Introduction.—The addition of chemotherapy and radiotherapy to local treatment for Ewing's sarcoma of bone (ES) significantly bettered its prognosis. Nonetheless, although with no signs of local recurrence some patients still relapse with lung metastases. These patients are generally treated with non-surgical procedures. The few reports in literature on surgical resection of metachronous pulmonary metastases do not allow any conclusions. This study aims to report the results achieved in 24 Ewing's sarcoma patients who relapsed only with lung metastases, and no local recurrence, treated with surgery at the authors' institution (Table 4).

► There are few reports on the surgical resection of pulmonary metastases for Ewing's sarcoma, as it is unusual for patients to solely relapse in the lungs. The authors have demonstrated that there is a role for pulmonary metastasec-

TABLE 4.—Overall Survival and Disease-Free Interval of the Two Groups

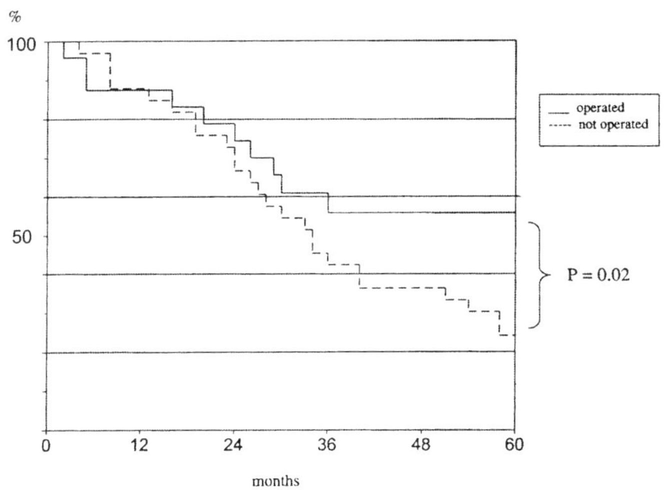

DFI (months) : *operated* = 37.4 *not operated* = 30.3

(Courtesy of Briccoli A, Rocca M, Ferrari S, et al: Surgery for lung metastases in Ewing's sarcoma of bone. *Eur J Surg Oncol* 30:63-67, 2004.)

tomy in patients with systemic relapse confined to the lungs. Again as in other sarcomas with lung metastasis, patient selection is critical. Patients who were treated with metastasectomy had a better overall survival than those who did not receive a thoracotomy. Metastasectomy, therefore, has a role in the management of patients with pulmonary disease in the absence of disease elsewhere.

C. P. Beauchamp, MD

Surgical Management and Outcome of Osteosarcoma Patients With Unilateral Pulmonary Metastases

Su WT, Chewning J, Abramson S, et al (Mem Sloan-Kettering Cancer Ctr, New York)

J Pediatr Surg 39:418-423, 2004 13–42

Purpose.—The surgical management of osteosarcoma patients with unilateral pulmonary nodules is controversial. The authors reviewed their institutional experience to evaluate the incidence of occult contralateral metastases.

Methods.—Data were obtained retrospectively on all consecutive osteosarcoma patients from 1980 to 2002. Eighty-four patients with pulmonary nodules were identified. Forty-one had bilateral disease, and 43 had unilateral involvement by computed tomography (CT) scan.

Results.—All 43 patients with unilateral nodules underwent ipsilateral thoracotomies. Fifteen patients had negative exploration findings, and only 1 had pulmonary relapse. Of the 28 patients with metastases confirmed at initial thoracotomies, 14 had extensive pleural or extrapulmonary disease at initial thoracotomy followed by disease progression. The other 14 are separated into early versus late metastases, using 2 years from diagnosis as the cutoff point. Seven of the 9 (78%) patients with early metastases had or subsequently had contralateral disease; 6 were identified at staged contralateral thoracotomy and 1 had relapsed in the unexplored lung a year later. Only 1 of the 5 patients with late unilateral metastases had relapse in the contralateral side.

Conclusions.—Our data indicate that there is a high rate of contralateral involvement in osteosarcoma patients with unilateral nodules diagnosed by CT scan. Staged bilateral thoracotomies should be considered in osteosarcoma patients presenting with unilateral pulmonary disease on imaging studies within 2 years of diagnosis.

► There is a rather small group of patients with osteosarcoma and pulmonary metastases who present with seemingly unilateral disease. The authors have followed this group and have noted a significant rate of contralateral involvement as well. The suggestion of staged bilateral thoracotomies is therefore recommended in these patients. It is our typical procedure that when patients present with either unilateral or bilateral pulmonary metastasis, we generally wait for a period of 4 to 6 weeks and repeat the scan to ensure that there isn't a development of massive pulmonary metastases in an effort to avoid attempted metastasectomy in patients who have a very poor prognosis. Perhaps with this technique, the diagnosis of unilateral metastatic disease could be made less frequently.

C. P. Beauchamp, MD

The Incidence and Prognosis of Osteosarcoma Skip Metastases

Sajadi KR, Heck RK, Neel MD, et al (Univ of Tennessee, Memphis; St Jude Children's Research Hosp, Memphis, Tenn; Univ of Chicago)

Clin Orthop 426:92-96, 2004 13–43

Introduction.—The poor prognosis for patients with osteosarcoma skip metastases has been established in the literature; however, most of the data in the literature concerning osteosarcoma skip metastases were collected before routine use of magnetic resonance imaging and before the use of modern multiagent chemotherapy regimens. This retrospective multiinstitutional study was done to evaluate the efficacy of magnetic resonance imaging to detect skip metastases and to evaluate the prognosis for these patients when treated with modern multiagent chemotherapy protocols. In a group of 155 patients who were younger than 26 years when diagnosed and treated for high-grade osteosarcoma of the long bones, 10 (6.5%) patients with skip metastases were identified. Eight of the 10 lesions were detected on pretreatment magnetic resonance imaging scans and two were detected only from the surgical pathology specimens. Five patients had concomitant pulmonary metastases at presentation and five patients had no other known site of diseases. All 10 patients died, with an average survival of 32.5 months (range 11-71 months). The five patients with only skip metastases at presentation survived an average of 27.2 months (range 15-44 months). Despite advances in the treatment of patients with osteosarcomas, those with skip metastases continue to have a poor prognosis, and they should be counseled regarding the limitations of current therapies.

► Patients with osteosarcoma and skip metastases have historically had a poor prognosis in comparison to patients with isolated unifocal disease. It has been postulated that with modern diagnostic methods and improved chemotherapy, an improvement in survival of this group could be realized. This, unfortunately, has not been shown in this group of patients with skip metastases. The prognosis of patients continues to be poor despite some advances in adjuvant chemotherapy.

C. P. Beauchamp, MD

Two Cases of Calcaneal Osteosarcomas Presenting as Aneurysmal Bone Cysts

Leithner A, Bodo K, Scheipl S, et al (Univ of Graz, Austria)

Foot Ankle Int 25:815-818, 2004 13–44

Introduction.—Aneurysmal bone cysts (ABC) are benign lesions of the bone that may arise as primary or secondary lesions. Osteosarcomas are bone-forming tumors. These tumors are different pathological entities that sometimes share strikingly similar clinical, radiological, and histological features. Described are 2 cases of osteosarcomas of the calcaneus that presented as ABC.

Case Report 1.—Female, 24, experienced a supination injury to the ankle in 1986 that recurred several times during the next 8 y. A radiograph in 1994 revealed a 4.7-cm × 2.5-cm lytic lesion of the right calcaneus. Since a simple bone cyst was suspected, trochar-directed, high-pressure lavage of the cyst was performed 3 times without histological evaluation. Pain worsened and another radiograph showed a persistent lytic lesion; 4 mo later, an extended biopsy with an intralesional curettage was performed. A local pathologist tentatively diagnosed ABC and sent specimens to the national reference pathologist; one pathologist diagnosed a high-grade osteosarcoma with secondary ABC; the other diagnosed ABC secondary to fibrous dysplasia. A second biopsy was deemed necessary. Of 2 reference pathologists who evaluated these specimens, 1 diagnosed an osteosarcoma and the other pathologist continued to diagnose an ABC secondary to fibrous dysplasia. The lesion recurred in 12 mo. Biopsy showed ABC secondary to fibrous dysplasia; this was verified via a reference pathologist. Four mo later, curettage and phenolization showed a grade 3 osteosarcoma accompanied by a secondary ABC; all pathologists agreed. Thorough staging showed no metastases. Neoadjuvant chemotherapy was administered. A wide below-knee amputation was performed, followed by adjuvant chemotherapy. Amputation specimen contained over 50% vital tumor cells corresponding to a histological regression grade 5 osteosarcoma. Revision was necessary once. At 39 mo follow-up, she had no evidence of disease.

Case Report 2.—Female, 23, seen for pain in her left calcaneus had magnetic resonance imaging and scintigraphy findings consistent with ABC. Primary ABC was reported on pathology. After recurrence, further evaluation revealed a grade 3 intramedullary osteosarcoma with secondary ABC. This patient also received neoadjuvant chemotherapy before wide amputation, which was followed by adjuvant chemotherapy. Amputation specimen consisted of over 50% vital tumor-cells corresponding to a histological regression grade 5. At 26 mo follow-up, she was alive with metastatic disease.

Conclusion.—Both cases presented support the concern that a biopsy specimen of aneurysmal bone cysts may conceal as osteosarcoma. When diagnosis is uncertain, definitive treatment should by delayed until all available data has been thoroughly examined by a pathologist, radiologist, and orthopedic surgeon; all should be specialized in the diagnosis and treatment of bone tumors.

▶ This report emphasizes the importance of caution in the diagnosis of ABC. Caution needs to be exercised if any of the radiographic or histologic features are not absolutely in keeping with the diagnosis of an ABC. Excellent representative sampling of the tumor needs to be obtained and the tissue needs to be evaluated by an experienced pathologist. And finally, close observation of patients who have undergone treatment for ABC needs to be done, especially in the first year.

C. P. Beauchamp, MD

Infection

Allograft Bone in Two-Stage Revision of the Hip for Infection: Is It Safe?
Ammon P, Stockley I (Northern Gen Hosp, Sheffield, England)
J Bone Joint Surg Br 86-B:962-965, 2003 13–45

Introduction.—A two-stage procedure was carried out on 57 patients with confirmed infection in a hip replacement. Allograft bone was used in the second stage. Pathogenic organisms were identified in all patients. In stage 1, the prosthesis was removed together with infected tissue. Antibiotics were added to customised cement beads. Systemic antibiotics were not used. At the second stage, 45 of the patients had either acetabular impaction grafting, femoral impaction grafting or a combination; 12 had a massive allograft.

Eight patients suffered recurrent infection (14%), in six with the original infecting organism. The risk factors for re-infection were multiple previous procedures and highly resistant organisms. We believe that systemic antibiotic therapy should be considered for these patients. Allograft bone is shown to be a useful adjunct in most infected hip replacements with considerable loss of bone stock.

▶ The authors share their results of 2-stage procedures for the management of infected hip replacements. They did not use systemic antibiotics and reported poor results with this method of treatment. There are a number of questions that need to be answered regarding how to manage an infected joint replacement. Some of the questions include: how long should the antibiotics be used, should systemic antibiotics be used, should antibiotics and cement be used at any stage, etc. I think this article provides suitable evidence to suggest that systemic antibiotic treatment is an essential component in the management of patients with periprosthetic infections.

C. P. Beauchamp, MD

Systemic Safety of High-Dose Antibiotic-Loaded Cement Spacers After Resection of an Infected Total Knee Arthroplasty

Springer BD, Lee G-C, Osmon D, et al (Mayo Clinic, Rochester, Minn; Florida Orthopedic Inst, Tampa; Insall Scott Kelly Inst, New York)

Clin Orthop 427:47-51, 2004 13–46

Introduction.—The purpose of this study was to assess the systemic safety and potential adverse effects of using a high-dose antibiotic-impregnated cement spacer after resection arthroplasty of an infected total knee replacement. Between October 2000 and December 2002, 36 knees (34 patients) had a resection arthroplasty of an infected total knee prosthesis with placement of a high-dose antibiotic impregnated cement spacer. There were 24 men and 10 women with a mean age of 66.5 years (range, 48-84 years). All spacers placed contained an average of 3.4 batches of cement with an average total dose of 10.5 g of vancomycin (range, 3-16 g) and 12.5 g of gentamicin (range, 3.6-19.2 g). All patients were followed up postoperatively until reimplantation for evidence of renal failure. The preoperative creatinine ranged from 0.7 to 1.8 mg/dL. All patients were concomitantly treated with 6 weeks of intravenous organism-specific antibiotics. One patient with normal preoperative renal function (Cr 0.7 mg/dL) had a perioperative 1-day transient rise in serum creatinine (1.7 mg/dL) postoperatively that subsequently normalized. No patients showed any clinical evidence of acute renal insufficiency, failure, or other systemic side effects of the antibiotics. Treatment of patients with an infected total knee arthroplasty with high-dose vancomycin and gentamicin antibiotic spacers seems to be clinically safe.

► Antibiotic impregnated cement has proven to be a useful adjuvant in the management of patients with failed infected joint arthroplasty. There are many unknowns in the management of patients with infections, most notably the dosage of antibiotics in the cement and the length of time it needs to be left in place before reimplantation. The specific issue of systemic safety of high-dose antibiotics in cement is addressed by this study. The patients were treated with an aggressive dose regimen of antibiotics and there was no clinical evidence of any significant acute renal insufficiency ascribed to the use of high-dose vancomycin and gentamicin antibiotic cement spacers.

C. P. Beauchamp, MD

Successful Treatment of Total Hip and Knee Infection With Articulating Antibiotic Components: A Modified Treatment Method

Evans RP (Cherry Creek Orthopaedic Specialists, Denver)

Clin Orthop 427:37-46, 2005 13–47

Introduction.—There are many problems associated with the use of articulating antibiotic cement spacer blocks and articulating components in the two-stage treatment of total hip replacement and total knee replacement infections. These include loss of motion during and after treatment, bone loss, generation of cement debris, inadequate dosing of cement with the appropriate antibiotic, and biologic failure. Forty-four patients with 54 consecutive periprosthetic hip and knee infections (31 septic total knee arthroplasties and 23 septic total hip arthroplasties) had treatment with a modified two-stage reimplantation protocol using articulating components made of antibiotic-cement-only prosthetic components and antibiotic–cement-covered prosthetic components between January 1995 and May 2002. Second-stage revision, after six weeks of parenteral antibiotics, was completed an average of 84 days after the first stage. A minimum two-year followup after final treatment is evaluated. One of the 23 total hip replacement infections persisted or recurred with the original organism(s) after treatment (95.7% success) as did two of the 31 total knee replacement infections (93.5% success). Combined success rate was 94.4%. This modified treatment method incorporates early range of motion during first-stage treatment with articulating components that provide local high-dose elution of broad-spectrum antibiotics, provides the flexibility of customizing the antibiotic cement components with culture-directed antibiotics, and results in a high biologic success rate.

► Articulated spacers for the management of infected TKA have been around for almost 20 years. This study emphasizes the safety and efficacy of this particular technique and outlines other treatment options available to achieve a mobile knee in the course of management of a periprosthetic infection. The authors cite a very acceptable success rate in not only managing the infection, but yielding a successful TKA. For those who look after patients with infected failed TKA, a spacer that allows mobility brings with it a lot of benefits, especially during the second stage as the exposure and execution of a revision TKA is greatly facilitated by an articulated spacer.

C. P. Beauchamp, MD

Alternative Materials to Acrylic Bone Cement for Delivery of Depot Antibiotics in Orthopaedic Infections

McLaren AC (Univ of Arkansas, Little Rock)

Clin Orthop 427:101-106, 2004 13–48

Introduction.—Acrylic bone cement has considerable laboratory and clinical data validating it as a delivery material for depot administration of antibiotics. However, an alternate material that does not require a secondary procedure for removal is desired. Many biodegradable materials have been evaluated as alternatives including protein-based materials (collagen, fibrin, thrombin, clotted blood), bone-graft, bone-graft substitutes and extenders (hydroxyapatite, beta-tricalcium phosphate, calcium sulfate, bioglass), and synthetic polymers (polyhanhydride, polylactide, polyglycolide, polyhydroxybutyrate-co-hydroxyvalerate, polyhydroxyalkanoate). Various forms and combinations of these materials have been investigated worldwide, characterizing their elution properties and performance in treating osteomyelitis in animal models. Many of these have had limited clinical evaluation. Outside the United States, some of these materials are used clinically. In the United States, none have been approved. None are commercially available for clinical use. Morselized cancellous bone and calcium sulfate are the two materials that have been used clinically in the United States on a physician-prescribed, hand-mixed, basis. Considering the limited clinical data that currently are available, the use of these materials still is experimental. Clinical application should be cautious, limiting the total antibiotic load. Until definitive data are available, a prudent dose would be no higher than one that would have acceptable toxicity risk if administered intravenously over 24 hours.

▶ This is an excellent review article outlining the current status of alternatives to polymethylmethacrylate to deliver antibiotics for orthopedic infections. We have been anxiously awaiting biodegradable materials, and the author shares with us some of the concerns utilizing these devices at the present time.

C. P. Beauchamp, MD

Two-Stage Revision Hip Arthroplasty for Infection: Comparison Between the Interim Use of Antibiotic-Loaded Cement Beads and a Spacer Prosthesis

Hsieh P-H, Shih C-H, Chang Y-H, et al (Chang Gung Mem Hosp, Taoyuan, Taiwan; Chung Shan Hosp, Taipei, Taiwan)

J Bone Joint Surg Am 86-A:1989-1997, 2004 13–49

Background.—A two-stage revision is a well-accepted method for the treatment of a deep infection of a hip with a joint implant. In the present study, the results associated with the interim use of antibiotic-loaded cement beads were compared with those associated with the interim use of an antibiotic-loaded cement prosthesis.

Methods.—One hundred and twenty-eight consecutive patients who were managed with a two-stage revision hip arthroplasty for the treatment of an infection were followed clinically and radiographically for an average of 4.9 years. Cement beads were implanted following resection arthroplasty in the first seventy hips, and a custom cement prosthesis was implanted in the subsequent fifty-eight hips.

Results.—There was no evidence of recurrent infection in 122 patients (95.3%); the infection-free rates in both groups were similar. The use of a spacer prosthesis was associated with a higher hip score, a shorter hospital stay, and better walking capacity in the interim period; a decreased operative time, less blood loss, and a lower transfusion requirement at the time of reimplantation; and fewer postoperative dislocations.

Conclusions.—The present study supports the safety and efficacy of the routine use of an antibiotic-loaded cement prosthesis in the interim between the stages of a two-stage revision procedure for the treatment of an infection at the site of a hip arthroplasty.

► Two-stage revision arthroplasty is the procedure of choice in the management of an infected failed total hip replacement. It carries with it, however, significant morbidity in the period between stages. The morbidity is even more with resection arthroplasty and beads compared with a functional spacer prosthesis. The authors have demonstrated an improvement utilizing a functional spacer prosthesis in that patients had a higher hip score, a shorter hospital stay, and a decrease in their morbidity during the interim period. This was all accomplished without noting an increased risk of persistent infection. The use of a functional antibiotic-loaded spacer prosthesis is the preferred method of treatment in our practice.

C. P. Beauchamp, MD

Subject Index

A

C

D

G

H

I

J

K

L

M

R

S

Author Index

E

F

G

H

I

J

Order your *Year Book* today! Simply complete and detach this card and drop it in the mail to receive the latest information in your field.

The year's best literature in one convenient volume!

YES! Please start my subscription to the ***Year Book(s)*** checked below with the current volume according to the terms described below.* I understand that I will have 30 days to examine each annual edition.

Please Print:

Name ______________________________

Address ______________________________

City ____________________ State __________ ZIP __________

Method of Payment

❑ Check (payable to **Elsevier**; add the applicable sales tax for your area)

❑ VISA ❑ MasterCard ❑ AmEx ❑ Bill me

Card number ____________________ Exp. date __________

Signature ______________________________

- ❑ **Year Book of Allergy, Asthma and Clinical Immunology (YALI)** $110.00 (Avail. November)
- ❑ **Year Book of Anesthesiology and Pain Management (YANE)** $115.00 (Avail. August)
- ❑ **Year Book of Cardiology® (YCAR)** $115.00 (Avail. August)
- ❑ **Year Book of Critical Care Medicine® (YCCM)** $110.00 (Avail. June)
- ❑ **Year Book of Dentistry® (YDEN)** $105.00 (Avail. August)
- ❑ **Year Book of Dermatology and Dermatologic Surgery™ (YDER)** $115.00 (Avail. October)
- ❑ **Year Book of Diagnostic Radiology® (YRAD)** $115.00 (Avail. November)
- ❑ **Year Book of Emergency Medicine® (YEMD)** $115.00 (Avail. May)
- ❑ **Year Book of Endocrinology® (YEND)** $115.00 (Avail. July)
- ❑ **Year Book of Family Practice™ (YFAM)** $99.00 (Avail. June)
- ❑ **Year Book of Gastroenterology™ (YGAS)** $110.00 (Avail. December)
- ❑ **Year Book of Hand Surgery® (YHND)** $115.00 (Avail. April)
- ❑ **Year Book of Medicine® (YMED)** $110.00 (Avail. July)
- ❑ **Year Book of Neonatal and Perinatal Medicine® (YNPM)** $115.00 (Avail. September)
- ❑ **Year Book of Neurology and Neurosurgery® (YNEU)** $110.00 (Avail. January)
- ❑ **Year Book of Nuclear Medicine® (YNUM)** $110.00 (Avail. June)
- ❑ **Year Book of Obstetrics, Gynecology, and Women's Health® (YOBG)** $115.00 (Avail. February)
- ❑ **Year Book of Oncology® (YONC)** $115.00 (Avail. November)
- ❑ **Year Book of Ophthalmology® (YOPH)** $115.00 (Avail. September)
- ❑ **Year Book of Orthopedics® (YORT)** $120.00 (Avail. October)
- ❑ **Year Book of Otolaryngology—Head and Neck Surgery® (YOTO)** $105.00 (Avail. July)
- ❑ **Year Book of Pathology and Laboratory Medicine® (YPAT)** $115.00 (Avail. March)
- ❑ **Year Book of Pediatrics® (YPED)** $105.00 (Avail. January)
- ❑ **Year Book of Plastic and Aesthetic Surgery® (YPRS)** $115.00 (Avail. March)
- ❑ **Year Book of Psychiatry and Applied Mental Health® (YPSY)** $105.00 (Avail. March)
- ❑ **Year Book of Pulmonary Disease® (YPDI)** $110.00 (Avail. April)
- ❑ **Year Book of Rheumatology, Arthritis, and Musculoskeletal Disease™ (YRHE)** $115.00 (Avail. January)
- ❑ **Year Book of Sports Medicine® (YSPM)** $110.00 (Avail. December)
- ❑ **Year Book of Surgery® (YSUR)** $110.00 (Avail. September)
- ❑ **Year Book of Urology® (YURO)** $115.00 (Avail. November)
- ❑ **Year Book of Vascular Surgery® (YVAS)** $115.00 (Avail. April)

**Your Year Book service guarantee:*

When you subscribe to a **Year Book**, you will receive notice of future annual volumes about two months before publication. To receive the new edition, do nothing—we'll send you the new volume as soon as it is available. (Applicable sales tax is added to each shipment.) If you want to discontinue, the advance notice allows you time to notify us of your decision. If you are not completely satisfied, you have 30 days to return any **Year Book**.